KU-184-934

To
Clinton, Gillian,
Kristian, Conner,
Gabrielle, Jayden, and Jaz:
"There are no limitations in life with the
exception of those we place on ourselves."

And to
Our colleagues at the
Duke University Medical Center,
Duke Clinical Research Institute, and
McMaster University:
"Knowledge that heals is among man's great quests."

Preface to the Second Edition

The origins of mammalian blood coagulation, carefully regulated by a network of integrated biochemical and cellular events, can be traced back over 400 million years. Despite its long history, only within the past century have some of the complexities of this pivotal teleologic system been understood. More recently the intricacies of hemostasis and pathologic thrombosis have come to light, leading the way toward new, more effective, and safer treatment modalities.

The second edition of *Fibrinolytic and Antithrombotic Therapy: Theory, Practice, and Management* highlights recent advances and a broadened understanding of coagulation, inflammation, and vascular medicine as an intricately linked triad of biochemical- and cellular-based phenomenology. It also underscores the importance of genomics, proteomics, and metabolomics as forming the basis for defining genotype–phenotype relationships, the natural history of disease, and patient-specific therapeutics.

The next decade promises to be filled with unparalleled opportunity for improved patient care through science, technology, and collaborative efforts among the field's thought leaders and visionaries.

Richard C. Becker, MD
Duke University School of Medicine

Frederick A. Spencer, MD
McMaster University

Contents

Part I
Fundamental Scientific Principles

Historical Perspectives in Hemostasis, Coagulation, and Fibrinolysis: A Foundation for Understanding Thrombotic Disorders and Developing Effective Treatment

Historical Perspectives on Thrombosis and Thrombolysis

Hemostasis, the prompt cessation of bleeding at a site of vascular injury, is among the most fundamental physiologic and teleologically vital defense mechanisms in nature. Without a functionally intact hemostatic mechanism, death could ensue rapidly even after minor traumas associated with everyday life.

A Brief History of Mammalian Hemostasis

In mammalian blood coagulation, regulated by a complex network of integrated biochemical events, five protease factors (f) (fIIa [thrombin], fVIIa, fIXa, fXa, and protein C) interact with five cofactors (tissue factor, fVIIIa, fVa, thrombomodulin, and protein S) to regulate the generation of fibrin (Davidson et al., 2003). Although each component of the mammalian coagulation network has unique functional properties, available data based on gene organizations, protein structure, and sequence analysis suggest that it may have resulted from the reduplication and diversification of two gene structures over 400 million years ago. A vitamin K–dependent serine protease is composed of a γ-carboxylated glutamic acid (GLA) epidermal growth factor-like (EGF) 1–EGF 2-serine protease domain structure common to fVII, fIX, fX, and protein C, and the A_1-A_2-B-AB-C1-C2 domain structure common to fV and fVIII. Prothrombin is also a vitamin K–dependent serine protease; however, it contains kringle domains rather than EGF domains (suggesting a replacement during gene duplication and shuffling). Analyses of active site function amino acid residues reveal distinguishing characteristics of thrombin from other serine proteases, supporting its position as the ancestral blood enzyme (Krem and Cera, 2002; McLysaght et al., 2002).

Early Observations

The rapid transformation of fluid blood to a gel-like substance (clot) has been a topic of great interest to scientists, physicians, and philosophers since the days of

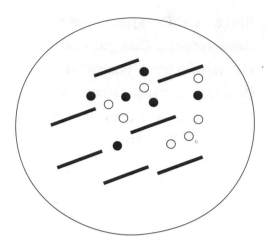

Figure 1.1 An early description of blood clots by Malpighi and others that included fibers, cells, and serum. The fibers were actually fibrin. It was later understood that coagulation proteins (thrombin in particular) and cellular components (predominately platelets) were essential contributors to blood clotting.

Plato and Aristotle (Jewett, 1892; Lee, 1952). However, it was not until the beginning of the 18th century that blood clotting (coagulation) was appreciated as a means to stem blood loss from wounds (hemostasis) (Petit, 1731).

As with other areas of science, the microscope played a pivotal role in the understanding of coagulation. In the mid-17th century, Marcello Malpighi separated the individual components of a blood clot into fibers, cells, and serum (Forester, 1956). The fibers were later found to be derived from a plasma precursor (fibrinogen) and given the name *fibrin* (Babington, 1830). Further developments in the mid-19th century included the recognition of an enzyme (later called thrombin) that was capable of coagulating fibrinogen (Buchanan, 1879) (Figure 1.1, Table 1.1).

Table 1.1 A Developmental Timeline for Hemostasis

Transformation of fluid blood to "gel-like" mass	Plato, Aristotle
Blood clots consist of fibers, cells, and serum	Malpighi, 1686
Blood clotting stems blood loss from wounds	Petit, 1731
"Fibers" given the name fibrin are derived from a plasma precursor "fibrinogen"	Babington, 1830
Thrombin converts fibrinogen to fibrin	Buchanan, 1879
Blood contains inactive precursors that are activated by a foreign surface (intrinsic coagulation) or exposed tissue (extrinsic coagulation)	Schmidt, 1892
Platelets aggregate and form the first line of defense in physiologic hemostasis	Osler, 1874
	Hayem, 1882

Thrombin

In the latter half of the 19th century, the scientific community began to appreciate that thrombin could not be a constituent of normal plasma (otherwise clotting would occur continuously and at random) (Schmidt, 1892). This concept was vital to our understanding of the complex "checks and balances" system of coagulation, wherein inactive precursors are activated precisely where and when they are needed. It also fostered the belief that blood contained many, if not all, of the necessary elements for intravascular coagulation (circulating predominantly in an inactive form). This hypothesis served as the basis for the theory of intrinsic coagulation (Schmidt, 1892).

Coagulation Cascades

Researchers were able to show that blood coagulated when it came into contact with a foreign surface and that some surfaces were more "thrombogenic" than others. This concept paved the way for an expanding knowledge of hereditary disorders of coagulation (Hay, 1813; Otto, 1803). Developments in defining extrinsic coagulation followed the pioneering work of several investigators (De Blainville, 1834; Howell, 1912; Mills, 1921; Thackrah, 1819), all of whom described blood coagulation following the infusion of tissue suspensions (later called tissue thromboplastin or tissue factor). A revised theory of extrinsic coagulation suggested that an exposed tissue surface (from a damaged blood vessel wall) was capable of stimulating blood clotting. Later discoveries included the direct contribution of calcium (Bordet, 1921), phospholipid (Chargaff et al., 1944), and other essential components of the prothrombinase complex (factors Va, Xa) (Hougie et al., 1957; Quick, 1957) to blood coagulation (Figure 1.2).

Cell-Based Models of Hemostasis

The "waterfall" or "cascade" model of coagulation, proposed almost simultaneously by MacFarlane (1964) and Davie and Ratnoff (1964), expanded earlier theories and provided both a structural and biochemical framework for understanding coagulation; however, its separation of the *intrinsic* and *extrinsic* pathways and the absence of platelets and other cellular elements from the working construct represented a clear limitation in application to in vivo hemostasis and thrombosis.

The cell-based model of hemostasis and thrombosis (Hoffman and Monroe, 2001) established a physiologic, integrated, and highly functional view of complex biochemical events on cellular surfaces rather than distinct and relatively independent cascades. It also provided a scientific underpinning for recognized variability between individuals regarding platelet procoagulant activity, thrombin gen-

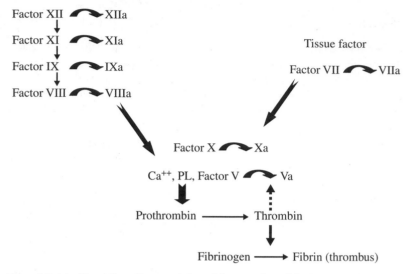

Figure 1.2 A traditional view of hemostasis (waterfall or cascade model). The *intrinsic coagulation cascade* is initiated following "contact" with an abnormal surface and, as the name implies, all of the coagulation proteins (clotting factors) are found within circulating blood. In contrast, the *extrinsic coagulation cascade* is initiated by tissue thromboplastin (tissue factor) that is found within damaged vessel walls. Both the intrinsic and extrinsic coagulation cascades lead to the generation of thrombin—an enzyme that is capable of converting fibrinogen to fibrin (the predominant constituent of blood clots/thrombus). PL, phospholipid.

eration in platelet-rich plasma (Brummel et al., 2001), platelet activation triggered by thrombin (Lasne et al., 1997), and the potential importance of specific platelet-binding sites for coagulation proteins (Monroe et al., 2002), as well as the non-hemostatic roles of the coagulation proteins, which include inflammation, vascular repair, and smooth muscle cell proliferation.

According to the cell-based model of coagulation, *initiation* takes place on tissue factor–bearing cells (monocytes, macrophages, activated endothelial cells). In the presence of fVIIa (complexed with tissue factor), activation of fIX and fXa (which subsequently activate fV) generates a small amount of thrombin (from prothrombin). In the *amplification* (or priming) phase, the small amount of thrombin generated activates platelets (causing release of α-granule contents), fV, fXI, and fVIII (by cleaving it from von Willebrand factor). During the *propagation* phase, fIXa binds to activated platelets and causes activation of fX (fXI provides an additional source of fIXa). The complexing of fXa and fVa leads to a "burst" of thrombin generation (Figure 1.3).

The remaining phases of hemostasis and thrombosis, *termination* and *elimination*, are overlooked frequently, yet provide a critical basis for understanding po-

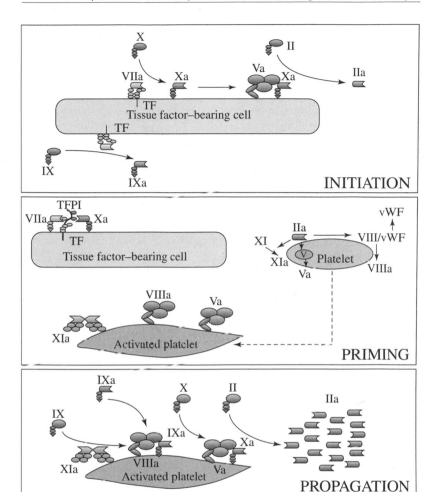

Figure 1.3 A current or cell-based model of coagulation. In this scheme, coagulation begins on tissue factor–bearing cells followed by platelets in three integrated phases: initiation, priming, and propagation. TF, tissue factor; TFPI, tissue factor pathway inhibitor; vWF, von Willebrand factor. (From Monroe DM, Hoffman M, Roberts HR. Platelets and thrombin generation. *Arterioscl Thromb Vasc Biol* 2002;22:1381–1389.)

tential focal points in dysregulated physiologic processes that characterize atherosclerosis and other vascular disorders associated with thrombosis. *Termination* of coagulation is regulated by (1) antithrombin III—a member of the serpin protease family that inhibits thrombin, fIXa, fXa, fXIa, and the fVIIa- tissue factor complex; (2) tissue factor pathway inhibitor—a modular protein that inhibits fXa and the fVIIa–tissue factor complex; and (3) activated protein C—generated in response to thrombin production (and thrombomodulin) and capable of inhibiting fVa and fVIIIa. *Elimination* is intricately linked to thrombin generation, fibrin homeostasis, and vascular repair. Tissue plasminogen activator (tPA) generates plasmin (from plasminogen) at the thrombus interface, where it digests fibrin. Urokinase plasminogen activator (uPA) binds to a cellular uPA receptor (uPAR), generating pericellular plasmin, which plays a pivotal role in tissue remodeling and cellular migration (Broze et al., 1988; Casu et al., 1991; Nesheim, 1998; Rapaport, 1991).

Platelets

The contribution of platelets to the coagulation process can be traced back to the mid-19th century and the original work of Alfred Donné, who discovered platelets with the help of a newly developed microscope lens (achromatic lens) (Donné, 1842). However, the clinical importance of platelets in normal hemostasis was not appreciated until the end of the 19th century, when Sir William Osler (1874) described platelet aggregation and Hayem (1882) cited the importance of platelet plugs in preventing blood loss after tissue injury (Figure 1.4).

The development of electron microscopy made it clear that platelets adhered to damaged blood vessels (Marcus, 1969) and subsequently were "activated" through a variety of pharmacologic (e.g., adenosine diphosphate, epinephrine, thrombin) or mechanical (e.g., shear stress) stimuli (Grette, 1962; Spaet and Zucker, 1964; Willis et al., 1974). More recent observations highlight the role of coagulation-binding sites on platelet surfaces in regulating thrombotic processes.

Fibrinolysis

The inability of blood to fully coagulate following death was observed centuries ago, possibly as early as the days of Hippocrates (Konttinen, 1968). Pioneering work

Figure 1.4 The vital role of platelets in providing the "first line of defense" or "hemostatic plug" after tissue (vessel wall) injury was described in the mid- to late-19th century.

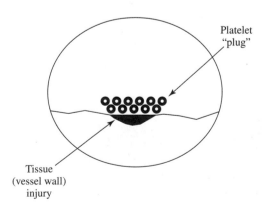

Platelet "plug"

Tissue (vessel wall) injury

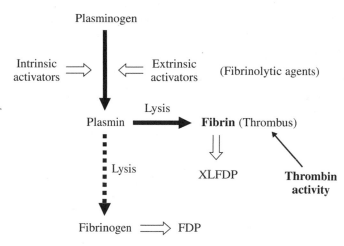

Figure 1.5 The fibrinolytic system consists of an inactive precursor (plasminogen) that is converted (by either intrinsic or extrinsic activators) to plasmin—an active enzyme that degrades (lysis) fibrin and, to a lesser degree, fibrinogen. FDP, fibrinogen degradation product; XL, cross-linked.

near the end of the 18th century described the process of fibrinolysis and a mechanism whereby a circulating precursor (plasminogen) generated (with the appropriate stimulus) an active enzyme (plasmin) capable of degrading clotted blood (Christensen and MacLeod, 1945; Hedin, 1904).

The potential clinical ramifications of fibrinolysis and its application in treating thrombotic disorders began with the work of Gratia in 1921, who observed that clots could be dissolved by staphylococcal extracts (Gratia, 1968). Tillet and Garner (1933) later reported that bacteria-free filtrates of β-hemolytic streptococci contained a substance (streptokinase) that was capable of dissolving blood clots. Soon thereafter, the groundbreaking work of Sherry et al. (1959) highlighted the potential use of fibrinolytics in humans. Plasminogen activators—found in many tissues of the body, including blood vessels themselves—were also discovered (MacFarlane and Pilling, 1947; Williams, 1951) and have served an important role in understanding natural thromboresistance as well as in the development of potent fibrinolytic agents for treating thrombotic disorders in humans (Figure 1.5).

Summary

Historical perspectives of hemostasis, coagulation, and fibrinolysis highlight fundamental and integrated constructs in genetics, biochemistry, and physiology, each carefully regulated to prevent life-threatening blood loss following vascular injury and to sustain vital organ perfusion. Recent observations underscore cell-based interactions that provide a basis for understanding hemostatic and thrombotic disorders as well as their management.

References

Babington BG. Some considerations with respect to the blood founded on one or two very simple experiments on that fluid. *Med Chir Trans* 1830;16:293–319.

Bordet J. The theories of blood coagulation. *Bull Johns Hopkins Hospital* 1921;32:213–218.

Broze GJ Jr, Warren LA, Novotny WF, et al. The lipoprotein-associated coagulation inhibitor that inhibits the factor VII-tissue factor complex also inhibits factor Xa: insight into its possible mechanism of action. *Blood* 1988;71:335–343.

Brummel KE, Paradis SG, Branda RF, Mann KG. Oral anticoagulation thresholds. *Circulation* 2001;104:2311–2317.

Buchanan A. On the coagulation of the blood and other fibriniferous liquids. *Lond Med Caz* 1845;1:617. Reprinted in *J Physiol* (Lond) 1879–1880;2:158–168.

Casu B, Oreste P, Torri G, et al. The structure of heparin oligosaccharide fragments with high anti-(factor Xa) activity containing the minimal antithrombin III-binding sequence. Chemical and ^{13}C nuclear-magnetic-resonance studies. *Biochem J* 1981; 197:599–609.

Chargaff E, Benedich A, Cohen SS. The thromboplastic protein: structure, properties, disintegration. *J Biol Chem* 1944;156:161–178.

Christensen LR, MacLeod CM. Proteolytic enzyme of serum: characterization, activation, and reaction with inhibitors. *J Gen Physiol* 1945;23:559–583.

Davidson CJ, Tuddenham EG, McVey JH. 450 million years of hemostasis. *J Thromb Haemost* 2003;1:1487–1494.

Davie EW, Ratnoff OD. Waterfall sequence for intrinsic blood clotting. *Science* 1964; 145:1310–1312.

De Blainville HMD. Injection de matiére cerebrale dans les veins. *Gaz Med Paris* 1834; 2:524.

Donné A. De l' origine des globules du sang, de leur mode de formation et leur fin. *C R Acad Sci* (Paris) 1842;14:366–368.

Forester JM (translator). Malpighi M: *De Polypo Cordis*, 1686. Uppsala, Almquist & Wiksels, 1956.

Gratia A. Quoted by Kontinnen YP. *Fibrinolysis: Chemistry, Physiology, Pathology and Clinics.* Tampere, Finland, Oy Star Ab, 1968.

Grette K. Studies on the mechanism of thrombin-catalyzed hemostatic reactions in blood platelets. *Acta Physiol Scand* [Suppl]1962;195:1–93.

Hay J. Account of a remarkable haemorrhagic disposition, existing in many individuals of the same family. *N Engl J Med* 1813;2:221–225.

Hayem G. Sur le méchanisme de l' arret des hemorrhagies. *C R Acad Sci* 1882;95:18–21.

Hedin SG. On the presence of a proteolytic enzyme in the normal serum of the ox. *J Physiol* (Lond) 1904;30:195–201.

Hoffman M, Monroe DM 3rd. The action of high-dose factor VIIa (FVIIa) in a cell-based model of hemostasis. *Sem Hem* 2001;38(Suppl 12):6–9.

Hougie C, Barrow EM, Graham JB. Stuart clotting defect. I. Segregation of an hereditary hemorrhagic state from the heterogenous group heretofore called "stable factor" (SPCA, proconvertin, factor VII) deficiency. *J Clin Invest* 1957;36:485–496.

Howell WH. The nature and action of the thromboplastin (zymoplastic) substance of the tissues. *Am J Physiol* 1912;31:1–21.

Jewett B (ed.). *The Dialogues of Plato,* 3rd ed., New York, Macmillan, 1892;3:339–543.

Konttinen YP. *Fibrinolysis: Chemistry, Physiology, Pathology and Clinics.* Tampere, Finland, Oy Star Ab, 1968.

Krem MM, Cera ED. Evolution of enzyme cascades from embryonic development to blood coagulation. *Trends Biochem Sci* 2002;27:67–74.

Lasne D, Krenn M, Pingault V, et al. Interdonor variability of platelet response to thrombin receptor activation: influence of PLA_2 polymorphism. *Br J Haematol* 1997;88:801–807.

Lee HDP (translator). *Aristotle: Meterologica.* Loeb Classical Library. Cambridge, Harvard University Press, 1952.

MacFarlane RG. An enzyme cascade in the blood clotting mechanism, and its function as a biological amplifier. *Nature* 1964;202:498–499.

MacFarlane RG, Pilling J. Fibrinolytic activity of normal urine. *Nature* 1947;159:779.

Marcus AJ. Platelet function. *N Engl J Med* 1969;280:1213–1220, 1278–1284, 1330–1335.

McLysaght A, Hokamp K, Wolfe KH. Extensive genomic duplication during early chordate evolution. *Nat Genet* 2002;31:200–204.

Mills CA. Chemical nature of tissue coagulants. *J Biol Chem* 1921;46:135–165.

Monroe DM, Hoffman M, Roberts HR. Platelets and thrombin generation. *Arterioscler Thromb Vasc Biol* 2002;22:1381–1389.

Nesheim M. Fibrinolysis and plasma carboxypeptidase. *Curr Opin Hematol* 1998;5:309–313.

Osler W. An account of certain organisms occurs in the liquor sanguinis. *Proc Roy Soc* 1874;22:391–398.

Otto JC. An account of an hemorrhagic disposition exists in certain families. *Med Repository* 1803;6:1–4.

Petit JL. Dissertation sur la manniére d'arrester le sang dans les hémorrhagies. *Mem Acad R Sci* 1731;1:85–102.

Quick AJ. *Hemorrhagic Diseases.* Philadelphia, Lea & Febiger, 1957.

Rapaport SI. The extrinsic pathway inhibitor: a regulator of tissue factor-dependent blood coagulation. *Thromb Haemost* 1991;66:6–15.

Schmidt A. *Zur Blutlehre.* Leipzig, Vogel, 1892.

Sherry S, Fletcher A, Alkjaersig N. Fibrinolysis and fibrinolytic activity in man. *Physiol Rev* 1959;39:343–381.

Spaet TH, Zucker MB. Mechanism of platelet plug formation and role of adenosine diphosphate. *Am J Physiol* 1964;206:1267–1274.

Thackrah CT. *An Inquiry into the Nature and Properties of the Blood.* London, Cox & Sons, 1819.

Tillett WS, Garner RL. The fibrinolytic activity of hemolytic streptococci. *J Exp Med* 1933;58:485–502.

Williams JRB. The fibrinolytic activity of urine. *Br J Exp Pathol* 1951;32:530–537.

Willis AL, Vane FM, Kuhn DC, et al. An endoperoxide aggregator (LASS) formed in platelets in response to thrombotic stimuli. *Prostaglandins* 1974;8:453–507.

Vascular Biology, Thromboresistance, and Inflammation

2

The delivery of vital substrate to metabolically active tissues and vital organs is achieved and maintained by the cardiovascular system including the heart, macrovasculature, and microvasculature. This life-sustaining process requires a normally functioning vascular endothelium—a multifunctional organ system composed of physiologically responsive cells responsible for vasomotion (vascular tone), thromboresistance, and inflammoresistance.

Vascular Endothelium

Simply by virtue of its anatomic location, the vascular endothelium is functionally complex. It defines the intra- and extravascular components, serves as a selectively permeable barrier, and provides a continuous lining to the cardiovascular system. The location of the vascular endothelium is vital to its biologic interactions with cells found within the circulation and to the vessel wall itself (Table 2.1). The surface activity is augmented in the microcirculation, also known as the resistance bed, where the ratio of endothelial surface to circulating blood is maximal.

Anatomic Features

In most vertebrates, vascular endothelial cells form a single layer of squamous lining cells (0.1–0.5 μm in thickness) joined by intercellular junctions. The cells themselves are polygonal (varying between 10 and 50 μm) and are positioned in the long axis of the vessel, orienting the cellular longitudinal dimension in the direction of blood flow.

The endothelial cell has three surfaces: luminal (nonthrombogenic), subluminal (adhesive), and cohesive. The luminal surface is devoid of electron-dense connective tissue. It does, however, possess an exterior coat (or glycocalyx), consisting primarily of starches and proteins secreted by the endothelial cells. Plasma proteins, including lipoprotein lipase, α_2-macroglobulin, heparin cofactor II, antithrombin, and albumin, as well as small amounts of fibrinogen and fibrin are adsorbed to the luminal surface. The surface membrane itself adds significantly to thromboresistance by carrying a negative charge that repels similarly charged circulating blood cells.

The subluminal (or abluminal) surface adheres to subendothelial connective tissues. Small processes penetrate through a series of internal layers to form myoendothelial junctions with subjacent smooth muscle cells.

Table 2.1 Anatomic and Biologic Features of the Vascular Endothelium

Vasoreactivity (maintain vascular tone)
Thromboresistance
Inflammoresistance
Metabolic activity (synthetic/secretory)
Inflammatory/immune regulation
Vascular growth and remodeling
Selective barrier

The cohesive component of the vascular endothelium connects individual endothelial cells to one another by cell junctions of two basic types: occluding (tight) junctions and communicating (gap) junctions. Occluding junctions represent a physical link between adjacent cells, sealing the intercellular space. Communicating junctions provide a means for cell–cell interactions and are instrumental in electronic coupling and intracellular exchange of ions and small metabolites.

Biologic Activity

The vascular endothelium is an active site of protein synthesis. Endothelial cells synthesize, secrete, modify, and internally regulate connective tissue components, vasoconstrictors, vasodilators, anticoagulants, procoagulants, prostanoids, fibrinolytic molecules, and modulators of inflammation, each contributing to the maintenance of normal vasomotion, thromboresistance, inflammoresistance and physiologic hemostasis (Figures 2.1 and 2.2).

Figure 2.1 The vascular endothelium is a major regulator of vasomotion. Vasodilation is mediated predominantly by NO and PGI$_2$, whereas vasoconstriction is driven by endothelin-1 and angiotensin II. AI, angiotensin I; AII, angiotensin II; ACE, angiotensin-converting enzyme; NO, nitric oxide; PGI$_2$, prostacyclin.

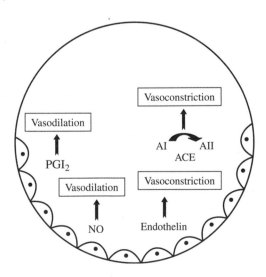

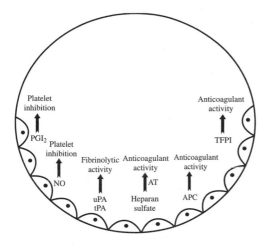

Figure 2.2 Thromboresistance is accomplished by a number of surface molecules that inhibit platelet aggregation (PGI$_2$, NO), prevent thrombus formation (heparan sulfate, AT, APC, TFPI), and promote clot dissolution (tPA, uPA). NO, nitric oxide; PGI$_2$, prostacyclin; AT, antithrombin; APC, activated protein C; TFPI, tissue factor pathway inhibitor; tPA, tissue plasminogen activator; uPA, urokinase plasminogen activator.

Vasoreactivity

Endothelium-dependent vasodilation, first described by Furchgott and Zawadski (1980), is direct and receptor-mediated (Table 2.2). It has been postulated that endothelium-dependent vasodilators stimulate the synthesis and/or release of nitric oxide (NO), which, in turn, activates guanylate cyclase and ultimately calcium release from smooth muscle cells. Endothelium-independent mediators activate guanylate cyclase directly.

Vasoconstriction is also mediated by endothelial cells that metabolize local and circulating vasoactive molecules. This process may involve uptake and subsequent intracellular metabolism or extracellular metabolizing by ectoenzymes present on the luminal surface.

Prostacyclin

Prostacyclin (PGI$_2$) is a potent vasodilating substance released locally in response to biochemical and mechanical stimulation, including thrombin, thromboxane A$_2$,

Table 2.2 Endothelium-Dependent and -Independent Vasodilation

Acetylcholine	Adenosine
Serotonin	Prostacyclin
Histamine	Nitroglycerin
Thrombin	Nitric oxide
Norepinephrine	Insulin
Leukotrienes (LTC$_4$, LTD$_4$)	Glucagon
	Bradykinin

histamine, bradykinin, high-density lipoproteins, tissue hypoxia, platelet-derived growth factor, and hemodynamic (shear) stress (Piper and Vane, 1971). Prostacyclin, by increasing intracellular cyclic adenosine monophosphate (cAMP), also inhibits platelet aggregation.

Nitric Oxide

Using strips of arteries in organ baths (i.e., an isolated system) Furchgott and Zawadski (1980) discovered that acetylcholine-mediated vasodilation required an intact vascular endothelium. Nitric oxide (Palmer et al., 1987) is an L-arginine derivative that causes smooth muscle relaxation by increasing intracellular cyclic guanosine monophosphate (cGMP). It is released locally in response to a number of pharmacologic mediators, including bradykinin, thrombin, histamine, thromboxane A_2, adenine nucleotides, and aggregating platelets. In addition to its vasoactive potential, NO is also a potent inhibitor of platelet adhesion and aggregation as well as leukocyte migration (Radomski et al., 1987 a, b).

Endothelin

The vascular endothelium, in addition to synthesizing and secreting potent vasodilators, also produces vasoconstricting substances (Miyanchi et al., 1990) that are essential for maintaining normal blood vessel tone and responsiveness. Endothelin is a potent vasoconstrictor that exists as three structurally and functionally distinct isopeptides; however, only endothelin-1 is synthesized by vascular endothelial cells (Yanagisawa et al., 1988). Following local mechanical or biochemical stimulation, endothelin-1 activates intracellular protein C, leading to smooth muscle contraction (vasoconstriction) (Stenflo and Fernlund, 1982). Endothelin may also have important thromboresistant properties.

Angiotensin II

Studied extensively since the late 1970s, angiotensin II is a potent vasoconstrictor that has a prominent role in maintaining blood vessel tone (Heeg and Meng, 1965). Although there has been some debate, most investigators in the field agree that angiotensin-converting enzyme (ACE), required for the conversion of angiotensin I to angiotensin II, is synthesized within vascular endothelial cells.

Thromboresistance

The hemostatic mechanism is among the most important defense mechanisms in humans; however, the maintenance of blood fluidity and vital organ perfusion is

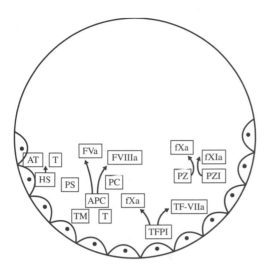

Figure 2.3
thrombin ge
through sever
nisms. Antithro
with heparin su
other heparin-like
facilitating the neut
thrombin (T). Small a
thrombin generated o
vascular surface combin
thrombomodulin (TM) and
C (PC) in the presence of pro
(PS) to cause its activation (A
which, in turn, neutralizes fact
(f) Va and VIIIa. Tissue factor pat
way inhibitor (TFPI) binds (and
neutralizes) fXa and the tissue
factor (TF)–fVIIa complex. And
last, protein Z (PZ) serves as a
cofactor for PZ inhibitor (PZI),
which neutralizes FXa and fXIa.

fundamental to life (Figure 2.3). The ultimate goal of thromboresistance is to prevent thrombin generation and subsequent fibrin formation.

Heparan Sulfate

Mast cells were previously thought to be the only cells capable of synthesizing anticoagulant-active heparin; however, studies by several prominent investigators (Marcum and Rosenberg, 1985; Teien et al., 1977; Thomas et al., 1979) have shown that vascular endothelial cells are capable of synthesizing heparin-like molecules. One in particular, heparan sulfate, has well-known anticoagulant properties. Accordingly, it is currently accepted that thromboresistance is maintained, at least in part, by the interaction of heparin-like substances with antithrombin and heparin cofactor II, both located on the vascular endothelial surface, accelerating the neutralization of hemostatic proteins.

Antithrombin

Antithrombin (AT) neutralizes thrombin (and other hemostatic proteins) by forming a 1:1 stoichiometric complex between two reactants (the interaction o   he-
tween arginine at the reactive site and serine at the active site). Comple
occurs slowly in the absence of heparin, but proceeds rapidly in it
causing an allosteric alteration in an AT arginine residue, making it
to thrombin. Coagulation factors IXa, Xa and XIa, and XIIa are
through a similar mechanism.

? for the important anticoagulation pro-

10) that is held together covalently
.o, 1982; Stenflo and Fernlund,
_ heavy chain, whereas the light chain
_s. Thus, the heavy chain is involved di-
.ty and the light chain participates in calcium-
_mbrane surfaces. Protein C differs from other vita-
₃ factors by inhibiting coagulation. The mechanism of
_ctive inactivation of factors Va and VIIIa (Kisiel et al., 1977;
₈82; Suzuki et al., 1983; Walker et al., 1979).
_ression of activated protein C (APC) anticoagulant activity is highly
_₄ and dependent on another vitamin K–dependent protein—protein S, a
₃.e-chain glycoprotein found on the endothelial surface. Physiologically, protein
C is activated by thrombin (APC) in the presence of protein S and thrombomodulin (an endothelial cell surface receptor). The interaction of thrombin and thrombomodulin also neutralizes thrombin's procoagulant potential.

Tissue Factor Pathway Inhibitor

Tissue factor pathway inhibitor (TFPI) is a protein that circulates bound to low-
density lipoprotein (LDL) and high-density lipoprotein (HDL). It can inhibit both
the VIIa tissue factor complex and factor Xa. In the coagulation cascade, TFPI inhibits the production of factor Xa generated by the extrinsic X^{ase} complex, thus inhibiting clot formation more "proximally" (in the coagulation cascade) than either
AT or APC. Although TFPI circulates bound to lipoproteins, a majority (nearly 90%)
is bound to heparin-like species on the endothelial surface (Broze et al., 1988) and
is released constitutively and following exogenous heparin administration. There is
evidence that endothelial cell depletion of TFPI may contribute to "rebound" thrombin generation following the sudden cessation of unfractionated heparin (Becker et
al., 1999).

Protein Z

Protein Z (PZ) is a vitamin K–dependent plasma protein that serves as a cofactor
for the inhibition of factor Xa by protein Z–dependent protease inhibitor. Inhibition of factor Xa by protein Z inhibitor (PZI) in the presence of phospholipid and
calcium is enhanced 1,000-fold by PZ, but PZI also inhibits factor XIa independently (Broze, 2001).

Fibrinolytic System

The primary fibrinolytic enzyme is plasmin, a serine protease generated from plasminogen by plasminogen activators found on the endothelial surface. Plasminogen activators are themselves highly specific serine proteases that have minimal effect on most proteins; however, they cleave plasminogen (a single-chain disulfide-linked glycoprotein of Mr 88000) at a single bond (Arg 560–Val 561), converting an inactive zymogen into the active trypsin-like enzyme plasmin. In turn, plasmin digests fibrin networks that bind platelets together and form the supporting meshwork for most clots (physiologic and pathologic).

There are at least two plasminogen activator systems: an intrinsic system and an extrinsic system. The intrinsic system defines a fibrinolytic pathway in which essential components exist in blood at relatively high concentrations, but in precursor forms. These components include factor XII, factor XI, high-molecular-weight kininogen, and prekallikrein. Urokinase is the predominant plasminogen activator in the intrinsic system. The extrinsic system consists of active enzymes extractable from tissues (tissue-type plasminogen activator). Vascular endothelial cells synthesize and secrete a single-chain form of tissue-type plasminogen activator.

Procoagulant Molecules

Because hemostasis is a vital function of blood vessels, for each molecule that prevents clot formation, there is a molecule that potentiates it, thereby illustrating the complex system of "checks and balances" that exists on the vascular endothelial surface. Some of the procoagulant substances include platelet activating factor, von Willebrand factor, tissue factor, and plasminogen activator inhibitor (PAI).

Anti-inflammatory Properties of the Normal Vessel Wall (Inflammoresistance)

The anti-inflammatory properties that characterize the normal vessel wall involve a variety of external signals and intracellular mediators (Kaene, 2000) (Figure 2.4). The external signals include anti-inflammatory cytokines, transforming growth factor-β, interleukin (IL)-10, IL-1 receptor agonist, and HDL cholesterol, as well as several angiogenic growth factors. Laminar shear stress, through the production of NO, is of particular importance in protecting endothelial cells against inflammation (Tedgui and Mallat, 2001).

A second line of defense is achieved by vascular endothelial cells and smooth muscle cells, which regulate chemokine-induced immunoinflammatory responses. Several antiapoptotic genes (cytoprotective genes) have also been shown to possess anti-inflammatory properties.

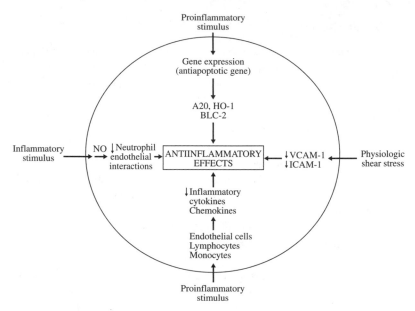

Figure 2.4 Anti-inflammatory properties, inherent to a normal vessel wall, are a vital defense against the proliferative, atherogenic, and prothrombotic effects of injurious agents. NO, nitric oxide; VCAM, vascular cell adhesion molecule; ICAM, intercellular adhesion molecule.

The importance of NO as an inhibitor of neutrophil–endothelial cell interactions has been demonstrated (Kubes et al., 1991). Transforming growth factor-β-1 significantly decreases monocyte chemotactic protein (MCP)-1 expression in human umbilical vein endothelial cells stimulated with tumor necrosis factor (TNF)-α. It also inhibits the synthesis of IL-8 by TNF-activated endothelial cells. IL-10 exerts its protective effect by attenuating NF(κ)B activity through both suppression of I(κ)B kinase activity and suppression of NF(κ)B DNA binding activity, inhibiting leukocyte–endothelial cell interactions and suppressing proinflammatory cytokine synthesis by macrophages and lymphocytes. IL-4 and IL-13 decrease monocyte-related chemokine production. High-density lipoprotein cholesterol inhibits cytokine-induced expression of E-selectin and intercellular adhesion molecule-1 (ICAM-1) on endothelial cells. It also inhibits TNF-induced sphingosine kinase activity.

Physiologic levels of shear stress play a pivotal role in maintaining a noninflammatory state. Prolonged exposure of endothelial cells to laminar flow causes down-regulation of vascular adhesion molecule-1 (VCAM-1) and ICAM-1, while low or oscillatory shear-stress conditions enhance monocyte adhesion and expression of E-selectin, ICAM, and VCAM-1. Laminar shear stress induces Cu/Zn superoxide dismutase, minimizing the production of superoxide radicals (Mohan et al., 1999; Sampath et al., 1995).

Endothelial Dysfunction

It has been recognized for some time that a denuded vascular endothelium can be a site for thrombus formation. There is also evidence that the functional status of endothelial cells may be as important as anatomic integrity in the maintenance of vasoreactivity, thromboresistance, and inflammoresistance.

Hypercholesterolemia, even in the absence of atherosclerosis, can adversely affect vascular endothelial cell function (Tagawa et al., 1991). Vascular relaxation in the coronary resistance bed is impaired (Selke et al., 1990). Furthermore, oxidized LDL reduces NO by disrupting the endothelial receptor signal transduction process (Galle et al., 1990). Even low concentrations of oxidized LDL have been shown to selectively impair G-proteins (or G-protein–dependent pathways) (Galle et al., 1990; Tagawa et al., 1991; Verbeuren et al., 1990).

Endothelial cell function can also be altered by cytokines and other humoral mediators that appear to participate in the atherosclerotic process (Pober and Gimbrone, 1982; Pober et al., 1983, a, b; Rodgers and Shuman, 1983).

Assembly of the complete coagulation pathway can take place on the endothelial surface of damaged or "dysfunctional" endothelial cells. The observed procoagulant potential may be the result of endothelial cell synthesis and expression of factors VIII, IX, and X and tissue factor (Stern et al., 1983, 1985), impaired thrombin–thrombomodulin interactions (APC-mediated anticoagulation), or impaired local fibrinolytic activity (Walker et al., 1977).

Once coagulation has been initiated, endothelial cells can promote prothrombinase assembly by binding factor Xa and expressing factor Va (endothelial cells have binding sites for factors Xa and Va). Further activation of coagulation is facilitated by the binding of thrombin and fibrinogen and through the release of von Willebrand factor (VWF; stored in Weibel-Palade bodies), potentiating platelet adherence (Rimm et al., 1987).

The failure of bone marrow–derived vascular endothelial progenitor cells to replenish damaged or dysfunctional senescent cells may contribute to a prothrombotic and proinflammatory environment (Rauscher et al., 2003).

Summary

The vascular endothelium is a metabolically active and physiologically diverse organ system that plays a pivotal role in maintaining normal tissue perfusion through distinct yet integrated processes, including vasoreactivity, thromboresistance, and inflammoresistance. Endothelial dysfunction in response to injury or inadequate bone marrow–derived precursors increases the propensity for atherosclerosis and thrombosis.

References

Becker RC, Spencer F, Li Y, et al. Thrombin generation after the abrupt cessation of intravenous unfractionated heparin among patients with acute coronary syndromes: potential mechanisms for heightened prothrombotic potential. *J Am Coll Cardiol* 1999;34:1020–1027.

Broze GJ Jr., Warren LA, Novotny WF, et al. The lipoprotein-associated coagulation inhibitor that inhibits the factor VII-tissue factor complex also inhibits factor Xa: insight into the possible mechanism of action. *Blood* 1988;71:335–343.

Broze GJ Jr. Protein Z-dependent regulation of coagulation. *Thromb Haemost* 2001; 86:8–13.

Fernlund P, Stenflo J. Amino acid sequence of the heavy chain of bovine protein C. *Biol Chem* 1982;257:12470–12479.

Furchgott RF, Zawadski JV. The obligatory role of endothelial cells in the relaxation of arterial smooth muscle cells by acetylcholine. *Nature* 1980;288:373–376.

Galle J, Bassenge E, Busse R. Oxidized low density lipoproteins potentiate vasoconstrictions to various agonists by direct interaction with vascular smooth muscle. *Circ Res* 1990;66:1287–1293.

Heeg E, Meng K. Die wirkung des bradykinins, angiotensins and vasopressins auf verhof papillarmusckel, undisoliert durstromte herzpraparate des meerchweinchens. Naunyn schmiedebergs. *Arch Pharmacol* 1965;250:35–41.

Kaene M, Strieter R. Chemokine signaling in inflammation. *Crit Care Med* 2000;28: N13–26.

Kisiel W, Canfield WM, Erisson EH, et al. Anticoagulant properties of bovine plasma protein C activation by thrombin. *Biochemistry* 1977;16:5824–5831.

Kubes P, Suzuki M, Granger DN. Nitric oxide: an endogenous modulator of leukocyte adhesion. *Proc Natl Acad Sci USA* 1991;88:4651–4655.

Marcum JA, Rosenberg RD. Heparin-like molecules with anticoagulant activity are synthesized by cultured endothelial cells. *Biochem Biophys Res Commun* 1985;123:365.

Miyanchi T, Tomobe Y, Shiba R, et al. Involvement of endothelin in the regulation of human vascular tonus: potent vasoconstrictor effect and existence in endothelial cells. *Circulation* 1990;81:1874–1880.

Mohan S, Mohan N, Valente AJ, Sprague EA. Regulation of low shear flow-induced HAEC VCAM-1 expression and monocyte adhesion. *Am J Physiol* 1999;276:C1100–C1107.

Nesheim ME, Canfield WM, Kisiel W, et al. Studies on the capacity of factor Xa to protect factor Va from inactivation by activated protein C. *Biol Chem* 1982;257: 1433–1447.

Palmer RMJ, Ferige AG, Moncada S. Nitric oxide release accounts for the biologic activity of endothelium-derived relaxing factor. *Nature* 1987;327:524–526.

Piper P, Vane JR. The release of prostaglandins from the vascular endothelium and other tissues. *Ann NY Acad Sci* 1971;180:363–385.

Pober JS, Gimbrone MA Jr. Expression of Ia-like antigens by human vascular endothelial cells inducible in vitro: demonstration by monoclonal antibody binding and immunoprecipitation. *Proc Natl Acad Aci USA* 1982;79:6641–6645.

Pober JS, Collins T, Gimbrone MA Jr, et al. Lymphocytes recognize human vascular endothelial and dermal fibroblast Ia antigens induced by recombinant immune interferon. *Nature* 1983a;305:726–729.

Pober JS, Gimbrone MA Jr, Cotran RS, et al. Ia expression by vascular endothelium is inducible by activated T-lymphocytes and human gamma interferon. *J Exp Med* 1983b;157:1339–1353.

Radomski MW, Palmer RM, Moncada S. Endogenous nitric oxide inhibits human platelet adhesion to vascular endothelium. *Lancet* 1987a;1:1057–1058.

Radomski MW, Palmer RM, Moncada S. The antiaggregatory properties of vascular endothelium: interactions between prostacyclin and nitric oxide. *Br J Pharmacol* 1987b; 92:639–646.

Rauscher FM, Goldschmidt-Clermont PJ, Davis BH, et al. Aging, progenitor cell exhaustion, and atherosclerosis. *Circulation* 2003;108:457–463.

Rimm S, Savior N, Scott T, et al. Identification of a factor IX and IXa binding protein in the endothelial cell surface. *J Biol Chem* 1987;262;6023–6031.

Rodgers GM, Shuman MA. Prothrombin is activated on vascular endothelial cells by factor Xa and calcium. *Proc Natl Acad Sci USA* 1983;80:7001.

Sampath R, Kukielka GL, Smith CW, Eskin SG, McIntire LV. Shear stress-mediated changes in the expression of leukocyte adhesion receptors on human umbilical vein endothelial cells in vitro. *Ann Biomed Eng* 1995;23:247–256.

Selke FW, Armstrong ML, Harrison DG. Endothelium-dependent vascular relaxation is abnormal in the coronary microcirculation of atherosclerotic primates. *Circulation* 1990;81:1586–1593.

Stenflo J, Fernlund P. Amino acid sequence of the heavy chain of bovine protein C. *Biol Chem* 1982;257:12180–12190.

Stern D, Drillings N, Nossel H, et al. Binding of factors IX and IXa to cultured endothelial cells. *Proc Natl Acad Sci USA* 1983;80:4119–4123.

Stern D, Knitter G, Kisiel W, et al. The binding of factor IXa to cultured bovine aortic endothelial cells. *J Biol Chem* 1985;260:6717–6722.

Suzuki K, Stenflo J, Dahlback B, et al. Inactivation of human coagulation factor V by activated protein C. *J Biol Chem* 1983;258:1914–1920.

23

Tagawa H, Tomoike H, Nakamura M. Putative mechanisms of the impairment of endothelium-dependent relaxation of the aorta with atheromatous plaque in heritable hyperlipidemic rabbits. *Circ Res* 1991;68:330–337.

Tedgui A, Mallat Z. Anti-inflammatory mechanism in the vascular wall. *Circulation* 2001;88:877–887.

Teien AN, Abildgaard U, Hook M, et al. The anticoagulant effect of heparan sulfate and dermatan sulfate. *Thromb Res* 1977;11:107.

Thomas DP, Merton RE, Barrowcliffe TW, et al. Antifactor Xa activity of heparan sulfate. *Thromb Res* 1979;14:501.

Verbeuren TJ, Jordaens FH, VanHove CE, et al. Release and vascular activity of endothelium-derived relaxing factor in atherosclerotic rabbit aorta. *Eur J Pharmacol* 1990;191: 173–184.

Walker ID, Davidson JF, Hutton I, et al. Disordered fibrinolytic potential in coronary heart disease. *Thromb Res* 1977;10:509–520.

Walker FJ, Sexton PW, Esmon CT. The inhibition of blood coagulation by activated protein C through the selective inactivation of activated factor V. *Biochim Biophys Acta* 1979;571:333–342.

Yanagisawa M, Kurihara H, Kimsura S, et al. A novel potent vasoconstrictor produced by vascular endothelial cells. *Nature* 1988;332:411–415.

Atherosclerosis and
Arterial Thrombosis

3

The development of atherosclerotic vascular disease represents a major risk for myocardial infarction, stroke, and occlusive peripheral vascular events. Although unique in their own right, atherosclerosis and arterial thrombosis share common origins and are linked by genetic, pathologic, and environmental factors. An increased knowledge base and in-depth understanding of vascular biology has laid the groundwork for prevention and targeted therapies.

Macroscopic Pathology

Coronary atherosclerosis has been described macroscopically over the past century and a half by renowned pathologists and clinicians ranging from Von Rokitansky and Virchow to Osler. The pathologic sequence of events includes an initiating step, defined as the fatty streak, followed by plaque maturation and transition, setting the stage for intravascular thrombosis. The progression of coronary atherosclerosis varies widely among individuals, as does the time course and influence of recognized risk factors (Figure 3.1).

Microscopic Pathology

Observations at the microscopic and cellular levels have contributed substantially to unraveling several of the mysteries that surround human atherosclerosis and fostering a clearer view of the mechanisms leading to intravascular thrombosis. It is now evident that the atherosclerotic plaque and its cellular components represent an ideal substrate for thrombus formation. Thus, the term "atherothrombosis" appears fitting.

Developmental Anatomy and Cellular Biology

In experimental animals, focal sites of predilection for either spontaneous or dietary-induced atherosclerosis can be determined reliably prior to plaque development. These areas are delineated by their in vivo uptake of the protein-binding azo dye Evans blue. Salient features of these lesion-prone areas include increased endothe-

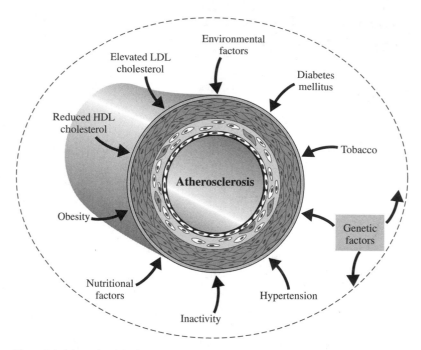

Figure 3.1 Atherosclerosis is the end result of numerous risk factors, acting either alone or, more often, in combination. The overall impact of any given risk factor is likely determined by genetic regulatory mechanisms. HDL, high-density lipoprotein; LDL, low-density lipoprotein.

lial permeability and intimal accumulation of plasma proteins, including albumin, fibrinogen, and low-density lipoproteins (LDLs). There is also increased endothelial cell turnover. Overall, the "prelesion" area within endothelial cells takes on a unique appearance, and the surface glycocalyx is two- to fivefold thinner than normal endothelial cells (Caplan et al., 1974).

Lesion-prone areas within blood vessel walls exhibit a unique property of blood monocyte recruitment, followed by accumulation of these cells in the subendothelial space, a process that is accelerated in the presence of hyperlipidemia. Based on the available information, it appears that at least two processes are pivotal in the initiation of atherosclerosis: (1) an enhanced focal endothelial transcytosis of plasma proteins, including LDLs, which accumulate in the widened proteoglycan-rich subendothelial space; and (2) the preferential recruitment of blood monocytes to the intima, a process that is markedly augmented by even a short period of hyperlipidemia. Thus, the lesion-prone subendothelial space has two key participants in atherosclerosis, namely, the monocyte (macrophage) and LDL.

Monocyte recruitment in the intimal space of lesion-prone areas is thought to be mediated by an enhanced generation of chemoattractants of which monocyte chemoattractant protein-1 (MCP-1), a cationic peptide synthesized and secreted by both arterial smooth muscle cells and endothelial cells, is of particular importance. It is also recognized that the production of MCP-1 is stimulated by minimally modified (oxidized) LDL, whereas oxidized LDL itself is chemotactic (Jauchem et al., 1982).

Atheromatous Plaque Growth, Evolution, and Ultrastructure

After monocytes attach to the morphologically intact but dysfunctional endothelium (receptive stage), there is a net directed migration of monocytes through the endothelium to the subendothelial space, where they undergo differentiation. The phenomenon of monocyte activation–differentiation plays an important role in atherosclerosis, particularly with regard to plaque remodeling and lesion progression. This complex process proceeds by means of at least two mechanisms: (1) the generation of reactive oxygen species (free radicals); and (2) the phenotypic modulation of expression of the scavenger receptor or family of receptors. The chemical modification of LDL results in its avid uptake of monocytes (now considered macrophages), and the subsequent transformation to foam cells follows. The specific receptor responsible for the uptake of modified LDL fails to down-regulate; as a result, a substantial amount of intracellular LDL cholesterol accumulates. When the influx of LDL particles exceeds the capacity of the macrophage scavenger receptors to remove them from the intracellular space, oxidized LDL particles accumulate within the arterial intima. These particles are cytotoxic, causing both injury and death to endothelial cells, smooth muscle cells, and macrophages. The net result is disruption of the relatively fragile macrophage-derived foam cells, leading to release of their intracellular lipid into the extracellular compartment of the intima; this sequence of events gives rise to the origin of the pultaceous cholesteryl ester-rich core of the atherosclerotic plaque (Table 3.1) (Figure 3.2 AB) (Stary, 1992; Swartz et al., 1985; Virmann et al., 2000).

Lipid (Necrotic) Core

The release of copious foam cell lipids to the extracellular compartment induces a second cascade of inflammatory responses within the vascular intimal layer. In particular, granulomatous foci involving macrophages, lymphocytes, and multinucleate giant cells surround and invade the extracellular lipid.

Several lines of evidence suggest that lipoproteins, particularly LDLs, aggregate and then fuse with one another in the extracellular space to form microscopi-

Table 3.1 Classification of Atherosclerosis and its Progression

Traditional Classification	Stary et al.	Virmani et al. Initial	Virmani et al. Progression
Early plaques	Type 1: Microscopic detection of lipid droplets in the intima and small groups of macrophage foam cells	Intimal thickening	None
	Type II: Fatty streaks visible on gross inspection, layers of foam cells, occasional lymphocytes and mast cells	Intimal xanthoma	None
	Type III (intermediate): Extracellular lipid pools present among layers of smooth muscle cells	Pathologic intimal thickening	Thrombus (erosion)
Intermediate plaques	Type IV: Well-defined lipid core; may develop surface disruption (fissure)	Fibrous-cap atheroma	Thrombus (erosion)[‡]
Late lesions		Thin fibrous-cap atheroma	Thrombus (rupture) Hemorrhage/fibrin[§]
	Type Va: New fibrous tissue overlying lipid core (multilayered fibroatheroma)*	Healed plaque rupture, erosion	Repeated rupture or erosion with or without total occlusion
	Type Vb: Calcification[†]	Fibrocalcific plaque (with or without necrotic core)	
Fibrous plaque	Type Vc: Fibrotic lesion with minimal lipid (could be result of organized thrombi)		
Miscellaneous/ complicated features	Type VIa: Surface disruption Type VIb: Intraplaque hemorrhage Type VIc: Thrombosis	Calcified nodule	Thrombus (usually nonocclusive)

*May overlap with healed plaque ruptures; [†]Occasionally referred to as type VII lesion; [‡]May further progress with healing (healed erosion); [§]May further progress with healing

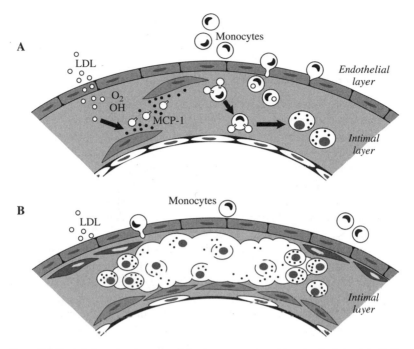

Figure 3.2 The initial step in atherosclerosis involves monocyte and low-density lipoprotein (LDL) binding to a dysfunctional endothelial surface (receptive stage). Monocyte activation and chemical modulation (oxidation) of LDL (modified LDL) results in avid uptake and transformation to macrophages (foam cells). Transformed smooth muscle cells synthesize and secrete monocyte chemoattractant proteins (MCPs) that participate in monocyte recruitment and migration within the intimal layer. The influx of modified LDL exceeds the capacity of macrophage surface receptors (impaired down-regulation), allowing accumulation of potentially cytotoxic LDL particles in the extracellular space. This step is a pivotal step in the development of a lipid core.

cally evident lipid deposits (Tirzui et al., 1995). Structures resembling lipoprotein aggregates have been visualized in human atherosclerosis by electron microscopy, and lipid aggregates containing apolipoprotein B (apo B) have also been isolated.

A number of proteins and peptides have been detected in relative abundance within or near the atherosclerotic core. Many of the proteins found in this region are relatively hydrophobic, including the apolipoproteins, C-reactive proteins (CRPs), and the 70- and 60-kDa heat shock proteins.

Cells that border and penetrate the atherosclerotic core not only participate in the deposition (or removal) of core lipids but can also be influenced by the accumulating lipids and proteins. Complement components have been found in relative abundance in the core, and both toxic and chemotactic responses may be generated via activation of complement. Antigenic markers of complement activation, including C3D and the terminal C5B-9 neoantigen, have been found in the atherosclerotic core, and terminal C5B-9 has been detected coincident with the cholesterol-rich vesicles in the subendothelium (Seifert et al., 1989).

Infection and Atherogenesis

The link between infection and atherosclerosis has been investigated with great enthusiasm given the potential for therapies that can be widely implemented (Table 3.2).

Chlamydia pneumoniae titers are increased among some individuals with atherosclerosis, and the organism has been isolated from atheromatous plaques. Although the pathobiologic relationships have not yet been elucidated fully, C. pneumoniae accelerates LDL uptake in monocytes and facilitates their transition to foam cells. Infected endothelial cells also become prothrombotic with decreased synthesis of tissue factor pathway inhibitor and plasminogen activator and increased tissue factor expression.

Cytomegalovirus (CMV) exhibits atherogenic effects through the synthesis of one or more proteins that stimulate smooth muscle cell proliferation and LDL uptake within monocytes. CMV also impairs fibrinolysis, increases production of lipoprotein-a ($LP_{(a)}$), and increases platelet adhesion.

The available evidence supports chronic rather than acute infection as a potential proatherogenic factor in genetically susceptible individuals. Infection has been linked to hypertriglyceridemia, hyperfibrinogenemia, reduced high-density lipoprotein levels, anticardiolipin antibodies, and elevated CRP levels, suggesting both direct and indirect effects on both atherogenesis and thrombogenesis (Gaydos et al., 1996; Gupta et al., 1997).

Arterial Thrombosis

Plaque Rupture

The clinical expression of atherosclerotic disease activity is determined by pathobiologic events leading to coronary thrombosis. In this regard, there are two key factors: (1) the propensity of plaques to rupture, and (2) the thrombogenicity of exposed plaque components.

The morphologic characteristics of plaques that determine their propensity to rupture have been determined. Pathology-based studies using necropsy and atherectomy tissue samples have shown convincingly that plaques associated with intraluminal thrombosis are rich in extracellular lipids and that the lipid core of these vulnerable or "rupture-prone" plaques occupies a large proportion of the overall plaque volume. The degree of cross-sectional stenosis involving the vessel lumen is typically less than 50%. In addition to the predominant lipid core, vulnerable plaques are characterized by a thin fibrous cap and high macrophage density. Whereas most individuals with atherosclerotic coronary artery disease exhibit a diversity of plaque types, most have a preponderance of one specific type (vulnerable or nonvulnerable). The genetic and acquired determinants of plaque types are subjects of intense investigation (Davies and Thomas, 1985) (Figure 3.3).

The lipid core of an advanced atherosclerotic plaque is bordered at its luminal aspect by a fibrous cap, at its edges by the shoulder region, and on its abluminal side by the plaque base. Because the lipid core contains a substantial amount of prothrombotic substrate (to be discussed in a subsequent section), the fibrous cap, separating the core from circulating blood components within the vessel's lumen, determines the overall stability of the plaque. In turn, the extracellular matrix of the fibrous cap, consisting of several proteinaceous macromolecules, including collagen (types I and III) and elastin secreted by transformed smooth muscle cells, determines its integrity.

The point should once again be made that core size and fibrous cap thickness are *not* related to absolute plaque size nor to the degree of luminal stenosis. Fibrous cap thickness appears to be related to macrophage and smooth muscle cell activity, particularly their production of metalloproteinases that degrade connective tissue.

Matrix metalloproteinases, part of a superfamily of enzymes that includes collagenases, gelatinases, and elastases, require activation from proenzyme precursors to attain enzymatic activity. Under normal circumstances, tissue inhibitors hold these enzymes in check; however, exposure of smooth muscle cells to the cytokines interleukin (IL)-1 and tumor necrosis factor-α (TNF-α) causes induction of interstitial collagenase and stromelysin. Macrophages exposed to inflammatory cytokines also stimulate the production of matrix-degrading enzymes (Moreno et al., 1994).

Coronary atherectomy specimens from patients with acute coronary syndromes contain a 92-kDa gelatinase that is produced predominantly by macrophages and smooth muscle cells. Within atherosclerotic plaques, the highest stress regions have a twofold greater matrix metalloproteinase (MMP-1) expression than the lowest stress regions. Overexpression of MMP-1 in vulnerable plaques is associated with a substantial increase in circumferential stress. Degradation and weakening of the collagenous extracellular matrix at critical points of high shear stress may play an important role in the pathogenesis of plaque rupture.

Fibrous cap thickness can be maintained by smooth muscle cell–mediated collagen synthesis (local repair); however, interferon-γ (IFN-γ), an inflammatory cytokine found within atherosclerotic plaques, decreases the ability of smooth muscle cells to express the collagen gene. Because only T lymphocytes can elaborate INF-γ, it has been suggested that chronic immune stimulation within atherosclerotic plaques leads to the production of IFN-γ from T cells that subsequently inhibits

Table 3.2 The Potential Link between Infectious Agents and Atherosclerotic Vascular Disease

Infectious Agent	Association Suggested in Animal Models	Comments	Association Suggested in Humans	Comments
Cytomegalovirus	0		+++	Detected in atheromatous tissue Serologic evidence for link with atherosclerosis Associated with allograft disease Potential role in restenosis Alters cellular function
Chlamydia pneumoniae	+++	Develop de novo atherosclerotic changes with infection in rabbits Azithromycin treatment prevents atherosclerosis	+	Often subclinical infection Detected in atheroma Serologic evidence for link with atherosclerosis Detected in subclinical atherosclerosis Alters cellular function
Helicobacter pylori	0		+	Associated with elevated inflammatory markers Limited serologic data Not detected in atheromatous plaques

Organism				
Herpes simplex virus	+++	Marek's disease (herpes virus in chickens) associated with atherosclerosis	+	Detected in atheroma Serologic data lacking
Coxsackie B virus	++	Acute coronary arteritis in mice	+++	No serologic data Not detected in atheroma
Pasteurella multicoda	++	Shown to enhance atherosclerotic changes in rabbits on high-cholesterol diets	0	
Periodontal disease: *Porphyromonas* *Streptococcus viridans* *Streptococcus anguis*	0		++	Epidemiologic associations observed S. viridans detected in atheroma
Hepatitis A	0		+/0	Seropositivity which may or may not be of pathologic significance

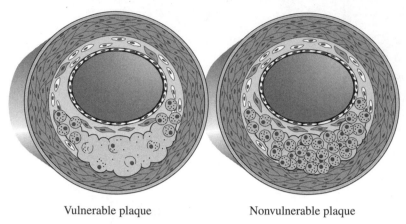

Vulnerable plaque   Nonvulnerable plaque

Figure 3.3 Vulnerable plaques are typified by (1) a prominent lipid core, (2) a thin fibrous cap, and (3) high-inflammatory cell density located at the plaque periphery. By contrast, nonvulnerable plaques contain few extracellular lipid particles and are fibrotic, making disruption a less common event.

collagen synthesis in vulnerable regions of the fibrous cap. IFN-γ can also contribute to apoptosis and, therefore, may be a key biochemical determinant of plaque vulnerability (Figure 3.4) (Amento et al., 1991).

Human mast cells contain proteoglycans and proteolytic enzymes, including chymase and tryptase. In normal coronary arteries, mast cells amount to 0.1% of all nucleated cells; however, within the fibrous cap, lipid core, and shoulder regions of atheromatous lesions, there are 5-, 5-, and 10-fold increased densities, respectively. Electron and light microscopic studies of mast cells in the plaque shoulder region have revealed evidence of degradation, a sign of activation that may contribute to matrix degradation and plaque rupture in acute coronary syndromes (Constantinides, 1995).

Models of Plaque Rupture

Shear Stress   The coronary arterial intimal surface is constantly exposed to the dynamic influences of circulating blood that creates shear stress. Assuming a constant viscosity, shear stress is described by the following formula: $\tau = [\mu 4(v_z)r]/R^2$, where U is viscosity, V_z is mean velocity, r is radial position, and R is vessel radius. Within arterial segments containing laminar flow, shear stress is described by $Re = 4pQ/\tau\mu D$, where Re is the Reynolds number, P is density of blood, Q is flow rate, and D is vessel diameter. Therefore, shear stress is directly proportional to flow (Q) and inversely proportional to the cube of the vessel's radius. In coronary atherosclerosis, the lumen is reduced in size and there is increased flow velocity, ultimately leading to increased shear stress.

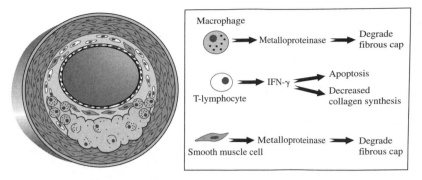

Figure 3.4 Plaque vulnerability is determined by both structure and intrinsic activity. Macrophages and smooth muscle cells synthesize and secrete matrix metalloproteinases that can degrade the fibrous cap. Interferon (IFN)-γ, an inflammatory cytokine secreted by T lymphocytes, participates in programmed cell death (apoptosis) and inhibits collagen synthesis, thereby weakening the plaque's supporting framework.

There is evidence that atherosclerosis typically develops in low flow/low shear stress segments of the coronary arterial tree. Low shear stress may also contribute, at least initially, to impaired vasoreactivity and thromboresistance by reducing the local stimulus to both prostaglandin and nitric oxide synthesis and release. It appears that unsteady (turbulent) flow is particularly detrimental to endothelial cell function (Davies et al., 1986).

In contrast to plaque development, plaque disruption occurs most often in regions of high shear stress.

Wall Stress   Plaque rupture occurs when the forces acting directly on the plaque exceed its tensile strength. Pressure generated within the arterial lumen exerts both radial and circumferential force, which must be countered by radial and circumferential wall tension. According to the law of Laplace, T (circumferential wall tension) $= pr/h$, where p is the intraluminal pressure, r is the vessel radius, and h is the wall thickness. Thus, atherosclerotic vessels with a thickened intima and small internal diameter maintain relatively low wall tension. This may explain why plaque rupture is more likely to occur in vessels with less severe stenosis.

Stress Distribution   Computer models have been developed to study the relative stress distribution within atherosclerotic coronary arteries. Overall, the circumferential stress is greatest at the intimal layer. In plaques that contain a large lipid pool, most of the stress is localized to the overlying fibrous cap. As the stiffness of the cap increases, the maximal circumferential stress shifts from the center of the cap to the lateral edges or "shoulder" region.

The thickness of the fibrous cap is a major determinant of circumferential stress and the plaque's predisposition to rupture. In the presence of a constant luminal dimension, there is increasing stress with enlargement of the lipid core. With increasing fibrous cap thickness, even in the presence of a decreasing luminal area, circumferential stress decreases. Another important feature is the lipid core itself, which, because of its semifluid nature, bears very little circumferential stress. Instead, stress is displaced to the fibrous cap (Loree et al., 1992).

Frequency of Stress   Much like fatigue fractures occurring in metal, the frequency, extent, and localization of stress play important roles in plaque rupture. Atherosclerotic plaques, particularly fibrous caps overlying large lipid cores, become progressively stiffer with increasing stress and frequency of stress. Elevations in heart rate have been shown to increase stiffness and circumferential stress at the plaque's shoulder regions.

Triggers for Plaque Rupture

Triggering events for plaque rupture are among the most contemplated and investigated areas in cardiovascular medicine. It has become clear, however, that triggers have less impact when they occur in the absence of a vulnerable plaque. This important feature allows for the development of several lines of prevention. Potential triggers include plasma catecholamine surges and increased sympathetic activity, blood pressure surges, exercise, emotional stress, changes in heart rate and myocardial contraction (angulation of coronary arteries), coronary vasospasm, and hemodynamic forces (Mittleman et al., 1993).

Cellular Plaque Components: Intrinsic Thrombogenicity

Pathologic studies performed on patients who died suddenly or who recently experienced an episode of unstable angina or myocardial infarction (MI) often reveal intraluminal thrombus anchored to a ruptured atherosclerotic plaque. Primarily based on the results of in vitro experiments and studies conducted in static systems, the thrombogenic capacity of atherosclerotic plaques has been attributed to collagen, fatty acids, and phospholipids. Fernandez-Ortiz and colleagues (1994) have investigated dynamic thrombus formation using an ex vivo perfusion chamber and reported that the greatest stimulus was, in fact, the atheromatous core, yielding a sixfold greater degree of platelet deposition and thrombus production over other substrates, including foam cell–rich matrix, collagen-rich matrix, collagen-poor matrix without cholesterol crystals, and segments of normal intima. There is mounting evidence that tissue factor is the predominant thrombogenic mediator found within the atheromatous core (Fernandez-Ortiz et al., 1994). This substrate will be discussed in a section to follow.

Cholesterol sulfate, present within human atherosclerotic plaques and plasma, is a substrate for platelet adhesion through a specific, but not yet defined, receptor. It, in all likelihood, plays a role in both atherosclerosis and prothrombotic potential of disrupted plaques (Merten et al., 2001).

Mild oxidation of LDL cholesterol (mox-LDL) forms lysophosphatidic acid, which accumulates within the intima of atheromatous plaques and is capable of activating platelets when exposed to circulating blood (Rother et al., 2003).

Regulatory Factors

In most instances, thrombosis occurring in the arterial system is composed of platelets and fibrin in a tightly packed network (white thrombus). By contrast, venous thrombi consist of a tightly packed network of erythrocytes, leukocytes, and fibrin (red thrombus).

The process of vascular thrombosis, particularly in the arterial system, is dynamic, with clot formation and dissolution occurring almost simultaneously. The overall extent of thrombosis and ensuing circulatory compromise is therefore determined by the predominant force that shifts the delicate balance. If local stimuli exceed the vessel's own thromboresistant mechanisms, thrombosis will occur. If, on the other hand, the stimulus toward thrombosis is not particularly strong and the intrinsic defenses are intact, clot formation of clinical importance is unlikely. In some circumstances, systemic factors contribute to or magnify local prothrombotic factors, shifting the balance toward thrombosis (Burke et al., 1997).

Overall, the site, size, and composition of thrombi forming within the arterial circulatory system are determined by (1) alterations in blood flow; (2) thrombogenicity of cardiovascular surfaces; (3) concentration and reactivity of plasma cellular components; and (4) effectiveness of physiologic protective mechanisms.

Cellular Interactions in Atherothrombosis

The traditionally held views of circulating platelets adhering to exposed subendothelial tissue to prevent bleeding and leukocytes responding to inflammatory stimuli to enhance tissue repair as separate and independent events must be modified to fully appreciate the dynamic environment that characterizes atherosclerosis and thrombosis (McEver, 2001). A new model involves (1) leukocyte adhesion to activated endothelial cells, (2) leukocyte adhesion to activated platelets, and (3) multicellular interactions between platelets, leukocytes, and endothelial cells on vascular surfaces (Figure 3.5). Each adhesive event is supported by the engagement of

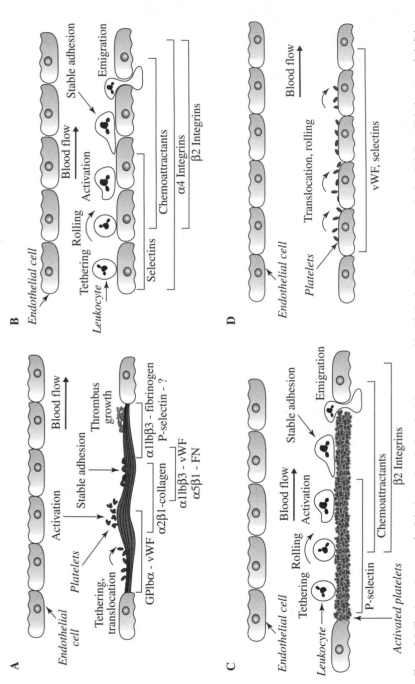

Figure 3.5 The dynamic nature of cellular interactions in thrombosis is represented by (A) platelet adhesion to exposed subendothelium, (B) leukocyte–endothelial cell interactions, (C) leukocyte adherence to aggregated platelets, and (D) platelet-activated endothelial cell interactions. FN, fibronectin; GP, glycoprotein; vWF, von Willebrand factor. (From McEver RP: Adhesive interactions of leukocytes, platelets, and the vessel wall during hemostasis and inflammation. *Thromb Haemost* 2001;86:746–756.)

an integrin with soluble or membrane-anchored ligands, which include p-selectin, von Willebrand factor, glycoprotein Ib, glycoprotein IIb/IIIa, P-selectin glycoprotein ligand-1, MAC-1, and a variety of intracellular vascular adhesion molecules (Maly et al., 1996).

Bloodborne Propensity for Arterial Thrombosis

Another traditionally held view that may require modification is the governance of arterial thrombosis solely on the basis of factors intrinsic to the vessel wall at sites of injury. It is widely recognized that tissue factor can be found in high concentrations within atheromatous plaques, activated endothelial cells, fibroblasts, and vascular smooth muscle cells; however, tissue factor antigen is also present within the circulating blood of patients with coronary artery disease and hematologic disorders characterized by heightened thrombogenicity. Tissue factor–containing neutrophils and monocytes circulating in peripheral blood may be delivered to sites of vascular injury when they contribute to both the initiation and subsequent propagation of thrombus. This construct also brings leukocytes into contact with activated endothelial cells, activated platelets, and the plaque matrix, where ample substrate for thrombin generation already exists (Giesen et al., 1999). Adherent leukocytes enhance fibrin deposition by CD18-dependent capture of fibrin protofibrils flowing in plasma and factor XII–dependent thrombin generation. They also activate platelets providing a fully functional platform for fibrin formation under flow conditions (Goel and Diamond, 2001).

A bloodborne propensity for thrombosis independent of vascular pathology may provide an explanation for observed disparities between "degree" or "extent" of atherosclerosis and the risk of thrombotic events, as well as a basis for individual thrombotic tendency (Karnicki et al., 2002; Rauch and Nemerson, 2000).

Atherosclerotic Plaque Imaging Modalities

The fine structure and composition of an atherosclerotic plaque, rather than the degree of stenosis, determines the likelihood of future clinical events. As a result, imaging modalities capable of characterizing the plaques' internal environment have strong appeal. Having information on both plaque composition and luminal features may also be useful during coronary interventions.

A majority of early imaging modalities were catheter-based; however, more generalizable techniques are being developed and studied. High-frequency intravascular ultrasound (20–40 MHz) provides tomographic images of the arterial wall and is able to quantitate luminal and plaque area as well as morphologic features, including calcification and intimal dissection. Axial resolution to approximately

150 MHz is possible, permitting identification of lipid-rich regions and features of the plaques' fibrous cap.

Intravascular ultrasound with elastography is a unique method that allows both visual characterization of the plaque and its mechanical properties. Tissue components behave differently in response to applied pressure determination of mechanical and structural integrity.

Coronary angioscopy, although not used frequently in North American catheterization laboratories, is a sensitive means to detect atherosclerotic plaques, grossly approximate their composition, determine the presence of fibrous cap disruption, and identify associated thrombosis formation.

Magnetic resonance imaging (MRI) (high-resolution fast spin echo) and computed tomography (CT) angiography represent promising tools for studying the progression and regression of atherosclerosis over time. In addition, recently developed intravascular techniques can accurately assess plaque size and vulnerability (for rupture).

A variety of innovative imaging modalities under development include optical coherence tomography, nuclear scintigraphy, thermometry, and Raman spectroscopy (MacNeill et al., 2003).

Emerging Concepts in Atherothrombosis

C-Reactive Protein

The link between inflammation and thrombosis in atherosclerotic vascular disease is complex; however, CRP may represent an important mediator given its association with both atherogenesis and thrombogenesis. In the Speedwell study, CRP cor-

Table 3.3 High Sensitivity (HS) C-Reactive Protein and Its Correlation with Atherothrombotic Events

	Endpoint				
	Coronary Heart Disease Death	Myocardial Infarction	Stroke	Peripheral Vascular Disease	Cardiovascular Death
Relative risk for future cardiovascular events					
5.0					
4.0	X				X
3.0		X		X	
2.0			X		
1.0					

Adapted from Ridker PM. High sensitivity C-reactive protein Circulation 2001;103:1813–1818.

related strongly with D-dimer levels, which is a marker of fibrin formation (and subsequent degradation). This observation is particularly relevant when one considers the ability of D-dimer (and other fibrin-related products) to activate neutrophils and monocytes, increase secretion of cytokines (IL-1, IL-6), and stimulate the hepatic synthesis of acute-phase proteins including CRP (Rus et al., 1996).

C-reactive protein can be found within macrophages of atheromatous plaques where it interacts with a specific cell surface receptor CD 32. The colocalization of CRP and LDL cholesterol suggest that it plays a major role in transport and atherosclerotic plaque development. Once present, CRP up-regulates adhesion molecule expression, activates complement, and induces monocyte tissue factor expression.

The strong correlation between elevated CRP concentrations (measured by a high-sensitivity assay) and vascular thrombotic events, while not proving cause and effect, provides, at the very least, a readily attainable prognostic marker. The potential relevance both pathologically and clinically is further underscored by the ability of therapeutic agents, including "statins" and aspirin, to reduce CRP (and predict treatment response) (Table 3.3; Figure 3.6) (Cermak et al., 1993; Crisby et al., 2001; Ridker, 2001).

Figure 3.6 C-reactive protein (CRP) is more than an "epiphenomenon" of atherosclerotic vascular disease. In response to cytokine stimulation, it colocalizes with low-density lipoprotein (LDL) cholesterol, facilitating monocyte entry via CD32, a cell surface receptor. Once internalized, the CRP–LDL–cholesterol complex incites complement activation, tissue factor expression, and surface adhesion molecule up-regulation.

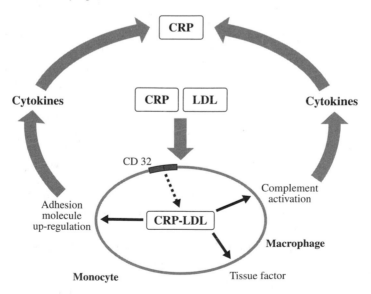

Summary

Atherosclerotic vascular disease, often involving the coronary, cerebral, and peripheral vasculature, represents a complex pathobiologic response (phenotype) to a variety of environmental conditions in the context of a permissive genetic profile (genotype). The plaque constituents, dysfunctional endothelium, and circulating cellular components each provide proinflammatory and prothrombotic stimuli, which must be considered in formulating targeted therapies.

References

Amento EP, Ehsani N, Palmer H, Libby P. Cytokines positively and negatively regulate interstitial collagen gene expression in human vascular smooth muscle cells. *Arterioscler Thromb* 1991;11:1223–1230.

Burke AP, Farb A, Malcom GT, Liang YH, Smialek J, Virmani R. Coronary risk factors and plaque morphology in men with coronary disease who died suddenly. *N Engl J Med* 1997;336:1276–1282.

Caplan BA, Gerrity RG, Schwartz CJ. Endothelial cell morphology in focal areas of in vivo Evans Blue uptake in the young pig aorta. I. Quantitative light microscopic findings. *Exp Mol Pathol* 1974;21:102–117.

Cermak J, Key NS, Bach RR, Balla J, Jacobs HS, Vercellotti GM. C-reactive protein induces human peripheral blood monocytes to synthesize tissue factor. *Blood* 1993; 82:513–520.

Constantinides P. Infiltrates of activated mast cells at the site of coronary atheromatous erosion or rupture in myocardial infarction. *Circulation* 1995;92:1084–1088.

Crisby M, Nordin-Fredriksson G, Shah PK, et al. Pravastatin treatment increases collagen content and decreases lipid content, inflammation, metalloproteinases, and cell death in human carotid plaques. *Circulation* 2001;103:926–933.

Davies MJ, Thomas AC. Plaque fissuring—the cause of acute myocardial infarction, sudden ischemic death and crescendo angina. *Br Heart J* 1985;53:363–373.

Davies PF, Remuzzi A, Gordon EJ, Dewey CF Jr, Gimbrone MA Jr. Turbulent fluid shear stress induces vascular endothelial cell turnover in vitro. *Proc Natl Acad Sci USA* 1986;83:2114–2117.

Fernandez-Ortiz A, Badimon JJ, Falk E, et al. Characterization of the relative thrombogenicity of atherosclerotic plaque components: implications for consequences of plaque rupture. *J Am Coll Cardiol* 1994;23:1562–1569.

Gaydos CA, Summersgil JT, Sahney NN, et al. Replication of Chlamydia pneumoniae in vitro in human macrophages, endothelial cells, and aortic artery smooth muscle cells. *Infect Immun* 1996;64:1614–1620.

Giesen PLA, Raugh U, Boheramm B, et al. Blood-borne tissue factor: another view of thrombosis. *Proc Natl Acad Sci USA* 1999;96:2311–2315.

Goel MS, Diamond SL. Neutrophil enhancement of fibrin deposition under flow through platelet-dependent and -independent mechanisms. *Arterioscler Thromb Vasc Biol* 2001;21:2093–2098.

Gupta S, Leathrm EW, Carrington D, et al. Elevated *Chlamydia pneumoniae* antibodies, cardiovascular events, and azithromycin in male survivors of myocardial infarction. *Circulation* 1997;96:404–407.

Jauchem JR, Lopez M, Sprague EA, Schwartz CJ. Mononuclear cell chemoattractant activity from cultured arterial smooth muscle cells. *Exp Mol Pathol* 1982;37:166–174.

Karnicki K, Owen WG, Miller RS, McBane RD II. Factors contribution to individual propensity for arterial thrombosis. *Arterioscler Thromb Vasc Biol* 2002;22:1495–1499.

Loree HM, Kamm RD, Stringfellow RG, Lee RT. Effects of fibrous cap thickness on peak circumferential stress in model atherosclerotic vessels. *Circ Res* 1992;71:850–858.

MacNeill BD, Loew HC, Takano M, Fuster V, Jang I-K. Intravascular modalities for detection of vulnerable plaque. Current status. *Arterioscler Thromb Vasc Biol* 2003;23:1333–1342.

Maly P, Thall AD, Petryniak B, et al. The $\alpha(1,3)$ fucosyltransferase Fuc-TVII controls leukocyte trafficking through an essential role in L-, E-, and P-selectin ligand biosynthesis. *Cell* 1996;86:643–653.

McEver RP. Adhesive interactions of leukocytes, platelets, and the vessel wall during hemostasis and inflammation. *Thromb Heamost* 2001;86:746–756.

Merten M, Dong JF, Lopez JA, Thiagarajan P. Cholesterol sulfate: a new adhesive molecule for platelets. *Circulation* 2001;103:2032–2034.

Mittleman MA, Maclure M, Tofler GH, Sherwood JB, Goldberg RJ, Muller JE. Triggering of acute myocardial infarction by heavy exertion: protection against triggering by regular exertion. *N Engl J Med* 1993;329:1677–1683.

Moreno PR, Falk E, Palacios IF, Newell JB, Fuster V, Fallon JT. Macrophage infiltration in acute coronary syndromes: implications for plaque rupture. *Circulation* 1994;90:775–778.

Rauch U, Nemerson Y. Circulating tissue factor and thrombosis. *Curr Opion Hematol* 2000;7:273–277.

Ridker PM. High sensitivity C-reactive protein. *Circulation* 2001;103:1813–1818.

Rother E, Brandl R, Baker DL, et al. Subtype-selective antagonists of lysophosphatidic acid receptors inhibit platelet activation triggered by the lipid core of atherosclerotic plaques. *Circulation* 2003;108:745–747.

Rus HG, Vlacicu R, Miculescu F. Interleukin-6 and interleukin-8 protein and gene expression in human arterial atherosclerotic wall. *Atherosclerosis* 1996;127:263–271.

Seifert PS, Hugo F, Hansson GK, Bhakdi S. Prelesional complement activation in experimental atherosclerosis. *Lab Invest* 1989;60:747–754.

Stary HC. Composition and classification of human atherosclerotic lessions. *Virchows Arch A Pathol Amat Histophthol* 1992;421:277–290.

Swartz CJ, Valente AJ, Sprague EA, et al. Atherosclerosis as an inflammatory process: the roles of the monocyte-macrophage. *Ann NY Acad Sci* 1985;454:115–120.

Tirzui D, Bobrain A, Tasca C, Simionescu M, Simionescu N. Intimal thickenings of human aorta contain modified reassembled lipoproteins. *Atherosclerosis* 1995;112: 101–114.

Virmann R, Koldgie FD, Burke AP, Farb A, Schwartz SM. Lessons from sudden coronary death: a comprehensive morphologic classification scheme for atherosclerotic lesions. *Arteriocler Thromb Vasc Biol* 2000;20:1262–1275.

Venous Thromboembolism

4

Blood clotting within the venous circulatory system, in contrast to arterial thrombosis, occurs at a relatively slow pace in response to stagnation of flow (stasis) and activation of coagulation. As with arterial thrombosis, vascular injury, either direct in the setting of trauma or indirect as a diffuse, systemic inflammatory response (that ultimately causes endothelial cell damage), represents an important stimulus.

Pathology

Venous thrombi are intravascular deposits composed predominantly of erythrocytes and fibrin, with a variable contribution of platelets and leukocytes. In a majority of cases, thrombosis begins in areas of slow flow within the venous sinuses of valve cusp pockets either in the deep veins of the calf or upper thigh or at sites of direct injury following trauma (Kakkar et al., 1969; Nicolaides et al., 1971).

Stasis predisposes to thrombosis most profoundly in the setting of inflammatory states and activated coagulation factors. Slowed blood flow impairs the clearance of coagulation proteases, which through bioamplification increases the local concentration of thrombin substrate. If local thromboresistance is impaired, as may be the case with inherited or acquired thrombophilias (see Chapter 24), thrombosis occurs. Blood flow velocity is reduced by indwelling catheters, which also causes

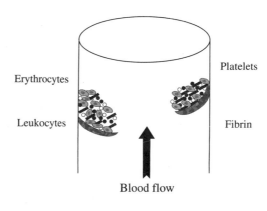

Figure 4.1 Venous thrombi, consisting of erythrocytes and fibrin and to a lesser degree leukocytes and platelets, form in areas of static blood flow. The stimulus for thrombosis often includes an increased systemic and local concentration of coagulation proteases, cytokine (inflammation)-mediated endothelial cell injury, and impaired thromboresistance (inherited or acquired). The combination of static blood flow, abnormalities of the vessel wall, and increased circulating procoagulant factors is known as Virchow's triad.

focal endothelial injury, peripheral edema, pregnancy, and valve cusp damage from prior venous thrombosis and/or chronic venous insufficiency (Trottier et al., 1995) (Figure 4.1).

Although venous thrombosis can occur in a variety of sites, the most common encountered in clinical practice is within the deep veins of the lower extremity. Thrombi developing within the veins of the calf or thigh can serve as a nidus for growth (propagation), which may cause complete venous obstruction, or embolize to the lungs (pulmonary embolism).

References

Kakkar VV, Howe CT, Flanc C, Clarke MB. Natural history of postoperative deep-vein thrombosis. *Lancet* 1969;2:230–232.

Nicolaides AN, Kakkar VV, Field ES, Renney JTG. The origin of deep vein thrombosis: a venographic study. *Br J Radiol* 1971;44:653–663.

Trottier SJ, Veremakis C, O'Brien J, Auer AL. Femoral deep vein thrombosis associated with central venous catheterization: results from a prospective, randomized trial. *Crit Care Med* 1995;23:52–59.

Cardiac Chamber, Aortic, and Valvular Thromboembolism

The left-sided cardiac chambers (left atrium, left ventricle) and heart valves (mitral valve, aortic valve) (native, prosthetic) serve as potential niduses for systemic thromboembolism, including fatal or debilitating stroke. The ascending aortic is also recognized as a source for embolism (aortoembolism) and should be considered when a comprehensive patient evaluation is being undertaken (Figure 5.1).

Cardiac Chamber Thromboembolism

The pathogenesis of intracavitary mural thrombosis, much like venous thromboembolism, follows the construct of Virchow's triad. The area of stasis is often provoked by chamber dilation, reduced performance, or impaired flow across an existing heart valve (e.g., left atrial dilation from mitral stenosis). Endothelial injury may follow either an acute (e.g., myocardial infarction) or chronic (e.g., dilated cardiomyopathy) cardiac process. In the case of aortoembolism, plaque rupture in areas of advanced atherosclerosis serves as the primary site for thrombus development. The third component, prothrombotic state, may be focal (areas of inflammation and necrosis) and/or systemic.

Left ventricular mural thrombosis is diagnosed either echocardiographically or at the time of autopsy among patients with myocardial infarction (MI), especially in those with anterior infarction involving the ventricular apex. In large, nonrandomized clinical trials of anticoagulant therapy, researchers have reported an incidence of cerebral embolism of 2% to 4% among nontreated patients, frequently causing either severe neurologic deficits or death. Of these trials, two showed a statistically significant reduction in stroke with early anticoagulation, whereas the third trial demonstrated a positive trend (Davis and Irelant, 1986).

A meta-analysis performed by Vaitkus and Barnathan (1993) supports the findings of three previous studies published in the early 1980s. The odds ratio for systemic embolism in the presence of echocardiographically demonstrated mural thrombus was 5.45 (95% confidence interval [CI] 3.02–9.83). The odds ratio of anticoagulation versus no anticoagulation in preventing embolism was 0.14 (95% CI 0.04–0.52) with an event rate difference of –0.33 (95% CI –0.50 to –0.16). The odds ratio of anticoagulation versus control in preventing mural thrombus formation was 0.32 (95% CI 0.20–0.52) and the event difference was –0.19 (95% CI 0.09–0.28).

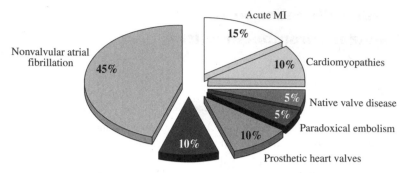

Figure 5.1 Cardiac and aortic sources of systemic emboli, including stroke. MI, myocardial infarction.

A more recent analysis of patients participating in the SAVE (Survival and Ventricular Enlargement) trial (Loh et al., 1997) suggests that ventricular dysfunction (ejection fraction <35%) increases the likelihood of thromboembolic stroke significantly, with increasing risk as ventricular performance worsens (Figure 5.2).

The available data from nonrandomized trials support the following four conclusions:

1. Mural thrombosis following acute MI increases the risk of systemic embolism.
2. The likelihood of cardioembolic events correlates inversely with left ventricular systolic performance.
3. Anticoagulation can reduce mural thrombus formation.
4. The risk of systemic embolism can be substantially reduced by anticoagulation.

Aortoembolism

Atheromatous plaques of the ascending aorta are recognized as a potential source of thromboemboli and atheroemboli. The former typically causes either stroke or peripheral embolic events, while the latter can lead to ischemic bowel, renal insufficiency, and/or microvascular occlusion of the lower extremities.

The prevalence of aortic atheromas in patients experiencing an embolic event based on autopsy series, transesophageal echocardiography, or intraoperative ultrasound during cardiac surgery is constantly in the 20% to 30% range (compared to 5–8% in control populations) (Amarenco et al., 1992; Khatibzadeh et al., 1996). Of added clinical relevance, atheromatous disease of the ascending aorta commonly coexists with advanced carotid artery disease, coronary artery disease, and atrial fibrillation.

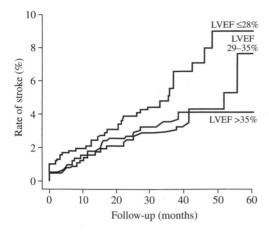

Figure 5.2 The occurrence of thromboembolic stroke according to left ventricular ejection fraction (LVEF). An LVEF below 35% was associated with an increased risk of stroke that persisted over time. (From Loh E, Sutton MS, Wun CC, et al. Ventricular dysfunction and the risk of stroke after myocardial infarction. *N Engl J Med* 1997;336:251–257.)

Aortic atherosclerosis, based on ultrasound imaging, can be graded as (1) mild (<3 mm intimal thickening), (2) moderate (intimal thickening ≥3 mm with diffuse irregularities and calcification), or (3) severe (>5 mm intimal thickening and one or more of the following: large protruding or mobile atheromatous debris, ulcerated plaques, and/or thrombi). Long-term follow-up studies have supported a relationship between the severity of atherosclerosis and the likelihood of a fatal or nonfatal neurologic event (Figure 5.3) (Dávila-Román et al., 1999).

Native Valve Thromboembolism

Clinical, pathologic, and experimental evidence supports two predominant mechanisms for the initiation of thrombosis (and risk for thromboembolism) in patients with valvular heart disease. The first involves disruption of the vascular endothelial surface and exposure of underlying prothrombotic substrate. The second is mediated by altered flow dynamics with areas of high and low velocity. The combination of localized tissue abnormalities and stasis (with accompanying high concentrations of coagulation proteases) represents a strong stimulus for thrombosis. There is also evidence that prolonged periods of stasis impair tissue perfusion, with resulting vascular damage and impaired fibrinolysis (Wessler, 1962).

Prosthetic Valve Thromboembolism

Despite the important contribution that surgical heart valve replacement has made over the past half-century, an existing propensity for localized thrombus formation

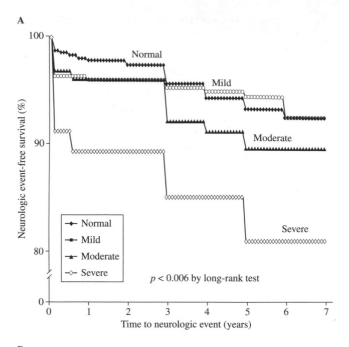

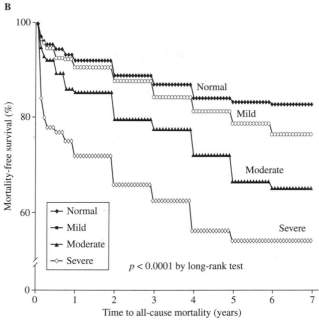

Figure 5.3 Kaplan-Meier analysis of survival without neurologic events (A) and without all-cause mortality (B), according to severity of atherosclerosis of the ascending aorta (normal, moderate, severe).

and systemic thromboembolic events, including fatal and disabling ischemic stroke, remains both an inherent limiting feature and a major concern for surgeons, clinicians, and patients alike.

Initial Observations

Surgeons have long recognized the potential devastating consequences of prosthetic heart valve–related thrombosis. The pioneering work of Frater and Ellis quickly brought the problem into full light. Observing valve thrombosis in 19 of 23 dogs receiving a flexible monocusp mitral valve prosthesis, they concluded that "clotting is the major problem" with this procedure (Frater and Ellis, 1961).

Over the past 25 years, more than 50 heart valve prostheses have been developed for clinical use, but only several have been approved by the Food and Drug Administration (FDA). Of these, approximately six are being implanted routinely by surgeons practicing in the United States. Although some prostheses are inherently more thrombogenic than others, (caged ball > monoleaflet > bileaflet; mitral > aortic > tricuspid), the occurrence of thromboembolism has decreased steadily over time. An advanced understanding of valve-related thrombogenicity, associated conditions predisposing to thromboembolism, and the important role of systemic anticoagulation are responsible for this favorable trend.

The FDA-approved mechanical and bioprosthetic valves as well as those currently available in other countries are summarized in Tables 5.1 and 5.2. Although annuloplasty rings are not considered true valve substitutes, they are made of pros-

---

Table 5.1 Mechanical Prosthetic Heart Valves

Caged-Ball
   Starr-Edwards
Monoleaflet (Tilting Disc)
   Medtronic Hall*
   Omniscience*
   Bjork-Shiley Monostrut*
   Sorin Monoleaflet Allcarbon
Bileaflet
   St. Jude Medical*
   CarboMedics*
   Edwards Techna
   ATS
   Sorin Bicarbon
   On-X Mechanical Prosthesis
   Carbomedics KineticUltracor Mechanical

---

*Food and Drug Administration–approved and currently in use in the United States.

Table 5.2 Bioprosthetic Heart Valves

Stented Porcine Valves
  Hanckock Porcine Valve*
  Carpentier-Edwards Porcine Valve*
  Medtronic Intact Porcine Valve
  Biocor Porcine Valve
  St. Jude Bioimplant Porcine Valve
  Medtronic Mosaic Porcine Valve
  Labcor Porcine Valve
  Tissue Med Porcine Valve
Stented Pericardial Valves
  Carpentier-Edwards Pericardial Valve*
  Mitroflow Pericardial Valve
  CarboMedics Photofix Pericardial Valve
  Biocor Pericardial Valve
  Sorin Pericarbon Valve
Stentless Porcine and Pericardial Valves
  St. Jude Medical; Toronto SPV Stentless Porcine Valve*
  Medtronic Freestyle Stentless Porcine Valve*
  Cryolife O'Brien Stentless Porcine Valve
  Cryolife O'Brien Stentless (Root) Porcine Valve
  Baxter Prima Stentless Porcine Valve
  Sorin Pericarbon Pericardial Valve
  Labcor Stentless Porcine Valve
  Tissue Med Heterograft Roots and Stentless Valve
Homografts
  Cryolife Allograft Root and Valve*
  LifeNET (St. Jude Medical)*
  American Red Cross (Baxter)*

Food and Drug Administration–approved and currently in use.

thetic materials and, through exposure to circulating blood, represent a potential site for thrombosis. The FDA-approved annuloplasty rings are listed in Table 5.3.

Thrombogenicity Inherent to Cardiac Prostheses

Although several patient-related factors, including atrial fibrillation, thrombophilic states, low cardiac output, ventricular chamber dilation, and left atrial enlargement, contribute to the risk of thrombosis and thromboembolic events in patients with prosthetic heart valves, the most obvious risk factor is the prosthetic valve itself. This inherent *thrombogenicity* is collectively determined by the *materials* used for construction of the prosthesis and the *flow conditions* through and adjacent to the valve, which are a function of *size* and *prosthetic design*.

Table 5.3 Annuloplasty Rings

Carpentier Edwards*
Duran*
Cosgrove-Edwards*
St. Jude Medical (tailor)*

*Food and Drug Administration–approved.

Interaction of Circulating Blood with Prosthetic Mechanical Components

Foreign materials provoke an immediate reaction when exposed to circulating blood. Protein adsorption to the housing and moving parts of the mechanical prosthesis represents the initial event, beginning immediately after implantation. Fibrinogen is the first and most prevalent protein involved in this process. Other plasma proteins such as fibronectin, von Willebrand factor, thrombospondin, factor XII, and kininogen quickly join fibrinogen as part of the "protein film." This initial process, known as *conditioning of the surface,* is characterized by a high degree of thrombogenicity.

After a brief period of dynamic flux, conditioning of the surface reaches a level of equilibrium where the protein coat has a fairly well-defined composition. The composition, in turn, is determined by the binding constants and plasma concentrations of several plasma proteins. The adsorbed proteins subsequently undergo changes in their molecular configuration, promoting variable degrees of platelet adhesion to the protein-coated surface.

The contribution of *platelet adhesion* to the thrombotic process is variable and influenced strongly by shearing force and flow conditions; however, most prosthetic materials are coated with a monolayer of platelets shortly after exposure to the circulating blood (Ruggeri, 1993).

The initial stage of maximal thrombogenicity is followed by a surface-related event known as *passivation.* Although the exact mechanism of this phenomenon is not completely understood, accumulating evidence suggests that the protein composition of the adsorbed film changes to a configuration that is less reactive to blood. In general, the greater the concentration of albumin on a protein-coated surface, the more passive the surface becomes. Once the surface has become passivated, it is less prone to thrombosis.

Experimental studies have demonstrated that "precoating" a given material with albumin accelerates the passivation process. Pyrolytic carbon induces surface passivation more rapidly than other materials, but the exact mechanism remains unclear. Minimal molecular alteration of the absorbed protein coat and a critical surface tension within the "biocompatible range" are some of the postulated mechanisms for its relative thromboresistance (Butchart, 1993).

Bioprosthetic Materials

The use of biologic tissue for valve replacement was undertaken to reduce thrombogenicity. It is known that native tissue thromboresistance is largely determined by endothelial cells. Unfortunately, during the processing of homografts and the preimplantation stages for bioprosthetic valve replacement, the endothelial layer is frequently injured.

With the exception of autografts, the surfaces of biologic valves are largely denuded of endothelial cells, exposing collagen and the basement membrane. This irregular surface is exposed to circulating blood and promptly becomes covered by a thin layer of platelets and fibrin. The concave surface of the valve cusps is most prone to these events because of low shear stress at this particular site. Although under ordinary circumstances platelet adhesion and aggregation would be heightened, manufactured bioprostheses do not initiate a strong platelet–collagen reaction compared with fresh tissue. Pretreatment with glutaraldehyde may, at least in part, be responsible for this weak response (Magilligan et al., 1984).

The endothelial cell layer is reconstituted to variable degrees over time. Although endothelial cells are typically absent during the first year, 70% of bioprostheses implanted for more than 5 years demonstrate an endothelial cell monolayer. The cells are typically grouped in islands and attached to host tissue (fibrin, thrombi, fibrous material). Platelet adhesion is *not* observed on surfaces containing endothelial cells. Late thrombosis of bioprosthetic valves is associated with structural valve degeneration and calcification of the leaflet, leading to increased shearing forces and resulting platelet adherence, activation, and aggregation.

Sewing Ring

A variety of materials including silastic and silicone rubber have been used for the fabrication of prosthetic valve sewing rings; however, only the material covering the sewing ring influences host reactions. The most common constituents of covering materials are synthetic polyethylene terephthalate (Dacron), polypropylene, polyester, and polytetrafluoroethylene (PTFE). Adequate tissue integration, structural stability, and low cost are the most attractive characteristics of these materials.

Plasma protein adsorption represents the host's initial response to implantation, followed soon thereafter by platelet deposition and initiation of the coagulation cascade. The resulting thrombus "organizes," ultimately forming a thin fibrous layer.

There appears to be a relationship between fibrous layer thickness and thromboembolic events. If the thickness is less than 0.5 mm, it is usually well nourished, carrying out physiologic/metabolic exchange directly with the bloodstream. In contrast, if the fibrous tissue layer exceeds 0.5 mm, the deeper portion is prone to ischemic necrosis and tissue sloughing. This explains why, despite the complete incorporation of the sewing ring, it remains a potential source for thromboembolism (Dewanjee, 1983). The thickness of the initial covering thrombus correlates directly with the thickness of the fibrous layer.

Annuloplasty Rings

Annuloplasty rings have been used in surgical practice for nearly 3 decades. Initially made with autologous pericardium or Dacron, they are currently industry manufactured and sized for more predictable and measured plication of the mitral and tricuspid annulus. Unlike sewing rings, the bulk of foreign material introduced by annuloplasty rings is relatively small. Nevertheless, the prosthetic material can trigger a similar host response. Incorporation of the annuloplasty ring begins with protein adsorption. Molecular alterations of the protein-coated surface activate several plasma enzymatic systems, including the complement pathway, coagulation, and the fibrinolytic system. Adsorbed proteins also stimulate platelet adhesion, platelet activation, platelet aggregation, and an acute inflammatory response.

Thrombogenicity Related to Flow Conditions

A comprehensive evaluation of prosthetic valve thrombogenicity must consider existing hemodynamic and hydrodynamic properties. Ideally, flow should be neither too fast (shear stress) nor too slow (stasis). Unfortunately, and despite substantial improvements in prosthetic heart valve design, abnormal flow patterns remain a concern. Some general abnormal flow conditions are common to all prostheses; however, specific abnormal flow conditions are typical of some mechanical prosthetic designs, particularly caged-ball valves and early monoleaflet tilting disc valves.

References

Amarenco P, Duychaerts C, Tzourio C, et al. The prevalence of ulcerated plaques in the aortic arch in patients with stroke. *N Engl J Med* 1992;326:221–225.

Butchart E. Thrombogenesis and anticoagulation in heart valve disease: toward a rational approach. *J Heart Valve Dis* 1993;1:1–6.

Dávila-Román VG, Murphy SF, Nickerson NJ, Kouchoukos NT, Schechtman KB, Barzilai B. Atherosclerosis of the ascending aorta is an independent predictor of long-term neurologic events and mortality. *J Am Coll Cardiol* 1999;33:1308–1316.

Davis MJ, Irelant MA. Effect of early anticoagulation on the frequency of left ventricular thrombi after anterior wall acute myocardial infarction. *J Am Coll Cardiol* 1986;57: 1244–1247.

Dewanjee M, TrastekV, Tago M, Torianni M, Kaye M. Non-invasive isotopic technique for detection of platelet deposition on bovine pericardial mitral valve prosthesis and in-vivo quantification of visceral microembolism in dogs. *Trans A Soc Artif Intern Organs* 1983;29:188–193.

Frater R, Ellis H Jr. Problems in the development of a mitral valve prosthesis. In: Merendino KA, ed. *Prosthetic Valves for Cardiac Surgery.* Springfield, IL: Charles C. Thomas; 1961.

Khatibzadeh M, Mitusch R, Stierle U, et al. Aortic atherosclerotic plaques as a source of systemic embolism. *J Am Coll Cardiol* 1996;27:664–669.

Loh E, Sutton MS, Wun CC, et al. Ventricular dysfunction and the risk of stroke after myocardial infarction. *N Engl J Med* 1997;336:251–257.

Magilligan D, Oyama C, Flein S, et al. Platelet adherence to bioprosthetic cardiac valves. *Am J Cardiol* 1984;53:945–949.

Ruggeri Z. Mechanisms of shear-induced platelet adhesion and aggregation. *Thromb Haemost* 1993;70:119–123.

Vaitkus PT, Barnathan ES. Embolic potential, prevention and management of mural thrombus complicating anterior myocardial infarction: a meta-analysis. *J Am Coll Cardiol* 1993;22:1004–1009.

Wessler S. Thrombosis in the presence of vascular stasis. *Am J Med* 1962;33:648–658.

Part II
Fibrinolytics and Platelet Antagonists

Fibrinolytic Agents

The fibrinolytic system plays a vital role in maintaining vital organ homeostasis. Fibrinolysis, defined as the dissolution of fibrin (the major scaffold for intravascular thrombus), is the process that regulates thrombus growth after hemostasis has been achieved, thus preserving tissue perfusion. An understanding of fibrinolysis has led to the development of pharmacologic agents that can be used in the treatment of arterial and venous thrombotic disorders, including acute myocardial infarction, acute ischemic stroke, and pulmonary embolism.

Fundamental Mechanisms of Fibrinolysis

Fibrinolytic therapy makes use of the vascular system's intrinsic defense mechanism by accelerating and amplifying the conversion of an inactive enzyme precursor (zymogen), plasminogen, to the active enzyme plasmin. In turn, plasmin hydrolyzes several key bonds in the fibrin (clot) matrix, causing dissolution (lysis) (Table 6.1 and Figure 6.1).

Plasminogen

A single-chain glycoprotein consisting of 790 amino acids, plasminogen is converted to plasmin by cleavage of the Arg560–Val561 peptide bond. The plasminogen molecule also contains specific lysine binding sites, which mediate its interaction with fibrin and α_2-plasmin inhibitor.

Plasmin

A serine protease with trypsinlike activity, plasmin attacks lysyl and arginyl bonds of fibrin at two principal sites: (1) the carboxyterminal portion α-chain (polar region) and (2) the coiled coil connectors containing α-, β-, and γ-chains.

Determinants of Fibrinolysis

The ability of a fibrinolytic agent to dissolve an occlusive thrombus is determined by several factors. After administration the agent must be delivered to, perfuse, and ultimately infiltrate the thrombus while concomitantly being provided with an ad-

Table 6.1 Components of Intrinsic Fibrinolytic System

	Molecular Weight	Activity
Plasminogen	88,000 (single chain)	Proenzyme form of fibrinolytic enzyme
Plasmin	88,000 (two chain)	Active fibrinolytic enzyme
tPA	70,000 (one/two chain)	Enzyme present in tissues that converts plasminogen to plasmin
uPA	54,000 (two chain)	Plasminogen activator (different from tPA)
α_2-PI	70,000 (single chain)	Specific fast-acting inhibitor in plasma
PAI-1	40,000 (single chain)	Fast-acting inhibitor of tPA (and uPA) secreted by endothelial cells

tPA, tissue plasminogen activator; uPA, urokinase plasminogen activator; α_2-PI, plasmin inhibitor; PAI-1, plasminogen activator inhibitor-1.

equate amount of substrate (plasminogen) and the appropriate metabolic environment for an enzymatic reaction (conversion of plasminogen to plasmin) to take place. The intrinsic composition or ultrastructure of a thrombus also affects its lysability.

Hemodynamic Factors

Changes in the total amount and distribution of blood flow determine oxygen delivery to metabolically active tissues. They also determine the delivery of enzymatic substrate and plasminogen activators to the occlusive thrombus. In the heart, coronary blood flow correlates directly with mean arterial pressure. The flow-pressure curve is relatively flat above 65 to 70 mmHg, but becomes steeper as the mean arterial pressure decreases below this point. The relationship within the brain is more complex.

Experimental data obtained by magnetic resonance imaging (MRI) and by photographing clot dissolution in vitro show that whole blood clots dissolve two orders of magnitude faster when fibrinolytic agents are introduced into the clot by pressure-induced permeation than when access is limited solely to diffusion. When a pressure gradient exists along an occlusive clot, plasma flows through pores in the fibrin network and distributes plasminogen activators (as well as other solvents) across the clot. In distinct contrast, without a pressure gradient, plasminogen activator molecules diffuse into the clot through the blood clot boundary plane. Over time, the boundary moves inward as a result of lysis that is spatially restricted to a relatively narrow zone. The velocity of lysis is thus limited by the diffusion constraints of both the plasminogen activator and plasmin.

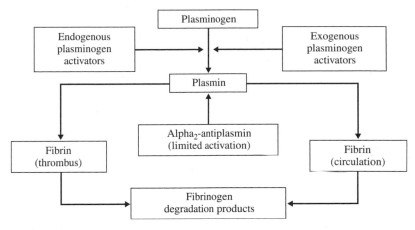

Figure 6.1 Pathways of Fibrinolysis. Endogenous or exogenous plasminogen activators convert plasminogen to the active serine protease plasmin, which degrades fibrin in thrombi and circulating fibrinogen. Plasmin in the circulation is rapidly inactivated by α_2-antiplasmin.

The importance of increased transport and bulk-flow delivery of fibrinolytic agents to an occlusive thrombus is illustrated by the slow rate of lysis of venous thrombi (Blomback and Okada, 1982; Marx, 1988).

Mechanical Factors

An existing arterial stenosis influences blood flow through and beyond the narrowed segment. Experimental studies performed in "flow-through" models demonstrate that the hemodynamic severity of a stenosis is determined by the reduction in luminal diameter, the velocity of blood flow, the length of the stenosis, and the viscosity of blood.

Coronary artery stenosis diminishes and, with increasing severity, eventually abolishes the peak reactive hyperemic response after transient complete vessel occlusion, suggesting that dynamic forces are at play.

Metabolic Factors

Thrombus Composition

Fibrin assembly is a complex process that is initiated by the proteolytic action of thrombin on fibrinogen. The gelation mechanism consists of two distinct polymerization stages. Initially, the activated fibrin monomers polymerize spontaneously in a linear mode to form staggered chains of protofibril oligomers. Subsequently,

61

the lateral assembly of linear segments allows generation of the three-dimensional network required for gelation.

For normal physiologic function, it is essential that the fibrin gel (thrombus) permit transport of both cells and macromolecules yet possess mechanical rigidity. The stiffness of the fibers and the number of contacts between fibers determine the mechanical rigidity of the gel. If many thin fibers with a high-fiber cross-link density are formed, the fibrin network pore size and, as a result, the mobility of a diffusion species within the gel are decreased.

A number of interrelated factors occurring in humans at a site of atheromatous plaque rupture may affect thrombus composition. The weight fraction of a fibrin gel is increased by fibrinogen concentration. As a result, the distance between fibers lessens, leading to decreased pore gel size and restricted transport of diffusion species. Increased thrombin concentration, observed commonly in the setting of myocardial infarction (MI), also decreases fiber diameter, as does thrombospondin, a large glycoprotein secreted from alpha granules of thrombin-stimulated platelets. Calcium concentration and pH also have been shown to affect fiber size (Carr and Powers, 1989; Dale et al., 1985; Shulman et al., 1952).

Restricted transport within a fibrin gel, either because of a reduced perfusion pressure or a "tightly packed" thrombus, limits the delivery of plasminogen, plasmin, and plasminogen activators, therefore compromising lysis. In contrast, increasing fiber size increases pore size and fibrinolytic agent–induced plasmin digestion of fibrin clots (Sabovic et al., 1989).

Plasminogen Activation

The physiologic regulation of plasmin formation in plasma depends primarily on (1) the plasma protein plasminogen, the zymogen precursor of plasmin; (2) the presence of plasminogen activators; and (3) protein inhibitors that inactivate plasmin. The mechanism of action of human plasminogens with activator species involves a specific cleavage of the single-chain Glu-1-plasminogen, a two-chain serine protease with trypsin-like specificity. The enzymatic conversion of plasminogen by urokinase and tissue plasminogen activator is directed by a single-step interaction, whereas streptokinase involves two steps. It is important to note that the transformation of plasminogen to plasmin occurs most efficiently at a pH of 7.4. Even with a slightly decreased pH (e.g., 7.2), the Michaelis constant (concentration of substrate at which the rate of end-product formation is equal to half the maximum velocity) is higher and the catalytic rate constant is lower than at a normal pH. Furthermore, the plasminogen–streptokinase complex can dissociate entirely at a low pH. Thus, in cardiogenic shock, alterations in blood pH may adversely affect the conversion of plasminogen to plasmin, impairing both physiologic thromboresistance and fibrinolytic efficacy (Wohl et al., 1980).

Fibrinolytic Agents

The evolution of fibrinolytic agents over the past several decades has focused on increased fibrinolytic potential, safety, and practical dosing strategies (Table 6.2).

First-Generation Agents

Streptokinase

Streptokinase is a nonenzymatic protein of β-hemolytic streptococci. It activates the fibrinolytic system indirectly by forming a 1:1 stoichiometric complex with plasminogen, which then activates plasminogen, converting it to the active enzyme plasmin.

Streptokinase is administered intravenously at a dose of 1.5 million U given over 1 hour. Patency (Thrombolysis in Myocardial Infarction (TIMI) grade 2 or 3 flow) occurs in approximately 60% of patients at 90 minutes, increasing to 80% to 90% by 24 hours. Full reperfusion, TIMI grade 3 flow, occurs in 35% of patients at 90 minutes, as demonstrated in the Global Use of Strategies to Open Occluded Arteries (GUSTO) angiographic substudy (The GUSTO Angiographic Investigators, 1993). Randomized clinical trials have demonstrated streptokinase's (SK) ability to reduce mortality, particularly when treatment is initiated within 6 hours of symptom onset. The Gruppo Italiano per lo Studio della Streptochinasi Nell' Infarcto Miocardico (GISSI) trial reported a 47% reduction in mortality when SK was administered within the first hour of symptom onset (GISSI, 1986). Clinical benefits with SK are substantially enhanced with the addition of aspirin at a dose of 160 mg

Table 6.2 Pharmacokinetic, Pharmacodynamic, and General Clinical Properties of Fibrinolytic Agents

Feature	SK	APSAC	tPA	rPA	TNKase
Half-life (minutes)	25	100	6	15	20
Method of administration	1 h IV	Bolus	1.5–h IV	2 boluses	Bolus
Dose	1.5 mU/ 60 min	30 U	15-mg bolus, up to 85 mg/ 90min	10 +10 mU	0.55 mg/kg (max 50 mg)
Mechanism of action	Indirect	Indirect	Direct	Direct	Direct
Fibrin specificity	NA	NA	+ +	+	+ + +
Antigenicity	+	+	NA	NA	NA
ICH rates	0.3%	0.7%	0.8%	0.8%	0.8%
Lives saved/1,000	2.5	2.5	3.5	3–3.5	3.5
Cost ($U.S.)	+	+ +	+ + +	+ + +	+ + +
90-min TIMI 3 flow	~30%	~50%	~60%	~60%	~60%

APSAC, anisoylated plasminogen–streptokinase activator complex; ICH, intracranial hemorrhage; NA, not applicable; rPA, reteplase; SK, streptokinase; TNKase, tenecteplase; tPA, alteplase; +, minimal; + +, moderate; + + +, high.

to 325 mg daily, as shown in the International Study of Infarct Survival (ISIS)-2 trial (ISIS-2 Collaborative Group, 1988). Antithrombotic therapy with subcutaneous heparin for patients at low risk for thromboemboli can be administered at a dose of 7,500 to 15,000 U every 12 hours, while patients at high risk for thromboemboli should receive IV heparin started 6 hours after SK therapy, when the activated partial thromboplastin time (aPTT) declines to 60 seconds or less. The initial infusion rate should not exceed 1,000 U/hour. After 48 hours, options include a change to subcutaneous heparin, warfarin, or aspirin alone.

Adverse reactions to SK include bleeding, hypotension, and allergic reactions. Hemorrhage occurs in approximately 5% to 10% of patients who do not undergo invasive procedures and in 15% to 20% who do. Serious bleeding occurs in 2% of patients, and intracranial hemorrhage is observed at a rate of approximately 0.5%. Transient hypotension occurs commonly (in 30–50% of patients), particularly when the SK infusion exceeds 750,000 U over 30 minutes. Because SK is a foreign protein, allergic reactions can and do occur in 2% to 5% of patients. Anaphylaxis, however, is rare (<0.3%). Readministration of SK is not recommended after 5 days and before 1 to 2 years of initial use or after recent streptococcal infection because of the high incidence of neutralizing antibodies, leading to reduced fibrinolytic activity or allergic reactions.

Urokinase

Urokinase is a trypsin-like serine protease composed of two polypeptide chains connected by a disulfide bridge. It activates plasminogen directly, converting it to the active enzyme plasmin.

Second-Generation Agents

APSAC

Streptokinase and the plasminogen–streptokinase activator complex are cleared rapidly from the circulation, with half-lives of 15 minutes and 3 minutes, respectively. By temporarily blocking the active center of plasminogen, the plasma half-life can be prolonged substantially. Therefore, acylation of plasminogen (APSAC) protects the molecule from autodigestion and also prevents its inactivation by circulating plasma inhibitors, resulting in a half-life of approximately 100 minutes. These features permit bolus dosing.

Anistreplase is administered as a 30-U bolus given over 5 minutes, which corresponds approximately to 1.1 million U of SK. In the circulation, gradual hydrolysis of the anisoyl group exposes the catalytic site of the complex, leading to generation of plasmin from plasminogen. The circulating half-life is approximately 90 minutes. The inactive, acyl form of the drug is thought to attenuate the generation of bradykinin, largely responsible for the hypotension seen with SK. Patency rates after anistreplase are slightly higher than with SK, in the range of 75%, with full perfusion (TIMI grade 3 flow) in approximately 50% of patients. Several large randomized trails have demonstrated reduction in mortality, improvement in left ventricular ejection fraction, and reduction in infarct size with anistreplase.

The largest comparative mortality trial, ISIS-3 (ISIS 3 Collaborative Group, 1992), demonstrated similar mortality rates for SK and anistreplase. Adverse reactions such as bleeding, hypotension, and allergic reactions also occurred with similar frequency. Recommendations for the administration of aspirin and unfractionated heparin parallel those for SK.

scuPA

scuPA (single-chain urokinase-like plasminogen activator) is a single-chain glycoprotein containing 411 amino acids that can be converted to urokinase by hydrolysis of the Lys148–149 peptide bond. Its fibrin specificity is not completely understood; however, the presence of intravascular fibrin, in and of itself, may neutralize a naturally occurring or inducible circulating scuPA inhibitor.

Tissue-Type Plasminogen Activator

Native tissue-type plasminogen activator (tPA) is a serine protease composed of one polypeptide chain containing 527 amino acids. The molecule is converted to a two-chain activator linked by one disulfide bond. This occurs by cleavage of the Arg 275-Ile 276 peptide bond yielding a heavy chain (Mr 31,000) derived from the aminoterminal part of the molecule and a light chain (Mr 28,000) comprising the carboxyterminal region.

Tissue-type plasminogen activator is a relatively weak enzyme in the absence of fibrin, but in its presence, plasminogen activation (and subsequent conversion to plasmin) is markedly enhanced. This unique property has been explained by an increased affinity of fibrin-bound tPA for plasminogen (without significant influence on the catalytic efficiency of the enzyme). Fibrin increases the local plasminogen concentration by creating an additional interaction between tPA and it substrate. This high affinity of tPA for plasminogen in the presence of fibrin thus allows efficient activation on the fibrin surface (fibrin specificity), with little plasminogen activation in plasma.

Evolution of Dosing Strategies

The dosing of tPA for the treatment of acute MI has evolved steadily since the late 1980s. Experience with a 12-hour infusion (designed with the goal of preventing arterial reocclusion) was followed by gradual abbreviated dosing schedules, initially 6 hours, then 3 hours, and, more recently, 90 minutes (accelerated or front-loaded strategy). Because a 90-minute infusion of tPA ($\leq$100 mg) provokes more rapid coronary thrombolysis than does a 3-hour infusion, interest turned to bolus and double-bolus tPA administration. The initial experience with double-bolus therapy was favorable, with angiographic TIMI grade 3 flow rates approaching 85%. With the goal of establishing an abbreviated (and easily implemented) dosing strategy that would be at least as effective as the traditional accelerated infusion, the Continuous Infusion vs. Double-Bolus Administration of Alteplase (COBALT) trial was undertaken (COBALT Investigators, 1997). A total of 7,169 patients with acute MI received either a weight-adjusted, accelerated infusion of alteplase ($\leq$100 mg over 90 minutes) or a double bolus of alteplase (50 mg followed 30 minutes later by a second 50 mg bolus; 40 mg for patients <60 kg). Mortality at 30 days was higher in the double-bolus treatment group (7.98% vs. 7.53%). The respective rates of hemorrhagic stroke were 1.12% and 0.81%.

A single-bolus strategy (50 mg) was employed in the Plasminogen Activator and Angioplasty Compatibility Trial (PACT). A total of 606 patients received a tPA bolus followed by coronary angiography or underwent primary angioplasty. Initial TIMI grade 3 flow rates were higher in the tPA-treated patients (33% vs. 15%), and there was no difference in postangioplasty perfusion. Perhaps most important, left ventricular function was preserved if coronary perfusion was present at the time of early coronary angiography (Lundergan et al., 1998).

Third-Generation Agents

A molecular approach to constructing superior fibrinolytic agents uses site-directed mutagenesis with an end-product that either lacks specific structural or functional domains or duplicates specific domains (Pannekoek et al., 1988). In this way, the most favorable properties of a given molecule can be used to their full potential, such as increasing fibrin specificity and prolonging the circulating half-life.

The wild-type (tPA) molecule (Figure 6.2 and Table 6.3) has served as the template for several third-generation molecules with the following distinct goals in mind: (1) more rapid restoration of TIMI grade 3 (normal) coronary arterial blood flow; (2) restoration of TIMI grade 3 flow in a larger proportion of patients; (3) a longer circulating half-life, permitting bolus administration; (4) a lower risk of intracranial hemorrhage; and (5) an acceptable cost (promoting wide-scale use).

Reteplase (Retavase)

Recombinant plasminogen activator (rPA) is a deletion mutant that contains the kringle-2 and protease domains of the parent tPA molecule. It has a prolonged half-

KRINGLE-KRINGLE

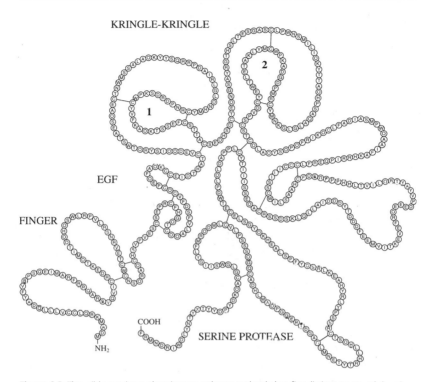

Figure 6.2 The wild-type tissue plasminogen activator molecule has five distinct structural domains that import specific biologic properties. EGF, epidermal growth factor.

life (18 minutes) and is given in two abbreviated intravenous infusions (2 minutes) 30 minutes apart. Reteplase is a Food and Drug Administration (FDA)-approved fibrinolytic for the treatment of acute MI.

The first phase II trial with rPA was an open-label, dose-finding study in patients with MI (Neuhaus et al., 1994). The initial dose (10 mg given as an IV bolus) was tested in a total of 42 patients, yielding a 90-minute angiographic patency rate of 67%. At an increased dose of 15 U (100 patients), the patency rate increased to 76%. As a means to increase efficacy further, the concept of double-bolus administration was investigated in an additional 50 patients. A regimen consisting of a 10-U bolus followed 30 minutes later by a 5-U bolus yielded a patency rate of 78% (Tebbe et al., 1993).

The 15-U bolus, 10 U followed 30 minutes later by 5 U (double bolus), and a new 10-U bolus followed 30 minutes later by a (double-bolus) regimen of rPA were compared with tPA (alteplase; 100 mg over 3 hours) in the Reteplase Angiographic Phase II International Dose Finding trial (RAPID-1; Smalling et al., 1995). The TIMI

Table 6.3 Structural–Function Relationship of the Wild-Type tPA Molecule

Domain/Region	Functional Property
Kringle-1	Receptor binding
Kringle-2	Fibrin binding (low affinity)
Fibronectin finger	Fibrin binding (high affinity)
Epidermal growth factor	Hepatic clearance
Protease	Catalytic activity; PAI-1 binding

PAI-1, plasminogen activator inhibitor-1.

grade 3 flow rates at 60 minutes and 90 minutes were 51% vs. 32.7% ($p <.01$) and 62.7% vs. 49.0% ($p <.01$) for the 10-U plus 10-U rPA- and alteplase-treated patients, respectively. The incidence of hemorrhage did not differ significantly between groups.

A second angiographic trial, Reteplase versus Alteplase Patency Investigation During Acute MI (RAPID-2; Bode et al., 1996) compared rPA and accelerated tPA administration. The TIMI grade 3 flow rates at 60 and 90 minutes were 51.2% vs. 37.4% ($p = 5 .03$) and 59.9% vs. 45.2% ($p = 5 .01$) for rPA- and tPA-treated patients, respectively.

To assess the safety and efficacy of rPA administration, a large-scale comparative, randomized trial with streptokinase was performed. The International Joint Efficacy Comparison of Thrombolytics (INJECT) trial was designed primarily as an equivalency study, and indeed failed to identify significant differences between rPA- and streptokinase-treated patients in 35-day mortality (primary endpoint) or the combined endpoint of death plus disabling stroke. The two treatments were associated with similar frequencies of in-hospital cardiac events, bleeding, and stroke (INJECT Study Group, 1995). A strong trend toward an improved clinical outcome among rPA-treated patients was observed at 6 months.

GUSTO III was a multicenter, randomized, open-label trial designed to test the primary hypothesis that rPA would significantly reduce 30-day mortality compared with an accelerated tPA infusion among patients with MI treated within 6 hours from symptom onset (GUSTO III Investigators, 1997). A total of 15,060 patients were enrolled at 822 hospitals in 20 countries. The 30-day mortality was 7.22% (95% confidence interval [CI] 6.5, 7.9) in tPA-treated patients, and 7.43 (95% CI 6.9, 7.9) in rPA-treated patients. There were no statistical differences in stroke or death/nonfatal disabling stroke. Several predefined patient subgroups, including those greater than 75 years of age, with anterior infarctions, and treatment initiation beyond 4 hours from symptom onset exhibited trends toward improved outcome with tPA.

The GUSTO V trial (GUSTO V Investigators, 2001) demonstrated similar 30-day mortality rates for full dose rPA and half-dose rPA combined with abciximab (5.9% and 5.6%, respectively); however, reinfarction and urgent revascularization occurred with reduced frequency in those receiving combination therapy (see Chapter 12).

TNK-tPA (Tenecteplase)

TNK-tPA is a multipoint mutation of the parent tPA molecule. In its mutant form, T103N, N117Q, KHRR (296–299), AAAA, threonine 103 has been changed to asparagine 103, creating a new glycosylation site (and a longer half-life) (Table 6.4). The change as ASP117 (to glutamine) also contributes to the molecule's prolonged half-life (18 minutes), while the protease sequence change renders TNK more resistant to plasminogen activator inhibitor-1 (PAI-1) (Refino et al., 1993).

The TIMI 10A trial was a phase I, dose-ranging pilot trial designed to evaluate the pharmacokinetics, safety, and efficacy of TNK-tPA in patients ($n = 113$) with acute MI presenting to the hospital within 12 hours of symptom onset. TIMI grade 3 flow at 90 minutes was achieved in 57% to 64% of patients at the 30- to 50-mg bolus doses. A total of seven patients (6.20%) experienced a major hemorrhagic event (vascular access bleeding in six of seven patients) (Cannon et al., 1997).

The TIMI 10B trial (Cannon et al., 1998) was a randomized, phase II trial that evaluated early coronary arterial patency rates with two TNK-tPA doses (30 mg and 40 mg) and an accelerated infusion of tPA. A total of 866 patients with MI presenting to the hospital within 12 hours of symptom onset were included in the study. A higher TNK-tPA dose (50 mg) yielded an excess number of hemorrhagic events and was terminated early in the study. The 30-mg dose was associated with a significantly lower rate of TIMI grade 3 flow than was tPA (55% vs. 63%; $p < .05$), and the 40-mg dose was associated with an identical rate (63%). The 50-mg dose

Table 6.4 Structure–Function Variations in TNK-tPA

Designation	Substitution	Description
T	T103N	Adds glycosylation site Decreases plasma clearance
N	N117Q	Removes glycosylation site Decreases plasma clearance Increases fibrin binding
K	KHRR (296–299) AAA	Increases fibrin specificity Increases resistance to PAI-1

PAI-1, plasminogen activator inhibitor-I; TNK-tPA, tenecteplase.

was associated with a slightly higher (66%), but not significantly different, rate of TIMI grade 3 flow. The rates of TIMI grades 2 and 3 flow combined did not differ significantly between groups. Based on a weight-based dosing analysis, the rate of TIMI 3 flow was determined to be highest at a TNK-tPA dose of ~0.5 mg/kg. This dose was also found to be safe.

The Assessment and Safety and Efficacy of a New Thrombolytic Agent (ASSENT) 1 trial was carried out simultaneously with TIMI 10B and was designed primarily to assess safety. A total of 3,325 patients were enrolled. A total of 1,705 patients received TNK-tPA (30 mg), 1,457 received 40 mg, and 73 received 50 mg. (The 50-mg dose was dropped from the study based on concerns of bleeding risk raised in TIMI 10B). The total stroke rate for the trial was 1.5%. The rate of intracranial hemorrhage was 0.77% (0.94% in the 30-mg group, 0.62% in the 40-mg group). The heparin dose did affect the rate of intracranial hemorrhage, particularly among patients weighing less than 67 kg. Corresponding 30-day death, disabling stroke, or severe bleeding rates for patients participating in the trial were 6.4%, 7.4%, and 2.8%, respectively (van de Werf et al., 1999).

The ASSENT 2 trial was a phase III, randomized, double-blind international trial designed to demonstrate equivalence in 30-day mortality between bolus administration of TNK-tPA (30- to 50-mg weight-adjusted dosing) and an accelerated infusion of tPA in patients with MI (≤6 hours from symptom onset). The secondary objectives of the study were to compare the in-hospital rate of death, stroke, intracranial hemorrhage, major bleeding, and nonfatal major cardiac events. A total of 16,949 patients were enrolled. All patients receiving aspirin and unfractionated heparin (adjusted aPTT target of 50–75 seconds). The incidence rates among TNK-tPA– and accelerated tPA-treated patients for the main endpoints were death (6.18% vs. 6.15%; risk ratio 1.00; 95% CI 0.91 to 1.10), intracranial hemorrhage (0.93% vs. 0.94%), total stroke (1.78% vs. 1.66%), and death or disabling stroke (6.21% vs. 6.05%). Major hemorrhage and transfusion rates were significantly lower in TNK-tPA–treated patients (4.7% vs. 5.9% and 4.3% vs. 5.5%, respectively) (van de Werf, 1999).

The ASSENT 3 trial (ASSENT-3 Investigators, 2001) has further characterized the benefits of tenecteplase in acute MI. In this trial, 6,095 patients were randomly assigned to full-dose TNK-tPA with weight-adjusted unfractionated heparin, TNK-tPA with enoxaparin, or reduced-dose tenecteplase with abciximab. Mortality at 30 days was similar among the three treatment groups (6.6%, 5.4%, and 6%, respectively), with a trend toward lower mortality in the TNK-tPA plus enoxaparin group. There were significantly fewer cumulative efficacy endpoints in the enoxaparin and abciximab groups (11.4% and 11.1%) than in the unfractionated heparin group (15.4%). Similar to observations made in GUSTO V, intracranial hemorrhage occurred more frequently in patients over the age of 75 who received the combination of a fibrinolytic agent and abciximab (Figure 6.3).

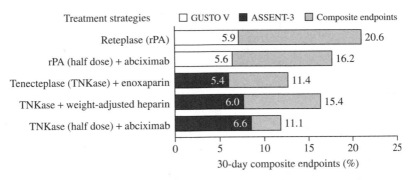

Figure 6.3 Clinical outcomes with third-generation fibrinolytics and combination pharmacotherapy for ST-segment elevation myocardial infarction. Composite endpoints included death, nonfatal myocardial infarction, and refractory ischemia. ASSENT, Assessment of the Safety and Efficacy of a New Thrombolytic Regimen; GUSTO, Global Use of Strategies to Open Occluded Arteries. (From ASSENT-3 Investigators. Efficacy and safety of tenecteplase in combination with enoxaparin, abciximab, or unfractionated heparin: the ASSENT-3 randomised trial in acute myocardial infarction. *Lancet* 2001;358:605–613.)

nPA (Lanoteplase)

nPA is a deletion and point mutant of wild-type tPA. The finger and epidermal growth factor domains have been deleted, and a point mutation within the kringle-1 domain (ASN117 Gln117) contributes to the molecule's long circulating half-life (30–45 minutes).

nPA was evaluated in a phase II, randomized, dose-ranging angiographic trial known as In Time I (den Heujer, 1998). A total of 602 patients were enrolled at 77 sites in Europe and North America and received 15, 30, 60, or 120 KU/kg of nPA or accelerated tPA within 6 hours of symptom onset. The proportion of patients achieving TIMI grade 2 or 3 infarct-related coronary artery at 90 minutes was significantly higher in the 120 KU/kg nPA group compared with the tPA group. The rate of TIMI grade 3 flow was also higher. Although a dose-related increase in major hemorrhage was observed with nPA, even at the highest dose (120 KU/kg) the overall rate was comparable with that seen with tPA.

In-TIME II was a randomized, double-blind, multicenter trial that determined whether a 120 KU/kg single-bolus dose of nPA was at least as effective as 100 mg of accelerated tPA in reducing mortality and major morbidity in patients with suspected MI presenting to the hospital within 6 hours of symptom onset. In this study, 15,078 patients were randomized between July 1997 and November 1998. All patients received aspirin and unfractionated heparin, titrated to an aPTT of 1.5 to 2.0 times control. The incidence of the primary endpoint (30-day mortality) was 6.7% with nPA and 6.6% with front-loaded tPA. Intracranial hemorrhage occurred more frequently with nPA (1.13%) than tPA (0.62%) and was likely influenced by the intensity of anticoagulation, particularly in older patients (Neuhaus, 1999). Further development of this compound has not been undertaken.

Other Plasminogen Activators

Staphylokinase is a single-chain polypeptide (136 amino acids) derived from *Staphylococcus aureus*. Like streptokinase, it is not an active enzyme, but forms a 1:1 stoichiometric complex with plasminogen that activates other plasminogen molecules (Lijinen et al., 1991). In animal models, staphylokinase has fibrinolytic potency similar to streptokinase (Collen et al., 1996). Small-scale clinical studies have yielded promising results with this agent; however, large-scale investigation has not been undertaken (Vanderschueren et al., 1995).

Importance of Bolus Dosing

The Institute of Medicine estimates that over 50,000 deaths yearly in the United States are attributable to medication errors. The available evidence suggests that nonbolus fibrinolytic therapy strategies are associated with a 15% to 20% error rate with potential catastrophic results, including intracranial hemorrhage and death (Gurwitz et al., 1998).

Summary

Fibrinolytic agents, taking advantage of scientific information and an understanding of endogenous fibrinolysis, have evolved considerably over the past 2 decades. Third-generation agents can be given as bolus or double-bolus dosing, reducing the potential for medication errors.

References

ASSENT-3 Investigators. Efficacy and safety of tenecteplase in combination with enoxaparin, abciximab, or unfractionated heparin: the ASSENT-3 randomised trial in acute myocardial infarction. *Lancet* 2001;358:605–613.

Blomback B, Okada M. Fibrin gel structure and clotting time. *Thromb Res* 1982;25: 51–70.

Bode C, Smalling RW, Berg G, et al. and the RAPID Investigators. Randomized comparison of coronary thrombolysis achieved with double bolus reteplase (r-PA) and front-loaded "accelerated" alteplase (rt-PA) in patients with acute myocardial infarction. *Circulation* 1996;94:891–898.

Cannon CP, McCabe CH, Gibson CM, et al. TNK-tissue plasminogen activator in acute myocardial infarction. Results of the Thrombolysis in Myocardial Infarction (TIMI) 10A dose-ranging trial. *Circulation* 1997;95:351–356.

Cannon CP, Gibson CM, McCabe CH, et al. for the TIMI 10B Investigators. TNK-tissue plasminogen activator compared with front loaded alteplase in acute myocardial infarction: results of the TIMI 10B Trial. *Circulation* 1998;98:2805–2814.

Carr ME, Powers PL. Effect of glycosaminoglycans on thrombin- and atroxin-induced fibrin assembly and structure. *Thromb Haemost* 1989;62:1057–1061.

COBALT Investigators. A comparison of continuous infusion of alteplase with double-bolus administration for acute myocardial infarction. *N Engl J Med* 1997;337: 1124–1130.

Collen D, Bernaerts R, Declerck P, et al. Recombinant staphylokinase variants with altered immunoreactivity. I: construction and characterization. *Circulation* 1996;94: 197–206.

Dale MD, Westrick LG, Mosher DF. Incorporation of thrombospondin into fibrin clots. *J Biol Chem* 1985;260:7502–7508.

den Heujer P, Vermeer F, Ambrosioni E, et al. For the In-TIME investigators evaluation of a single-bolus plasminogen activator in patients with myocardial infarction: a double-blind, randomized angiographic trial of lanoteplase versus alteplase. *Circulation* 1998;98:2117–2125.

GISSI Investigators. Effectiveness of intravenous thrombolytic treatment in acute myocardial infarction. *Lancet* 1986;1:397–402.

Gurwitz JH, Gore JM, Goldberg RJ, et al. Risk for intracranial hemorrhage after tissue plasminogen activator treatment for acute myocardial infarction. Participants in the National Registry of Myocardial Infarction 2. *Ann Int Med* 1998;129.597-604.

GUSTO Angiographic Investigators. The effects of tissue plasminogen activator, streptokinase, or both on coronary-artery patency, ventricular function, and survival after acute myocardial infarction (published correction appears in *N Engl J Med* 1994; 330:516). *N Engl J Med* 1993;329:1615–1622.

GUSTO III Investigators. A comparison of reteplase with alteplase for acute myocardial infarction. *N Engl J Med* 1997;337:1118–1123.

GUSTO V Investigators. Reperfusion therapy for acute myocardial infarction with fibrinolytic therapy or combination reduced fibrinolytic therapy and platelet glycoprotein IIb/IIIa inhibition: the GUSTO V randomised trial. *Lancet* 2001;357:1905–1914.

INJECT Study Group. Randomized, double-blind comparison of reteplase double-blind administration with streptokinase in acute myocardial infarction (INJECT): trial to investigate equivalence. *Lancet* 1995;346:329–336.

ISIS-2 Collaborative Group. Randomised trial of intravenous streptokinase, oral aspirin, both, or neither among 17,187 cases of suspected acute myocardial infarction: ISIS-2. *Lancet* 1988;2:349–360.

ISIS-3 Collaborative Group. A randomised comparison of streptokinase vs tissue plasminogen activator vs anistreplase and of aspirin plus heparin vs aspirin alone among 41,299 cases of suspected acute myocardial infarction: ISIS-3. *Lancet* 1992; 339:753–770.

Lijinen HR, Stassen JM, Vanlinthout I, et al. Comparative fibrinolytic properties of staphylokinase and streptokinase in animal models of venous thrombosis. *Thromb Haemost* 1991;66:468–473.

Lundergan CF, Reiner JS, Coyne KS, et al. Effect of delay of successful reperfusion on ventricular function outcome: the case for prior thrombolytic therapy with PTCA in acute myocardial infarction. *Circulation* 1998;98(Suppl):I-281.

Marx G. Divalent citations induce protofibril gelation. *Am J Hematol* 1988;27:104–109.

Neuhaus K-L, von Essen R, Vogt A, et al. Dose finding with a novel recombinant plasminogen activator (BM 06.022) in patients with acute myocardial infarction: results of the German Recombinant Plasminogen Activator Study. *J Am Coll Cardiol* 1994;24:55–60.

Neuhaus K-L, for the In-TIME Investigators. In-TIME results. *Circulation* 1999;100:574.

Pannekoek H, de Vries C, Van Zonnerveld A-J. Mutants of human tissue-plasminogen activator (tPA): structural aspects and functional properties. *Fibrinolysis* 1988;2: 123–133.

Refino CJ, Paoni NF, Keyt BA, et al. A variant of tPA (T103N, KHRR-269–299 AAA) that, by bolus, has increased potency and decreased systemic activation of plasminogen. *Thromb Haemost* 1993;70:313–319.

Sabovic M, Lijnen HR, Keber D, et al. Effect of retraction on the lysis of human clots with fibrin specific and nonfibrin specific plasminogen activators. *Thromb Haemost* 1989;62:1083–1087.

Shulman S, Ferry JD, Tinoco I Jr. The conversion of fibrinogen to fibrin. XII. Influence of pH, ionic strength and hexamethylene glycol concentration on the polymerization of fibrinogen. *Univ Wis J* 1952;42:245–256.

Smalling RW, Bode C, Kalbfleisch J, et al. and the RAPID Investigators. More rapid, complete, and stable coronary thrombolysis with bolus administration of reteplase compared with alteplase infusion in acute myocardial infarction. *Circulation* 1995; 91:2725–2732.

Tebbe U, von Essen R, Smolarz A, et al. Open, noncontrolled dose-finding study with a novel recombinant plasminogen activator (BM 06.022) given as a double bolus in patients with acute myocardial infarction. *Am J Cardiol* 1993;72:518–524.

Vanderschueren S, Barrios L, Kerdsinchai P, et al. for the STAR Trial Group. A randomized trial of recombinant staphylokinase versus alteplase for coronary artery patency in acute myocardial infarction. *Circulation* 1995;92:2004–2049.

Van de Werf F, for the ASSENT II Investigators. Results of the ASSENT II trial. *Circulation* 1999;100:574.

Van de Werf F, Cannon CP, Luyter A, et al. for the ASSENT-1 investigators. Safety assessment of single-bolus administration of tnk tissue plasminogen activator in acute myocardial infarction: the ASSENT-1 Trial. *Am Heart J* 1999;137:786–791.

Wohl RC, Summaria L, Robbins KC. Kinetics of activation of human plasminogen by different activator species at pH 7.4 and 37 C. *J Biol Chem* 1980;255:2005–2013.

Aspirin

Aspirin, considered the prototypic platelet antagonist, has been available for over a century and currently represents a mainstay both in the prevention and treatment of vascular events that include stroke, myocardial infarction, peripheral vascular occlusion, and sudden death.

Mechanism of Action

Aspirin irreversibly acetylates cyclooxygenase (COX), impairing prostaglandin metabolism and thromboxane A_2 (TXA_2) synthesis. As a result, platelet aggregation in response to collagen, adenosine diphosphate (ADP), and thrombin (in low concentrations) is attenuated (Roth and Majerus, 1975).

Because aspirin more selectively inhibits COX-1 activity (found predominantly in platelets) than COX-2 activity (expressed in tissues following an inflammatory stimulus), its ability to prevent platelet aggregation is seen at relatively low doses, compared with the drug's potential antiinflammatory effects, which require much higher doses (Patrono, 1994).

Several alternative mechanisms of platelet inhibition by aspirin have been proposed, including: (1) inhibition of platelet activation by neutrophils and (2) enhanced nitric oxide production.

In addition, aspirin may prevent the progression of atherosclerosis by protecting low-density lipoprotein (LDL) cholesterol from oxidation and scavenging hydroxyl radicals.

Pharmacokinetics

Following oral ingestion, aspirin is promptly absorbed in the proximal gastrointestinal (GI) tract (stomach, duodenum), achieving peak serum levels within 15 to 20 minutes and platelet inhibition within 40 to 60 minutes. Enteric-coated preparations are less well absorbed, causing an observed delay in peak serum levels and platelet inhibition to 60 and 90 minutes, respectively. The antiplatelet effect occurs even before acetylsalicylic acid is detectable in peripheral blood, probably from platelet exposure in the portal circulation.

The plasma concentration of aspirin decays rapidly with a circulating half-life of approximately 20 minutes. Despite the drug's rapid clearance, platelet inhibition persists for the platelet's life span (7 ± 2 days) due to aspirin's irreversible inactivation of COX-1. Because 10% of circulating platelets are replaced every 24 hours, platelet activity (bleeding time, primary hemostasis) returns toward normal ($\geq$50% activity) within 5 to 6 days of the last aspirin dose (O'Brien, 1968). A single dose of 100 mg of aspirin effectively reduces the production of TXA_2 in many (but not all) individuals.

Adverse Effects

The adverse-effect profile of aspirin in general and its associated risk for major hemorrhage in particular are determined largely by (1) dose, (2) duration of administration, (3) associated structural (peptic ulcer disease, *Helicobacter pylori* infection) defects, (4) hemostatic (inherited, acquired) abnormalities, and (5) concomitant use of other antithrombotic agents.

Aspirin is usually well tolerated when given in low doses ($\leq$325 mg) for brief periods of time (6 to 8 weeks) to patients at low risk for bleeding complications. Unfortunately, a majority of conditions for which aspirin is considered the standard of care persist over time (e.g., atherosclerotic vascular disease), requiring prolonged treatment. For this reason, aspirin, like all antithrombotic drugs that can also compromise hemostatic capacity, should only be given after a comprehensive evaluation of an individual patient's thrombotic and hemorrhagic risk has been established.

Enteric coating of aspirin has *not* been shown to reduce the likelihood of adverse effects involving the GI tract. Patients with gastric erosions or peptic ulcer disease who require treatment with aspirin should concomitantly receive a proton pump inhibitor to minimize the risk of hemorrhage.

The impact of aspirin use on the hemodynamic properties of angiotensin-converting enzyme (ACE) inhibitors is a subject of clinical relevance. Because COX-1 participates in prostaglandin production, which, in turn, influences vascular tone, drugs with preferential COX-1 activity would be expected to interact with ACE inhibitors to a greater extent than COX-2 antagonists. The available evidence, derived from retrospective analyses, suggests that antihypertensive and hemodynamic benefits are attenuated when doses of aspirin in excess of 100 mg are administered daily. This effect may be particularly important in patients with poor ventricular performance and clinical heart failure. In this setting, alternative vascular/hemodynamic (e.g., angiotensin II receptor antagonist) and antithrombotic (e.g., clopidogrel) therapies should be considered. The interaction of aspirin and ACE inhibitors does not influence short-term outcome following acute myocardial infarction (MI) (Latini et al., 2000).

Aspirin Administration in Clinical Practice

Aspirin's beneficial effect is determined largely by the absolute risk of vascular events. Patients at low risk (healthy individuals without predisposing risk factors for vas-

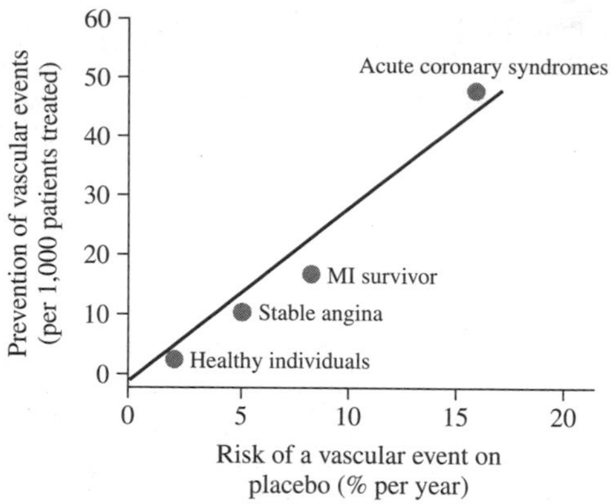

Figure 7.1 The risk–benefit relationship for aspirin administration is influenced by the overall likelihood of suffering a vascular event. Patients at greatest risk (for thrombosis) derive the greatest benefit. MI, myocardial infarction.

cular disease) derive minimal benefit, while those at high risk (unstable angina, prior MI, stroke) derive considerable benefit (Figure 7.1) (Awtry and Loscalzo, 2000). A risk-based approach to aspirin administration is recommended to avoid subjecting individuals who are unlikely to benefit from aspirin administration to its potential adverse effects.

Primary Prevention of Vascular Events

Aspirin had been tested in three primary prevention trials involving over 30,000 healthy individuals (Medical Research Council, 1998; Peto et al., 1988; Steering Committee of the Physicians' Health Study Research Group, 1989). Considering those trials collectively, the data show strongly that aspirin reduces the risk of vascular events. With increasing risk (for thrombosis) there is further benefit (Hansson et al., 1998).

The Women's Health Study (Ridker, 2005) randomly assigned 39,876 initially healthy women 45 years of age or older to receive either 100 mg aspirin on alternate days or placebo. During a follow-up of 10 years, cardiovascular events (MI, nonfatal stroke, or death from cardiovascular causes) were reduced by 9% in women receiving aspirin ($p = .13$). There was a significant reduction in ischemic stroke with aspirin use (24% relavitve risk reduction; $p = .009$), as well as a nonsignificant increase in hemorrhagic stroke (relative risk 1.24). Women 65 years of age or older derived the greatest overall benefit from aspirin, with a significant reduction in the risk of major cardiovascular events, ischemic stroke, and MI.

Secondary Prevention of Vascular Events

The Antiplatelet Trialists' Collaboration, based on a comprehensive evaluation of existing data, provides convincing evidence in support of aspirin's ability to prevent

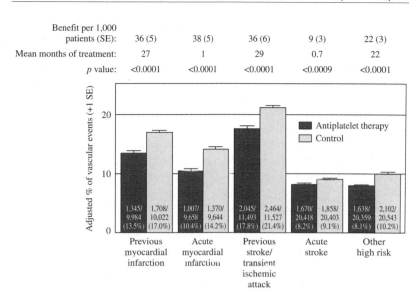

Benefit per 1,000 patients (SE):	36 (5)	38 (5)	36 (6)	9 (3)	22 (3)
Mean months of treatment:	27	1	29	0.7	22
p value:	<0.0001	<0.0001	<0.0001	<0.0009	<0.0001

Figure 7.2 Absolute effects of antiplatelet therapy on vascular events (myocardial infarction, stroke, or vascular death) in five high-risk categories

vascular events (vascular death, nonfatal MI, nonfatal stroke) in a wide variety of high-risk patients. Overall, antiplatelet therapy (predominantly aspirin therapy) reduces nonfatal MI by one third, nonfatal stroke by one third, and vascular death by one quarter (Figure 7.2).

Aspirin Dosing

The updated meta-analysis of the Antiplatelet Trialists' Collaboration provides additional information on the effects of different doses of aspirin (Antiplatelet Trialists' Collaboration, 2002). Overall, among 3,570 patients in three trials directly comparing aspirin (≥75 mg daily vs. <75 mg daily), there were significant differences in vascular events (two trials compared 75–325 mg of aspirin daily vs. <75 mg daily and one trial compared 500–1500 mg of aspirin daily vs. <75 mg daily). Considering both direct and indirect comparisons of aspirin dose, the proportional reduction in vascular events was 19% with 500 to 1500 mg daily, 26% with 160 to 325 mg daily, and 32% with 75 to 150 mg daily. Whether the greater reductions observed with decreasing doses are clinically meaningful will require a large, randomized comparison of aspirin doses in patients with coronary heart disease. Similarly, the relative benefits for patients with non–ST-segment elevation acute coronary syndrome compared with other subsets must be more clearly defined through large-scale studies.

The effects of antiplatelet drugs other than aspirin (vs. control) were assessed in 166 trials that included 81,731 patients. Indirect comparisons provided no clear evidence of differences in reducing serious vascular events (χ^2 for heterogenicity between any aspirin regimen and other antiplatelet drugs = 10.8; ns). Most direct comparisons assessed the effects of replacing aspirin with another antiplatelet agent.

The effect of adding another antiplatelet drug to aspirin (vs. aspirin alone) was assessed in 43 trials including 39,205 patients. Overall, a 15% reduction in serious vascular events was observed (p = .0001). The benefits of adding an intravenous glycoprotein (GP) IIb/IIIa receptor antagonist to aspirin were particularly evident among patients undergoing percutaneous coronary intervention (PCI).

Coronary Artery Bypass Grafting

Patients undergoing coronary artery bypass surgery are unique for several reasons. First, a majority of patients have advanced coronary atherosclerosis. Second, many individuals have concomitant peripheral vascular and cerebrovascular disease. Finally, conduits (bypass grafts) provide a strong stimulus for atherothrombosis. Over 20 clinical trials have been conducted to determine the effectiveness of antiplatelet therapy in preventing early ($\leq$10 days) and late (6–12 months) saphenous vein graft occlusion. Ten of the trials investigated aspirin in doses ranging from 100 mg to 975 mg daily. Several also evaluated patients receiving internal mammary coronary bypass grafts (Goldman et al., 1990; Lorenz et al., 1984).

Considered collectively, and aided by the Antiplatelet Trialists' Collaboration overview, the data reveal improved saphenous vein graft patency with aspirin administration. Although a direct benefit on internal mammary bypass grafts has not been established, treatment is recommended given the common coexistence of vascular disease (and the risk for thrombotic events). A majority of evidence supporting the use of aspirin after bypass grafting is based on clinical trials using a dose of at least 325 mg daily. Accordingly, the benefit derived from lower doses is less well established. Patients unable to take aspirin should be given clopidogrel 300 mg (loading dose) 6 hours after surgery followed by 75 mg daily. The potential benefit of combination therapy requires prospective evaluation.

Transient Ischemic Attacks/Stroke

The International Stroke Trial and Chinese Acute Stroke Trial (CAST) (CAST Collaborative Group, 1997; International Stroke Trial Collaborative Group, 1997) evaluated the efficacy and safety of aspirin given in a daily dose of 300 mg and 160 mg, respectively, in nearly 40,000 patients with acute ischemic stroke. Treatment was initiated within 48 hours of symptom onset and continued for 2 to 4 weeks. The combined results suggest an absolute benefit of 10 fewer deaths or nonfatal strokes per 1,000 patients in the first month of treatment. The risk of hemorrhagic stroke was also increased (two excess events per 1,000 patients).

Long-term aspirin administration reduces the likelihood of stroke (and other vascular events) in patients with transient ischemic attacks and completed minor strokes. Although there is an ongoing debate within the neurology community concerning the optimal daily dose, 75 mg to 325 mg is considered an acceptable range.

The combination of aspirin (25 mg) and extended-release dipyridamole (200 mg bid) is more effective that aspirin alone for the prevention of stroke. Patients unable to take aspirin should be treated with clopidogrel (75 mg daily) (Albers et al., 2004).

Percutaneous Coronary Intervention

PCI, including standard balloon angioplasty, rotational atherectomy, and laser angioplasty, with or without stent placement, is associated with vascular injury, atheromatous plaque disruption, platelet activation, and at times, coronary thromboembolism. Several studies performed over the past decade have documented reduced periprocedural complication, including thrombus formation, abrupt closure, and MI, with antiplatelet therapy given prior to PCI (relative risk reduction, 60%) (Barnathan et al., 1987; Schwartz et al., 1988).

The current recommendations for PCI include aspirin (80 to 325 mg daily) for secondary prevention of cardiovascular events; for patients unable to tolerate aspirin, pretreatment with clopidogrel (300–600 mg) followed by 75 mg daily is suggested. Aspirin desensitization should be considered if true aspirin allergy is documented given the potential for benefit. Combination antiplatelet therapy will be discussed in Chapter 12 (Schunemann et al., 2004).

Aspirin Response Variability

Aspirin's ability to inhibit platelet aggregation is discordant and upward of 30% of individuals who are either nonresponders or, less often, exhibit a paradoxical increase in platelet aggregation and activation following high-dose (325 mg) administration.

It has been recognized that patients with anemia and thrombocytopenia experience a shortening of their bleeding time following red blood cell transfusion, raising the possibility that platelet behavior is influenced directly by erythrocytes. In vitro, erythrocytes augment platelet activation through several mechanisms, including (1) physical interactions, (2) adenosine diphosphate–mediated agonism; and (3) facilitated TXA_2 production.

The interplay between erythrocytes and platelets has important clinical implications with regard to aspirin dosing. Low-dose aspirin (80 mg) inhibits TXA_2 production; however, the relationship between TXA_2 concentration and platelet activation is nonlinear, suggesting one or more alternative pathways of platelet activation that includes thrombin, serotonin, and platelet-activating factor. Erythrocytes can activate platelets in the presence of low-dose aspirin, but Santos and colleagues have shown that the acute administration of higher doses (500 mg) suppresses residual red blood cell–facilitated platelet performance (Santos et al., 1997).

Thromboxane A_2, a potent platelet agonist, must be suppressed by 90% or more for complete inhibition. Aspirin's ability to reduce COX activity varies considerably among individuals and, in addition, atherosclerosis is associated with increased tissue level expression due to cytokine-mediated induction. It is important to recognize that an acquired form of aspirin resistance may be induced by concomitant administration of ibuprofen (Catella-Lawson et al., 2001). Lastly, genetic polymorphisms and resulting gene expression of COX and thromboxane synthase could limit aspirin effectiveness (Figure 7.3) (Nair et al., 2001).

A classification scheme for aspirin response variability has been proposed (Patrono, 2003; Weber et al., 2002) that includes three categories: type 1, inhibition of platelet TXA_2 formation in vitro but not in vivo; type 2, inability of aspirin to inhibit TXA_2 formation in vitro and in vivo (biochemical resistance); and type 3, TXA_2 independent platelet activation (pseudoresistance).

Figure 7.3 Aspirin reduces platelet activation by limiting the synthesis of thromboxane A_2, a potent agonist. The platelet can be activated through other means (in the presence of aspirin). In addition, local COX (cyclooxygenase) concentrations are elevated with atherosclerotic vascular disease. ADP, adenosine 5' diphosphate.

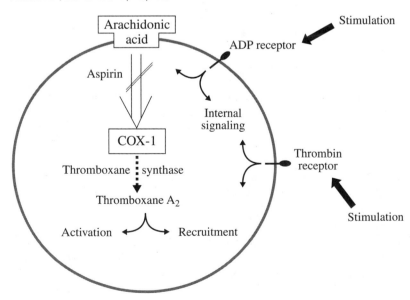

Clinical Impact of Aspirin Response Variability and Failures (Clinical Resistance)

Despite its proven benefit, aspirin does have inherent limitations. A critical review of the existing literature reveals a sizable proportion of events in patients receiving aspirin. If one were to adopt a "half empty" view toward aspirin, between 60% and 70% of patients experience MI, stroke, or cardiovascular death during periods of treatment. Thus, aspirin response variability has clinical relevance to current practice (Eikelboom et al., 2002; Gum et al., 2003) and requires further investigation in the form of a large-scale randomized trial.

Summary

Aspirin is a time-tested platelet antagonist that is widely available, inexpensive, and well tolerated by most individuals at low doses, even with long-term administration. High-risk patients enjoy the greatest overall benefit, with a relative reduction in major vascular event rates approaching 25% to 30%. The discordant effects of aspirin on platelet aggregation, aspirin response variability, aspirin failures, and the added benefit of combined pharmacotherapy must be investigated through large-scale clinical trials.

References

Albers GW, Amarenco P, Easton D, et al. Antithrombotic and thrombolytic therapy for ischemic stroke. *Chest* 2004;126:483S–512S.

Antiplatelet Trialists' Collaboration. Collaborative meta-analysis of randomised trials of antiplatelet therapy for prevention of death, myocardial infarction, and stroke in high risk patients. *BMJ* 2002;324:71–86.

Awtry EH, Loscalzo J. Aspirin. *Circulation* 2000;101:1206–1218.

Barnathan ES, Schwartz JS, Taylor L, et al. Aspirin and dipyridamole in the prevention of acute coronary thrombosis complicating coronary angioplasty. *Circulation* 1987; 76:125–134.

CAST Collaborative Group. CAST: randomised placebo-controlled trial of early aspirin use in 20,000 patients with acute ischaemic stroke. *Lancet* 1997;349:1641–1649.

Catella-Lawson F, Reilly MP, Capoor SC, et al. Cyclooxygenase inhibitors and antiplatelet effects of aspirin. *N Engl J Med* 2001;345:1809–1817.

Eikelboom JW, Hirsh J, Weitz JI, et al. Aspirin resistant thromboxane biosynthesis and the risk of myocardial infarction, stroke or cardiovascular death in patients at high risk for cardiovascular vents. *Circulation* 2002;105:1650–1655.

Goldman S, Copeland J, Moritz T, et al. Internal mammary artery and saphenous vein graft patency. Effects of aspirin. *Circulation* 1990;82(Suppl):IV237–IV242.

Gum PA, Kottl ke-Marchant K, Welsch PA, White J, Topol EJ. A prospective, blinded determination of the natural history of aspirin resistance among stable patients with cardiovascular disease. *J Am Coll Cardiol* 2003;41:961–965.

Hansson L, Zanchetti A, Carruthers SG, et al. Effects of intensive blood-pressure lowering and low-dose aspirin in patients with hypertension: principle results of the Hypertension Optimal Treatment (HOT) randomized trial. HOT Study Group. *Lancet* 1998;351:1755–1762.

International Stroke Trial Collaborative Group. The International Stroke Trial (IST): a randomized trial of aspirin, subcutaneous heparin, both or neither among 19,435 patient's with acute ischaemic stroke. *Lancet* 1997;349:1569–1581.

Latini R, Tognoni G, Maggioni AP, et al. Clinical effects of early angiotensin-converting enzyme inhibitor treatment for acute myocardial infarction are similar in the presence and absence of aspirin: systemic overview of individual data from 96,712 randomized patients. Angiotensin-converting Enzyme Inhibitor Myocardial Infarction Collaborative Group. *J Am Coll Cardiol* 2000;35:1801–1807.

Lorenz RL, Schacky CV, Weber M, et al. Improved aortocoronary bypass patency by low-dose (100 mg daily). Effects of platelet aggregation and thromboxane formation. *Lancet* 1984;1:1261–1264.

The Medical Research Council's General Practice Research Framework. Thrombosis Prevention Trial: randomized trial of low intensity oral anticoagulation with warfarin and low-dose aspirin in the primary prevention of ischaemic heart disease in men at increased risk. *Lancet* 1998;351:233–241.

Nair GV, Davis CJ, McKenzi ME, Lowry DR, Serebruany VL. Aspirin in patients with coronary artery disease: is it simply irresistible? *J Thromb Thrombolysis* 2001;11: 117–126.

O'Brien JR. Effects of salicylates on human platelets. *Lancet* 1968;1:779–783.

Patrono C. Aspirin as an antiplatelet drug. *N Engl J Med* 1994;330:1287–1294.

Patrono C. Aspirin resistance: definition, mechanisms and clinical read-outs. *J Thromb Haemost* 2003;1:1710–1713.

Peto R, Gray R, Collins R, et al. Randomized trial of prophylactic daily aspirin in British male doctors. *Br Med J* 1988;926:313–316.

Ridker PM, Cook NR, Lee I-M, et al. A randomized trial of low-dose aspirin in the primary prevention of cardiovascular disease in women. *N Engl J Med* 2005;352: 1293–1304.

Roth GJ, Majerus PW. The mechanism of the effect of aspirin on human platelets. I. Acetylation of a particular fraction protein. *J Clin Invest* 1975;56:624–632.

Santos MT, Balles J, Aznar J, Marcus AJ, Broekman MJ, Safier LB. Prothrombotic effects of erythrocytes on platelet reactivity. Reduction by aspirin. *Circulation* 1997;95:63–68.

Schunemann HJ, Cook D, Grimshaw J, et al. Antithrombotic and thrombolytic therapy: from evidence to application: the Seventh ACCP Conference on Antithrombotic and Thrombolytic Therapy. *Chest* 2004;126:688S–696S.

Schwartz L, Bourassa MG, Lesperance J, et al. Aspirin and dipyridamole in the prevention of restenosis after percutaneous transluminal coronary angioplasty. *N Engl J Med* 1988;318:1714–1719.

Steering Committee of the Physicians' Health Study Research Group. Final report on the aspirin component of the ongoing Physicians' Health Study. *N Engl J Med* 1989; 321:129–135.

Weber A-A, Przytukski B, Schanz A, et al. Towards definition of aspirin resistance: a typological approach. *Platelets* 2002;13:37–40.

Clopidogrel

8

Clopidogrel, a thienopyridine derivative, is a novel platelet antagonist that is several times more potent than ticlopidine but associated with fewer adverse effects.

In Vitro and Ex Vivo Effect on Platelets

After repeated 75-mg oral doses of clopidogrel, plasma concentrations of the parent compound, which has no platelet-inhibiting effect, are very low. Clopidogrel is extensively metabolized in the liver. The main circulating metabolite is a carboxylic acid derivative with a plasma elimination half-life of 7.7 ± 2.3 hours. Approximately 50% of an oral dose is excreted in the urine and the remaining 50% in feces over the following 5 days.

Dose-dependent inhibition of platelet aggregation is observed 2 hours after a single oral dose of clopidogrel, with a more significant inhibition achieved with loading doses (≥300 mg) by approximately 6 hours. Repeated doses of 75 mg of clopidogrel per day inhibit adenosine diphosphate (ADP)-mediated aggregation, with steady state being reached between day 3 and day 7. At steady state, the average inhibition to ADP is between 40% and 60%.

Based on ex vivo studies, clopidogrel is approximately 100-fold more potent than ticlopidine. There are no cumulative antiplatelet effects with prolonged oral administration.

The combined administration of clopidogrel (300 mg loading dose) and aspirin yields a readily discernible platelet-inhibiting effect within 90 to 120 minutes.

Clopidogrel selectively inhibits the binding of ADP to its platelet receptor ($P2Y_{12}$) and the subsequent G-protein–linked mobilization of intracellular calcium and activation of the glycoprotein (GP)IIb/IIIa complex (Gachet et al., 1992). The specific receptor has been cloned and is abundantly present on the platelet surface (Hollopter et al., 2001). Clopidogrel has no direct effect on cyclooxygenase, phosphodiesterase, or adenosine uptake.

Absorption

Clopidogrel is rapidly absorbed following oral administration with peak plasma levels of the predominant circulating metabolite occurring approximately 60 minutes later. Administration with meals does not significantly modify the bioavailability of clopidogrel.

Safety

The available information suggests that clopidogrel offers safety advantages over ticlopidine, particularly with regard to bone marrow suppression and other hematologic abnormalities. Although thrombotic thrombocytopenic purpura (TTP) has been reported with clopidogrel (Bennett et al., 2000), its occurrence (11 cases per 3 million patients treated) is rare, and has not been reported in randomized clinical trials performed to date.

Clinical Experience

Vascular Disease

The well-documented benefit derived from platelet inhibition in patients with vascular disease, coupled with a concerning adverse-effect profile witnessed with aspirin (particularly at daily doses ≥ 325 mg) and ticlopidine, fostered the rapid development of clopidogrel as a potential alternative to existing therapies. The Clopidogrel versus Aspirin in Patients at Risk for Ischemic Events (CAPRIE) study (CAPRIE Steering Committee, 1996) was designed to test the hypothesis that clopidogrel (75 mg daily) would reduce vascular events in high risk patients by approximately 15% compared with aspirin (325 mg daily). The study population consisted of patients with atherosclerotic vascular disease manifested as recent ischemic stroke, recent myocardial infarction (MI), or symptomatic peripheral arterial occlusive disease. A total of 19,185 patients were enrolled in the international trial. The mean follow-up was 1.91 years. Patients treated with clopidogrel (by intention-to-treat analysis) had a 5.32% annual risk of ischemic stroke, MI, or vascular death compared with 5.83% among aspirin-treated patients (relative risk reduction 8.7%; 95% confidence interval [CI] 0.3 to 16.5; $p = .043$) (Figure 8.1).

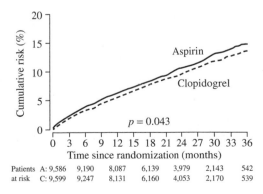

Figure 8.1 Cumulative risk of ischemic stroke, myocardial infarction, or vascular death in the CAPRIE study. Event rates were lower with clopidogrel than with aspirin (relative risk reduction 8.7%). (From CAPRIE Steering Committee. A randomised, blinded, trial of clopidogrel versus aspirin in patients at risk for ischaemic events (CAPRIE). *Lancet* 1996;348:1329–1339.)

Although CAPRIE was not powered to identify differences in specific subsets, for patients experiencing a stroke, the average event rate per year was 5.03% in the clopidogrel group compared with 4.84% in the aspirin group (relative risk increase 3.7%; $p = .66$). In contrast, patients with peripheral vascular disease experienced a 3.71% annual event rate with clopidogrel and a 4.86% rate with aspirin (relative risk reduction 23.8%; $p = .002$).

There were no major differences in safety between treatment groups; however, a greater proportion of patients receiving aspirin had the study drug permanently discontinued because of gastrointestinal hemorrhage, indigestion, nausea, or vomiting. Approximately 1 out of every 1,000 patients treated with clopidogrel experienced neutropenia ($<1.2 \times 10^9$/L) (similar to aspirin treatment).

In the CAPRIE study (Bhatt et al., 2001), all-cause mortality, vascular death, MI, stroke, and rehospitalization were determined for 1,480 patients who had previously undergone bypass grafting. Those randomized to clopidogrel had a 31.2% relative risk reduction of events compared with aspirin treatment (Figure 8.2). Considering the composite endpoint used in the main CAPRIE trial—vascular death, MI, or ischemic stroke—a 36.3% relative reduction was seen with clopidogrel (5.8% per year) compared with aspirin (9.1% per year; $p = .004$).

Coronary Arterial Stenting

A multicenter, randomized, controlled trial, Clopidogrel Aspirin Stent Intervention/ Aspirin Cooperative Study (CLASSICS) (Bertrand, 2000) included 1,020 patients

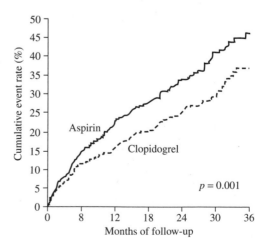

Figure 8.2 Kaplan-Meier curves for clopidogrel vs. aspirin for composite of vascular death, myocardial infarction, stroke, or rehospitalization for ischemia or bleeding, with cumulative event rates. (From Bhatt DL, Chew DP, Hirsch AT, et al. Superiority of clopidogrel versus aspirin in patients with prior cardiac surgery. *Circulation* 2001;103:363–368.)

undergoing coronary stent placement who received either aspirin (325 mg qd) plus ticlopidine (250 mg bid), aspirin plus clopidogrel (75 mg daily), or aspirin plus front-loaded clopidogrel (300 mg as an initial dose followed by 75 mg qd). Treatment was continued for 28 days after stent placement. Intravenous GPIIb/IIIa antagonists were not administered to patients enrolled in the trial. The primary safety endpoint was a composite of neutropenia, thrombocytopenia, bleeding, and drug discontinuation for adverse events (noncardiac). The secondary efficacy endpoint was a composite of MI, target vessel revascularization, and cardiovascular death.

The primary endpoint was experienced by 9.1% of ticlopidine-treated patients, 6.3% of clopidogrel-treated patients, and 2.9% of front-loaded clopidogrel-treated patients. Early drug discontinuation occurred in 8.2%, 5.1%, and 2.0% of patients, respectively. The most commonly reported adverse effects prompting drug discontinuation were allergic reactions, gastrointestinal distress, and skin rashes. The secondary cardiovascular endpoints were reached by 0.9%, 1.5%, and 1.3% of patients, respectively.

In patients undergoing coronary arterial stent placement, clopidogrel (plus aspirin) compared favorably with ticlopidine in preventing thrombotic closure; however, it was associated with fewer noncardiac adverse events that caused discontinuation of treatment (Muller et al., 2000).

The importance of adequate platelet inhibition both preceding and following percutaneous coronary intervention (PCI) (with stenting) was supported in the PCI-CURE study (Mehta et al., 2001). A total of 2,658 patients undergoing PCI were randomized to double-blind treatment with clopidogrel or placebo (aspirin alone) for, on average, 6 days before the procedure followed by 4 weeks of open-label thienopyridine (after which the study drug was resumed for 8 months). The primary endpoint (cardiovascular death, MI, or urgent target vessel revascularization within 30 days) was reached in 4.5% of clopidogrel-treated patients and 6.4% of placebo-treated patients (30% relative risk reduction) (Figure 8.3). Long-term

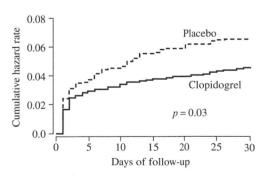

Figure 8.3 Cumulative hazard rates for the composite outcome of cardiovascular death, myocardial infarction, or target vessel revascularization at 30 days in the PCI-CURE Study. (From Mehta SR, Yusuf S, Peters RJ, for the CURE Investigators. Effects of pretreatment with clopidogrel and aspirin followed by long-term therapy in patients undergoing percutaneous coronary intervention: the PCI-CURE Study. *Lancet* 2001;358:527–533.)

Figure 8.4 Kaplan-Meier cumulative hazard rates for cardiovascular death or myocardial infarction from randomization to follow-up following percutaneous coronary intervention. (From Mehta SR, Yusuf S, Peters RJ, for the CURE Investigators. Effects of pretreatment with clopidogrel and aspirin followed by long-term therapy in patients undergoing percutaneous coronary intervention: the PCI-CURE Study. *Lancet* 2001;358:527–533.)

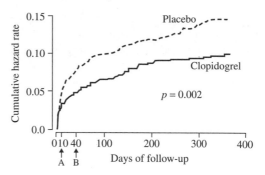

administration of clopidogrel was associated with a lower rate of death, MI, or any revascularization without increased bleeding complications (Figure 8.4).

Intracoronary radiation therapy has been used to treat in-stent restenosis; however, late stent thrombosis is a serious complication with rates approaching 10% to 15%. Prolonged treatment with clopidogrel and aspirin (6 months or more) is a more effective means to prevent late thrombosis than an abbreviated course (1 month) (Waksman et al., 2001).

At least 3 months of treatment is recommended following placement of a sirolimus drug-eluting stent (DES) and 6 months with paclitaxal DES.

Acute Coronary Syndromes

The potential benefit of combination platelet-directed therapy with aspirin and clopidogrel was investigated in the Clopidogrel in Unstable Angina to Prevent Recurrent Events (CURE) trial (CURE Investigators, 2001). A total of 12,562 patients experiencing an acute coronary syndrome without ST-segment elevation received clopidogrel (300 mg immediately, 75 mg daily) plus aspirin (75 to 325 mg daily) or aspirin alone for 3 to 12 months. The composite of death, MI, or stroke occurred in 9.3% and 11.4 % of patients, respectively (relative risk reduction 20%). In-hospital refractory ischemia, congestive heart failure, and revascularization procedures were also less likely in clopidogrel-treated patients (Figure 8.5). Although there was a greater risk of major hemorrhage with combination therapy (3.7% vs. 2.7%; relative risk 1.38), life-threatening bleeding and hemorrhagic stroke occurred at similar rates between groups.

The potential benefit of clopidogrel among patients with ST segment MI receiving fibrolytic therapy was investigated in CLARITY (Clopidogrel as Adjunctive Reperfusion Therapy)-TIMI 28. A total of 3,491 patients, 18 to 75 years of age, were

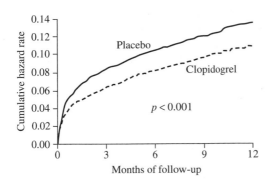

Figure 8.5 Cumulative hazard rates for the first primary outcome of death (cardiovascular), nonfatal myocardial infarction, or stroke during the 12-month follow-up of the CURE Trial. (From The Clopidogrel in Unstable Angina to Prevent Recurrent Events Trial Investigators. Effects of clopidogrel in addition to aspirin in patients with acute coronary syndromes without ST-segment elevation. *N Engl J Med* 2001;345:494–502.)

randomly assigned withing 12 hours of symptom onset to either clopidogrel (300 mg oral load, 75 mg daily) or placebo. There was a 36% reduction (15.0% versus 21.7%) in the composite of an occluded coronary artery, death, or recurrent MI (before angioplasty) in the clopidogrel group. By 30 days clopidogrel-treated patients had a 20% reduction in the composite of cardiovascular death, recurrent MI, or recurrent ischemia requiring urgent revascularization. There was no difference in major hemorrhage between groups (Sabatine et al., 2005).

Pretreatment and Duration of Therapy

The CREDO (Clopidogrel for the Reduction of Events During Observation) trial (Steinhubl et al., 2002) evaluated the long-term benefit (12 months) of treatment with clopidogrel after PCI as well as the potential benefit of initiating clopidogrel with preprocedure loading dose (both in addition to aspirin therapy). A total of 2,116 patients scheduled for elective PCI were randomly assigned to receive clopidogrel (300 mg) or placebo 3 to 24 hours before PCI. All patients received aspirin (325 mg). Greater than two thirds of the patients had either a recent MI or unstable angina as an indication for PCI. Thereafter, all patients received clopidogrel (75 mg daily) through day 28. From day 29 through 12 months, patients in the loading dose group received clopidogrel (75 mg daily) or placebo. Both groups continued to receive standard therapy including aspirin (81–325 mg daily). Pretreatment with clopidogrel was associated with a nonsignificant 18.5% relative risk reduction for the combined endpoint of death, MI, or target vessel revascularization at 28 days. Larger loading doses (600 mg) or more prolonged pretreatment may yield greater benefit.

In the ARMYDA-2 (Antithrombotic Therapy for Reduction of Myocardial Damage during Angioplasty) study (Patti et al., 2005), 255 patients undergoing PCI were randomized to a 600 mg or 300 mg clopidogrel loading regimen given 4 to 8 hours before the procedure. The primary end point (30 days to death, or to MI or target vessel revascularization) occurred in 4% and 12% of patients, respectively (due entirely to a reduction in peri-procedural MI).

Treatment of Patients Receiving Chronic Therapy

Two series of 20 consecutive patients with coronary artery disease received 600 mg of clopidogrel. The first patient group had not received clopidogrel previously, while the second group took 75 mg previously for at least 30 days. Six hours after loading, platelet aggregation in response to ADP (20 µmol/L) was inhibited by 31% and 51%, respectively. Clopidogrel inhibited ADP-induced expression of platelet GPIIb/IIIa and P-selectin receptors as well (Kastrati et al., 2004).

Clopidogrel Response Variability

Although the incidence rates and mechanisms likely differ, clopidogrel and aspirin response variability may have cumulative clinical relevance. The available evidence suggests that clopidogrel resistance (<10% inhibition of ADP-mediated platelet aggregation) exists in upward of 20% of patients following a 300-mg loading dose (Gurbel et al., 2003) and may identify patients at risk for coronary arterial events (Matetzky et al., 2004). Patients with heightened platelet activity (prior to treatment) appear to be at greatest risk for clopidogrel resistance (Gurbel and Bliden, 2003) (Figure 8.6). Although the mechanism(s) underlying clopidogrel response variability have not been elucidated, GI drug absorption alterations in cytochrome (CYP) 3A4 metabolic activity (conversion of prodrug to active drug), polymorphisms of the platelet ADP receptor, or individual differences in postreceptor signaling pathways are likely contributors.

Summary

Clopidogrel, a thienopyridine derivative that is structurally and functionally distinct from other platelet antagonists, exerts modest benefit when used alone in patients at risk for vascular events. In contrast, the combination of aspirin and clopidogrel offers considerable benefit in patients with non–ST-segment elevation acute coronary syndromes and following coronary arterial stent placement. The potential mechanism for clopidogrel response variability and its overall clinical relevance requires further investigation, as does more potent ADP receptor inhibition with novel pharmaceutical agents.

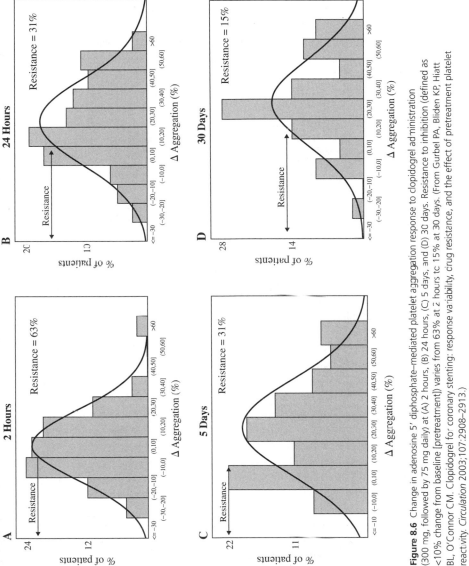

Figure 8.6 Change in adenosine 5' diphosphate–mediated platelet aggregation response to clopidogrel administration (300 mg, followed by 75 mg daily) at (A) 2 hours, (B) 24 hours, (C) 5 days, and (D) 30 days. Resistance to inhibition (defined as <10% change from baseline [pretreatment]) varies from 63% at 2 hours to 15% at 30 days. (From Gurbel PA, Bliden KP, Hiatt BL, O'Connor CM. Clopidogrel for coronary stenting: response variability, drug resistance, and the effect of pretreatment platelet reactivity. *Circulation* 2003;107:2908–2913.)

References

Bennett CL, Connors JM, Carwile JM, et al. Thrombotic thrombocytopenia purpura associated with clopidogrel. *N Engl J Med* 2000;342:1773–1777.

Bertrand ME. Double-blind study of the safety of clopidogrel with and without a loading dose in combination with aspirin compared with ticlopidine in combination with aspirin after coronary stenting: the Clopidogrel Aspirin Stent International Cooperative Study (CLASSICS). *Circulation* 2000;102:624–629.

Bhatt DL, Chew DP, Hirsch AT, et al. Superiority of clopidogrel versus aspirin in patients with prior cardiac surgery. *Circulation* 2001;103:363–368.

CAPRIE Steering Committee. A randomised, blinded trial of clopidogrel versus aspirin in patients at risk for ischaemic events (CAPRIE). *Lancet* 1996;348:1329–1339.

CURE Trial Investigators. Effects of clopidogrel in addition to aspirin in patients with acute coronary syndromes without ST-segment elevation. *N Engl J Med* 2001;345: 494–502.

Gachet C, Savi P, Ohlmann P, et al. ADP receptor induced activation of guanine nucleotide binding proteins in rat platelet membranes—an effect selectively blocked by the thienopyridine clopidogrel. *Thromb Haemost* 1992;68:79–83.

Gurbel PA, Bliden KP. Interpretation of platelet inhibition by clopidogrel and the effect of non-responders. *J Thromb Haemost* 2003;1:1318–1319.

Gurbel PA, Bliden KP, Hiatt BL, O'Connor CM. Clopidogrel for coronary stenting: response variability, drug resistance, and the effect of pretreatment platelet reactivity. *Circulation* 2003;107:2908–2913.

Hollopter G, Jantzen HM, Vincent D, et al. Identification of the platelet ADP receptor targeted by antithrombotic drugs. *Nature* 2001;409:202–207.

Kastrati A, von Beckerath N, Joost A, Pogatsa-Murray G, Gorchakova O, Schomig A. Loading with 600 mg clopidogrel in patients with coronary artery disease with and without chronic clopidogrel therapy. *Circulation* 2004;110:1916–1919.

Matetzky S, Shenkman B, Guetta V, et al. Clopidogrel resistance is associated with increased risk of recurrent atherothrombotic events in patients with acute myocardial infarction. *Circulation* 2004;109:3171–3175.

Mehta SR, Yusuf S, Peters RJ, for the CURE Investigators. Effects of pretreatment with clopidogrel and aspirin followed by long-term therapy in patients undergoing percutaneous coronary intervention: the PCI-CURE study. *Lancet* 2001;358:527–533.

Muller C, Buttner HJ, Peterson J, Roskamm H. A randomized comparison of clopidogrel and aspirin versus ticlopidine and aspirin after placement of coronary-artery stents. *Circulation* 2000;101:590–593.

Patti G, Colona AG, Pasceri V, et al. Randomized trial of high loading dose of clopidogrel for reduction of periprocedural MI in patients undergoing coronary intervention. *Circulation* 2005;111:2099–2106.

Sabatine M, Cannon CP, Gibson CM, et al., for the CLARITY-TIMI 28 Investigators. Addition of clopidogrel to aspirin and fibrolytic therapy for myocardial infarction with ST-segment elevation. *N Engl J Med* 2005;352:1179–1189.

Steinhubl SR, Berger PB, Mann JT III, Fry ETA, DeLago A, et al. Early and sustained dual oral antiplatelet therapy following percutaneous coronary intervention: a randomized controlled trial. *JAMA* 2002;288:2411–2420.

Waksman R, Ajani AE, White RL, et al. Prolonged antiplatelet therapy to prevent late thrombosis after intracoronary-radiation in patients with restenosis: Washington Radiation for In-Stent Restenosis Trial plus 6 months of clopidogrel (WRIST PLUS). *Circulation* 2001;103:2332–2335.

Platelet Glycoprotein IIb/IIIa
Receptor Antagonists

9

The glycoprotein (GP) IIb/IIIa (α_{IIb}/β_3) receptor totalling 50,000 to 70,000 copies per platelet represents a common pathway for platelet aggregation in response to a wide variety of biochemical and mechanical stimuli. Accordingly, it represents an attractive target for pharmacologic inhibition that can be applied to patients with acute coronary syndromes.

Intravenous Platelet GPIIb/IIIa Receptor Antagonists

The evolution of GPIIb/IIIa receptor antagonists began with murine monoclonal antibodies and subsequently expanded to include small peptide or nonpeptide molecules with structural similarities to fibrinogen (Figure 9.1). There are three intravenous GPIIb/IIIa receptor antagonists that have been approved by the U.S. Food and Drug Administration:

- Abciximab (ReoPro)
- Tirofiban (Aggrastat)
- Eptifibatide (Integrilin)

Abciximab

Abciximab (ReoPro) is the Fab fragment of the chimeric human–murine monoclonal antibody c7E3.

Pharmacokinetics

Following an intravenous bolus, free plasma concentrations of abciximab decrease rapidly with an initial half-life of less than 10 minutes and a second-phase half-life of 30 minutes, representing rapid binding to the platelet GPIIb/IIIa receptor. Abciximab remains in the circulation for 10 or more days in the platelet-bound state.

Pharmacodynamics

Intravenous administration of abciximab in doses ranging from 0.15 mg/kg to 0.3 mg/kg produces a rapid dose-dependent inhibition of platelet aggregation in response to adenosine diphosphate (ADP). At the highest dose, 80% of platelet

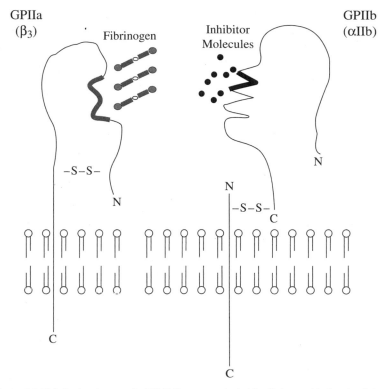

Figure 9.1 The platelet glycoprotein (GP) IIb/IIIa receptor is vital for fibrinogen binding that links adjacent platelets to one another. GPIIb/IIIa receptor inhibitors compete with fibrinogen-preventing therapy, platelet aggregation.

GPIIb/IIIa receptors are occupied within 2 hours and platelet aggregation, even with 20 µM ADP, is completely inhibited. Sustained inhibition is achieved with prolonged infusions (12 to 24 hours) and low-level receptor blockade is present for up to 10 days following cessation of the infusion; however, platelet inhibition during infusions beyond 24 hours has not been well characterized. Platelet aggregation in response to 5 µM ADP returns to greater than or equal to 50% of baseline within 24 hours of drug cessation.

Clinical Experience

In nearly 2,100 patients undergoing either balloon coronary angioplasty or atherectomy at high risk for ischemic (thrombotic) complications, a bolus of abciximab

(0.25 mg/kg) followed by a 12-hour continuous infusion (10 µg/min) reduced the occurrence of death, the occurrence myocardial infarction (MI), or the need for an urgent intervention (repeat angioplasty, stent placement, balloon pump insertion, or bypass grafting) by 35% (EPIC Investigators, 1994). At 6 months (Topol et al., 1994), the absolute difference in patients with a major ischemic event or elective revascularization was 8.1% comparing patients who received abciximab (bolus plus infusion) with those given placebo (35.1% vs. 27.0%; 23% reduction). All patients received aspirin and unfractionated heparin during the procedure. At 3 years (Topol et al., 1997), the composite endpoint occurred in (1) 41.1% of those receiving an abciximab bolus plus infusion, (2) 47.4% of those receiving an abciximab bolus only, and (3) 47.2% of those receiving placebo.

The Evaluation in PTCA to Improve Long-Term Outcome with Abciximab GPIIb/IIIa Blockade (EPILOG) study (EPILOG Investigators, 1997) included 2,792 patients undergoing elective or urgent percutaneous coronary revascularization who received either abciximab with standard, weight-adjusted unfractionated heparin (initial bolus 100 U/kg, target activated clotting time [ACT] ≥300 seconds) or placebo with standard-dose, weight-adjusted heparin. At 30 days, the composite event rate was observed in both high-risk and low-risk patients.

The c7E3 Fab Antiplatelet Therapy in Unstable Refractory Angina (CAPTURE) study (CAPTURE Investigators, 1997) was designed to investigate whether abciximab, given during the 18 to 24 hours before coronary angioplasty, could improve outcome in patients with refractory (myocardial ischemia despite nitrates, heparin, and aspirin) unstable angina. A total of 1,265 patients were randomly assigned to abciximab or placebo. By 30 days, the primary endpoint (death, MI, urgent revascularization) occurred in 11.3% of abciximab-treated patients and in 15.9% of placebo-treated patients ($p = .012$). The rate of MI was lower *before* and *during* coronary interventions in those given abciximab.

Patients participating in the Global Use of Strategies to Open Occluded Arteries (GUSTO) IV-ACS trial (GUSTO IV Investigators, 2001) had chest pain and either ST-segment depression or elevated troponin levels. They were randomized to receive placebo, abciximab for 24 hours, or abciximab for 48 hours with recommended avoidance of revascularization during the initial 48 hours. Neither abciximab group fared better than placebo with respect to death or MI at 30 days. In addition, early mortality rates were higher with a prolonged abciximab infusion, suggesting a prothrombotic (or other adverse) effect.

The Abciximab before Direct Angioplasty and Stenting in Myocardial Infarction Regarding Acute and Long-Term Follow-Up (ADMIRAL) trial (Montalescot et al., 2001) included 300 patients with acute percutaneous coronary intervention (PCI) (plus stenting) and who received either abciximab or placebo. At 30 days, a composite of death, reinfarction, or urgent revascularization (target vessel) had occurred in 6% of abciximab-treated and 14.6% of placebo-treated patients; at 6 months, the corresponding figures were 7.4% and 15.9%, respectively. The early administration of abciximab improved coronary patency before stenting, the success rate of the procedures, and the rate of patency 6 months after the procedure.

In the GUSTO V study (Topol and the GUSTO V Investigators, 2001) 16,588 patients with acute ST-segment elevation MI received either reteplase (standard dose) or half-dose reteplase plus abciximab. Although the 30-day mortality rates did not differ significantly, there were fewer nonfatal ischemic complications of MI with reteplase plus abciximab compared with reteplase alone. Intracranial hemorrhage rates did not differ between treatments; however, moderate to severe bleeding was more likely with combined therapy, and patients greater than 75 years of age were at increased risk for hemorrhagic stroke (odds ratio 1.91). All patients in the GUSTO V study received unfractionated heparin and aspirin.

Tirofiban

Tirofiban (Aggrastat), a tyrosine derivative with a molecular weight of 495 kd, is a nonpeptide inhibitor (peptidomimetic) of the platelet GPIIb/IIIa receptor.

Pharmacodynamics

Tirofiban, like other nonpeptides, mimics the geometric, stereotactic, and charge characteristics of the RDG sequence (of fibrinogen), thus interfering with platelet aggregation.

Three doses of tirofiban were evaluated in a phase I study of patients undergoing coronary angioplasty who received one of three regimens intravenously with a bolus dose of 5, 10, or 15 µg/kg and a continuous (16- to 24-hour) infusion of 0.05, 0.10, or 0.15 µg/kg/min (Kereiakas et al., 1996). A dose-dependent inhibition of ex vivo platelet aggregation was observed within minutes of bolus administration and was sustained during the continuous infusion.

Clinical Experience

The Randomized Efficacy Study of Tirofiban Outcomes and Restenosis (RESTORE) trial (RESTORE Investigators, 1997) was a randomized, double-blind, placebo-controlled trial of tirofiban in patients with acute coronary syndrome (ACS) undergoing PCI.

Patients ($n = 2,139$) received tirofiban as a 10 µg/kg intravenous bolus over a 3-minute period and a continuous infusion of 0.15 µg/kg/min over 36 hours. All patients received unfractionated heparin and aspirin. The primary composite endpoint (death, MI, angioplasty, failure requiring bypass surgery or unplanned stent placement, recurrent ischemia requiring repeat angioplasty) at 30 days was reduced from 12.2% in the placebo group to 10.3% in the tirofiban group (16% relative reduction).

The Platelet Receptor Inhibition in Ischemic Syndrome Management (PRISM) trial (PRISM Study Investigators, 1998) included 3,231 patients with non–ST-segment elevation ACS. All patients received aspirin and were randomized to treatment with either unfractionated heparin or tirofiban, given as a loading dose of 0.6 μg/kg/min over 30 minutes followed by a maintenance infusion of 0.15 μg/kg/min for 48 hours (angiography/revascularization was discouraged during the infusion period). The primary composite endpoint (death, MI, refractory ischemia) at 48 hours was 5.6% in tirofiban-treated patients and 3.8% in placebo (aspirin/heparin)-treated patients (risk reduction 33%). Benefit was maintained but overall was more modest at 7 and 30 days.

The PRISM in Patients Limited by Unstable Signs and Symptoms (PLUS) trial (PRISM PLUS Study Investigators, 1998) included 1,915 patients with non–ST-segment elevation ACS who were treated with aspirin and unfractionated heparin and subsequently randomized to either tirofiban (0.4 μg/kg/min × 30 min; then 0.1 μg/kg/min for a minimum of 48 hours and a maximum of 108 hours) or placebo (unfractionated heparin). Angiography and revascularization were performed at the discretion of the treating physician. Tirofiban-treated patients had a lower composite event rate of 7 days than the placebo group, 12.9% vs. 17.9% (risk reduction 34%). The benefit was mainly due to a reduced incidence of MI (47% risk reduction) and refractory ischemia (30% risk reduction). The benefit was maintained at 30 days (22% risk reduction in composite event rate) and at 6 months. The trial originally included a tirofiban-alone arm (no heparin) that was dropped because of excess mortality at 7 days.

The importance of early PCI among patients with non–ST-segment elevation ACS was underscored in the Treat Angina with Aggrastat and Determine Cost of Therapy with an Invasive or Conservative Strategy (TACTICS)–Thrombolysis in Myocardial Infarction (TIMI) 18 trial (Cannon et al., 2001), as was the benefit of aggressive pharmacologic therapy (GPIIb/IIIa receptor antagonist) in combination with PCI for patients at greatest risk for adverse ischemic outcomes (prior MI, ST-segment changes, elevated cardiac biomarkers).

Eptifibatide

Eptifibatide (Integrilin) is a nonimmunogenic cyclic heptapeptide with an active pharmacophore that is derived from the structure of barbourin, a platelet GPIIb/IIIa inhibitor from the venom of the southeastern pigmy rattlesnake (Phillips and Scarborough, 1997).

Pharmacokinetics

The plasma half-life of eptifibatide is 10 to 15 minutes and clearance is predominantly renal (75%) and to a lesser degree hepatic (25%). The antiplatelet effect has a rapid onset of action and is rapidly reversible.

Pharmacodynamics

In a pilot study of PCI, patients were randomized to one of four eptifibatide dosing schedules:

- 180 µg/kg bolus, 1 µg/kg/min infusion
- 135 µg/kg bolus, 0.5 µg/kg/min infusion
- 90 µg/kg bolus, 0.75 µg/kg/min infusion
- 135 µg/kg bolus, 0.75 µg/kg/min infusion

All patients received aspirin and unfractionated heparin and were continued on the study drug for 18 to 24 hours. The two highest bolus doses produced greater than 80% inhibition of ADP-mediated platelet aggregation within 15 minutes of administration in a majority of patients (>75%). A constant infusion of 0.75 µg/kg/min maintained the antiplatelet effect, whereas an infusion of 0.50 µg/kg/min allowed gradual recovery of platelet function. In all dosing groups, platelet function returned to greater than 50% of baseline within 4 hours of terminating the infusion (Harrington et al., 1995).

Clinical Experience

The Integrilin to Minimize Platelet Aggregation and Coronary Thrombosis (IMPACT-II) trial (IMPACT-II Investigators, 1997) enrolled 4,010 patients undergoing elective, urgent, or emergent PCI. Patients were assigned to either placebo, a bolus of 135 µg/kg eptifibatide followed by an infusion of 0.5 µg/kg/min for 20 to 24 hours, or a 135 µg/kg bolus with a 0.75 µg/kg/min infusion. By 30 days, the composite endpoint (death, MI, unplanned revascularization, stent placement for abrupt closure) occurred in 11.4%, 9.2%, and 9.9% of patients respectively. Although the benefit of treatment was maintained at 6 months, the differences between groups were not statistically significant.

The IMPACT-After Myocardial Infarction (AMI) study (Ohman et al., 1997) was designed to determine the effect of eptifibatide on coronary arterial patency when used adjunctively with alteplase (tPA). A total of 132 patients with MI received tPA, heparin, and aspirin, and were randomized to receive a bolus and continuous infusion of one of six eptifibatide doses or placebo. The doses ranged from 36 to 180 µg/kg (bolus) to 0.2 to 0.75 µg/kg/min (infusion). The study drug was

Table 9.1 Clinical Trials of GPIIb/IIIa Receptor Antagonists in Patients with Coronary Artery Disease

Trial	Patients	GPIIb/IIIa Antagonist	UFH	Death	Nonfatal MI	Repeat PCI	Unplanned Surgery	Major Bleeding	Time
CAPTURE	630	Abciximab bolus + infusion 18–24 h before PCI, 1 h after	Heparin to aPTT 2–2.5 × control before PCI; ACT 300 sec; 1 h post	1.0	4.1[d]	4.5	1.0	3.8	30 d
	635			1.3	8.2	6.6	1.7	1.9	
EPILOG	918	Abciximab bolus + infusion (12 h)	100 U/kg target ACT 300 sec	0.4	3.8[a]	1.5[b]	0.9	3.5	30 d
	935	Abciximab bolus + infusion (12 h)	70 U/kg target ACT 200 sec	0.3	3.7[b]	1.2[b]	0.4	20	
	939	Placebo	100 U/kg target ACT 300 sec	0.8	8.7[b]	3.8	1.7	3.1	
	4,739	Placebo	aPTT 50–70 sec[b] ACT 300–350 sec[b]	3.7	12.0	—	—	9.3	
EPIC	708	Abciximab + infusion (12 h)	10–12 K bolus add. bolus up to 20 K ACT 300–350 sec	1.7	5.2[a]	0.8[a]	2.4	14	30 d
	695	Abciximab bolus	ACT 300–350 sec	1.3	6.2	3.6	2.3	11	
	696	Placebo	Postprocedure to aPTT 1.5–2.5 × control for 12 h	1.7	8.6	4.5	3.6	7	
EPIC	708	Abciximab bolus + infusion (12 h)	10–12 K bolus add. bolus up to 20 K ACT 300–350 sec	3.1	6.9	14.4[b]	9.4		1 yr
	695	Abciximab bolus	Postprocedure to aPTT 1.5–2.5 × control for 12 h	2.6	8.0	19.9	9.9		
	696	Placebo		3.4	10.5	20.9	10.9		

Trial	N	Treatment	Heparin						
EPIC	708	Abciximab bolus + infusion (12 h)	10–12 K add. bolus up to 20 K ACT 300–350 sec	6.8	10.7	—	34.8[d]	—	3 yr
	698	Abciximab bolus	Postprocedure to aPTT 1.5–2.5 × control for 12 h	3.0	12.2	—	38.6	—	
	696	Placebo		8.6	13.6	—	40.1	—	
IMPACT II	1,333	Eptifibatide bolus + infusion for 20–24 h (high)	100 U/kg bolus	0.8	5.9	2.9	2.0	5.2	30 d
	1,349	Eptifibatide bolus + infusion (low)	Target ACT 300–350 sec	0.5	6.6	2.6	1.6	5.1	
	1,328	Placebo	No heparin after PCI	1.1	2.8	2.8	2.8	4.8	
PRISM	1,616	Tirofiban bolus + infusion × 48 h	No	0.2	0.9	3.5[a]	—	0.4	48 h
	1,616	UFH × 48 h	—	0.4	1.4	5.3[a]	—	0.4	
PRISM-PLUS	773	Tirofiban bolus + infusion × 72 h	aPTT 2 × control	1.9	3.9	9.3[a]	—	4.0	7 d
	797	UFH × 72 h	aPTT 2 × control	1.9	7.0	12.7[a]	—	3.0	
PURSUIT	4,722	Eptifibatide	aPTT 50–70 sec[b] ACT 300–350 sec[b]	3.5	10.7	—	—	10.8	30 d

a = 0.01—refractory ischemia.

b ≤ 0.001—heparin use at discretion of physician.

c = 0.02

d = 0.002

e <80 kg 60 U/kg, 12 U/kg/h

ACT, activated clotting time; aPTT, activated partial thromboplastin time; GP, glycoprotein; MI, myocardial infarction; PCI, percutaneous coronary intervention; UFH, unfractionated heparin.

started within 24 hours. The highest-dose eptifibatide groups had more complete reperfusion (TIMI grade 3 flow) and shorter mean time to ST-segment recovery than placebo-treated patients. The composite clinical event rate (death, reinfarction, revascularization, heart failure, hypertension, stroke) was relatively high in all groups: 44.8% in eptifibatide-treated patients and 41.8% in placebo-treated patients.

The Platelet Glycoprotein IIb/IIIa in Unstable Angina Receptor Suppression Using Integrilin Therapy (PURSUIT) trial (PURSUIT Trial Investigators, 1998) included patients with non–ST-segment elevation ACS with symptoms within 24 hours and electrocardiographic changes within 12 hours (of ischemia). A total of 10,948 patients were randomized to eptifibatide: 180 µg/kg bolus plus 1.3 µg/kg/min infusion, 180 µg/kg bolus plus 2.0 µg/kg/min infusion, or placebo for up to 3 days (in addition to unfractionated heparin [in most patients] and aspirin). The 30-day event rate of death or nonfatal MI was 14.2% with eptifibatide and 15.7% with placebo (1.5% absolute reduction). A reduction in MI or death (composite) with eptifibatide was observed at later time points.

The Enhanced Suppression of the Platelet GPIIb/IIIa Receptor with Integrilin Trial (ESPRIT) was designed to test the hypothesis that a minimum threshold of 80% GPIIb/IIIa receptor blockade was required for benefit (ESPRIT Investigators, 2000). A total of 2,064 patients received either eptifibatide (180 µg/kg boluses [× 2] 10 minutes apart or continuous infusion of 2.0 µg/kg/min for 18 to 24 hours) or placebo prior to PCI. The trial was terminated early for efficacy as patients receiving eptifibatide had a 4% absolute reduction in death, MI, urgent target vessel revascularization, or "bailout" GPIIb/IIIa antagonist use within 48 hours compared with placebo. Major events were significantly lower at 30 days as well (Table 9.1).

GPIIb/IIIa Receptor Antagonists and Diabetes Mellitus

Patients with diabetes mellitus suffer increased mortality in the setting of acute coronary syndromes. A meta-analysis of diabetic populations enrolled in six large-scale clinical trials ($n = 6,458$ patients) revealed a 30-day mortality reduction with GPIIb/IIIa receptor antagonist use from 6.2% to 4.6% (26% relative risk reduction). The benefit was greatest in those undergoing PCI (70% relative risk reduction) (Roffi et al., 2001).

Agent-Specific Characteristics

Although considered collectively as GPIIb/IIIa receptor antagonists, abciximab, tirofiban, and eptifibatide differ at several levels, including their:

- Molecular weight
- Binding characteristics

- Route of clearance
- Plasma half-life
- Platelet-bound and biologic half-life
- Potential reversibility (Table 9.2; Figure 9.2 A,B)

The approved indications and use in clinical practice also differ (Table 9.3). The duration of platelet inhibition following drug discontinuation and the potential for reversing the pharmacologic effect are particularly important properties in cases of emergent surgery and major hemorrhagic complications. In general, a return of platelet function toward a physiologic state ($\leq$50% inhibition) occurs within 4 hours following the cessation of tirofiban and eptifibatide. In contrast, 12 hours are required for abciximab (Figure 9.3). Some of the delayed return of physiologic platelet function following abciximab termination may be counterbalanced by its low free plasma concentrations and drug-to-receptor ratio. These properties are responsible for the rapid return of hemostatic potential following platelet transfusions (and may also limit platelet-inhibiting potential with marked mobilization of GPIIb/IIIa receptors from intraplatelet storage pools). In contrast, the high plasma concentrations observed with the small-molecule inhibitors limit the effectiveness of platelet transfusions. Fibrinogen supplementation (fresh frozen plasma, cryoprecipitate) is the more logical choice for restoration of hemostatic potential, given the competitive nature of binding and relative availability of platelet GPIIb/IIIa receptors (Becker et al., 2001).

Comparing Clinical Endpoints

The intravenous GPIIb/IIIa receptor antagonists have been shown to reduce cardiac event rates in patients with ACS who are treated by pharmacologic means alone or

Table 9.2 Agent-Specific Characteristics for GPIIb/IIIa Receptor Antagonists

Characteristic	Abciximab	Eptifibatide	Tirofiban
Type	Antibody	Peptide	Nonpeptide
Molecular weight (daltons)	~50,000	~800	~500
Platelet-bound half-life	Long (H)	Short (sec)	Short (sec)
Plasma half-life	Short (min)	Extended (2 h)	Extended (2 h)
Drug-to-GPIIb/IIIa receptor ratio	1.5–2.0	250–2,500	>250
50% return of platelet function (without transfusion)	12 h	~4 h	~4 h
Route of clearance	RES	Renal/hepatic	Renal
Dose adjustment required with renal insufficiency	No	Yes	Yes

GP, glycoprotein; RES, reticuloendothelial system.

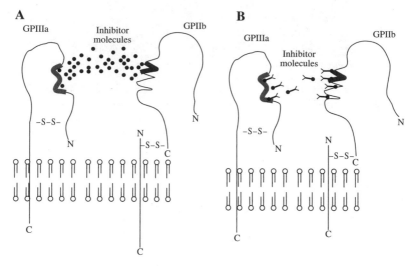

Figure 9.2 The small molecule (competitive) glycoprotein (GP) IIb/IIIa receptor inhibitors (tirofiban, eptifibatide) are characterized by a relatively high plasma–to–bound receptor ratio (A). In contrast, the monoclonal antibody abciximab is highly bound to the platelet GPIIb/IIIa receptor (B).

undergo PCI. The available data suggest, however, that the greatest overall benefit occurs in high-risk patients, particularly those undergoing mechanical revascularization.

Methodologic differences between the major clinical trials make it difficult to compare the GPIIb/IIIa receptor antagonists; however, there is clear consistency among the agents with regard to efficacy and safety (Kong et al., 1998). The Do Tirofiban and ReoPro Give Similar Efficacy Trial (TARGET) randomized 5,308 patients to either tirofiban (RESTORE trial dosing strategy) or abciximab before PCI

Table 9.3 Intravenous GPIIb/IIIa Receptor Antagonists: Approved Indications and Use in Clinical Practice

Agent	Medical Treatment ACS	PCI	PCI STEMI	Fibrinolytic Combination STEMI	Facilitated PCI
Abciximab	++*	+++	++	+	0
Eptifibatide	++	+++	+	+	0
Tirofiban	++	++	+	+	0

*Refractory angina if PCI performed within 12 hours.
+++, clear benefit; ++, modest benefit; +, risk–benefit not fully defined; 0, no clear benefit.
ACS, acute coronary syndrome; GP, glycoprotein; PCI, percutaneous coronary intervention; STEMI, ST-segment elevation myocardial infarction.

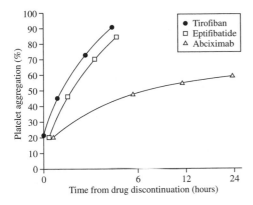

Figure 9.3 Restoration of platelet aggregability following cessation of glycoprotein (GP) IIb/IIIa receptor antagonists.

(with the intent to perform stenting). The primary endpoint, a composite of death, nonfatal MI, or urgent revascularization at 30 days, was reached in 7.6% and 6.0% of tirofiban-treated and abciximab-treated patients, respectively (hazard ratio 1.26) (Topol et al., 2001). There were no differences in the rates of major bleeding complications or transfusions, but tirofiban was associated with a lower rate of minor bleeding episodes and thrombocytopenia (Figure 9.4).

The ideal dosing strategy for tirofiban has become a topic of considerable interest. In the COMPARE (Comparison of Measurement of Platelet Aggregation with Aggrastat, ReoPro, and Eptifibatide) study (Batchelor et al., 2002), a tirofiban dose of 10 mg/kg (bolus) was associated with a lower degree of platelet inhibition 15 and

Figure 9.4 The TARGET trial is the only comparative study of glycoprotein (GP) IIb/IIIa receptor antagonists. The 30-day clinical outcomes were more often experienced by patients receiving tirofiban than those randomized to receive abciximab. Hazard ratios for the individual end points in Tirofiban and ReoPro give similar efficacy outcomes trial (TARGET). MI, myocardial infarction. (From Topol EJ, Moliterno DJ, Herrmann HC, et al., for the TARGET Investigators. Comparison of two platelet glycoprotein IIb/IIIa inhibitors, tirofiban and abciximab, for the prevention of ischemic events with percutaneous coronary revascularization. *N Engl J Med* 2001;344:1888–1894.)

Endpoint	p	Hazard ratio	Tirofiban (%)	Abciximab (%)
Composite	0.038		7.6	6.0
Death	0.66		0.5	0.4
Nonfatal MI	0.04		6.9	5.4
Death or nonfatal MI	0.04		7.2	5.7
Urgent target vessel revacularization	0.49		0.8	0.7

0.0 0.5 1.0 1.5 2.0 2.5 3.0
Tirofiban   Abciximab
better   better

30 minutes after drug infusion than with abciximab or eptifibatide. A trial of 202 patients undergoing high-risk PCI employing a larger tirofiban bolus dose (25 mg/kg) identified a 50% reduction in ischemic/thrombotic events compared to placebo (Valgimigli et al., 2004).

A large-scale, randomized trial will be required to define the comparative benefit (and safety) of high-dose tirofiban in the setting of PCI.

Do Platelet GPIIb/IIIa Receptor Antagonists Reduce Mortality Rates?

When considering the potential benefits of treatment, a clinician must carefully consider the inherent risk for adverse outcomes. A meta-analysis of 19 randomized placebo-controlled trials including over 20,000 patients with acute coronary syndromes (ST-elevation and non–ST-elevation ACS) reported a 31% risk reduction (for mortality) at 30 days and 21% at 6 months in those receiving a platelet GPIIb/IIIa receptor antagonist (vs. those not treated) in the setting of PCI (Karvouni et al., 2003). Major bleeding was increased only in trials where anticoagulant therapy (unfractionated heparin) was continued after the procedure (relative risk 1.70).

Thrombocytopenia

The administration of a GPIIb/IIIa receptor antagonist, particularly abciximab, is associated with thrombocytopenia (platelet count <100,000/mm^3) in approximately 2% to 3% of patients (Giugliano, 1998). A more marked reduction (<50,000/mm^3) is seen in less than 1% of patients, but can be profound (<10,000/mm^3) and observed within several hours of treatment (Berkowitz et al., 1997).

The binding of GPIIb/IIIa antagonists to their platelet surface receptor has been shown to alter the structure, exposing potential antigens (neoepitopes) also known as ligand-induced binding sites (LBS). The binding of preexisting antibodies (typically IgG) to those expressed sites (or to the nonmodified receptor) may be responsible for thrombocytopenia and, in some cases, a prothrombotic effect mediated by platelet activation (Abrams and Cines, 2002).

Oral GPIIb/IIIa Receptor Antagonists

To date, more than 30,000 patients have been enrolled in four large-scale, double-blind, placebo-controlled clinical trials. Individually, each trial failed to identify a reduction in ischemic outcomes. Collectively, a significant excess in mortality with three different oral GPIIb/IIIa antagonists was observed (Figure 9.5) (Chew et al., 2001).

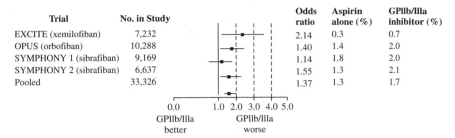

Trial	No. in Study		Odds ratio	Aspirin alone (%)	GPIIb/IIIa inhibitor (%)
EXCITE (xemilofiban)	7,232		2.14	0.3	0.7
OPUS (orbofiban)	10,288		1.40	1.4	2.0
SYMPHONY 1 (sibrafiban)	9,169		1.14	1.8	2.0
SYMPHONY 2 (sibrafiban)	6,637		1.55	1.3	2.1
Pooled	33,326		1.37	1.3	1.7

Figure 9.5 The pooled results of four large-scale, randomized trials including over 30,000 patients revealed a higher mortality with oral glycoprotein (GP) IIb/IIIa receptor antagonists (compared to aspirin alone). Odds ratio and 95% confidence intervals for death beyond 30 days in trials of oral GPIIb/IIIa receptor antgonists. EXCITE, evaluation of oral Xemilofiban in controlling thrombotic events; OPUS, Orbonfiban in patients with unstable coronary syndromes; SYMPHONY, Sibrafiban versus Aspirin to yield maximum protection from ischemic heart events post acute coronary syndromes. (From Chew DP, Bhat DL, Sapp S, Topol EJ. Increased mortality with oral platelet glycoprotein IIb/IIIa antagonist. *Circulation* 2001;103:201–206.)

Summary

The platelet GPIIb/IIIa receptor represents an important target for pharmacologic intervention. A large experience with GPIIb/IIIa receptor antagonists underscores their benefit, particularly in high-risk patients undergoing PCI, as well as unique characteristics among the individual agents. The benefit of "upstream" use in ACS requires further investigation.

References

Abrams CS, Cines DB. Platelet glycoprotein IIb/IIIa inhibitors and thrombocytopenia: possible link between platelet activation, autoimmunity and thrombosis. *Thromb Haemost* 2002;88:888–889.

Batchelor WB, Tolleson TR, Huang Y, et al. Randomized comparison of platelet inhibition with abciximab, tirofiban and eptifibatide during percutaneous coronary intervention in acute coronary syndromes: the COMPARE trial. *Circulation* 2002; 106:1470–1476.

Becker RC, Spencer FA, Liu T. Fibrinogen exerts varying effects on GPIIb/IIIa receptor-directed platelet inhibition in vitro. *Am Heart J* 2001;412:204–210.

Berkowitz SD, Harrington RA, Rund MM, Tcheng JE. Acute profound thrombocytopenia after c7E3 Fab (abciximab) therapy. *Circulation* 1997;95:809–813.

Cannon CP, Weintraub WS, Demopoulos LA, et al., for the TACTICS-TIMI 18 Investigators. Comparison of early invasive and conservative strategies for patients with unstable coronary syndromes treated with the glycoprotein IIb/IIIa inhibitor tirofiban. *N Engl J Med* 2001;344:1879–1887.

CAPTURE Investigators. Randomized placebo-controlled trial of abciximab before and during coronary intervention in refractory unstable angina: the CAPTURE study. *Lancet* 1997;349:1429–1435.

Chew DP, Bhat DL, Sapp S, Topol EJ. Increased mortality with oral platelet glycoprotein IIb/IIIa antagonist. *Circulation* 2001;103:201–206.

EPIC investigators. Use of a monoclonal antibody directed against the platelet glycoprotein IIb/IIIa receptor in high-risk coronary angioplasty. *N Engl J Med* 1994;330: 956–961.

EPILOG Investigators. Platelet glycoprotein IIb/IIIa receptor blockade and low-dose heparin during percutaneous coronary revascularization. *N Engl J Med* 1997;336: 1689–1696.

ESPRIT Investigators. Novel dosing regimen of eptifibatide in planned coronary stent implantation (ESPRIT): a randomized, placebo-controlled trial. *Lancet* 2000;356: 2037–2044.

Giugliano RP. Drug-induced thrombocytopenia—is it a serious concern for glycoprotein IIb/IIIa receptor inhibitors? *J Thromb Thrombolysis* 1998;5:191–202.

GUSTO IV Investigators. Effect of glycoprotein IIb/IIIa receptor blocker abciximab on outcome in patients with acute coronary syndromes without early coronary revascularization: the GUSTO IV-ACS randomized trial. *Lancet* 2001:357:1915–1924.

Harrington RA, Kleiman NS, Kottke-Marchant K, et al. Immediate and reversible platelet inhibition after intravenous administration of a peptide glycoprotein IIb/IIIa inhibitor during percutaneous coronary intervention. *Am J Cardiol* 1995;76:1222–1227.

IMPACT-II Investigators. Randomised placebo-controlled trial of effect of eptifibatide on complications of percutaneous coronary intervention: IMPACT-II. *Lancet* 1997;349: 1422–1428.

Karvouni E, Katritsis DG, Ioannidis JPA. Intravenous glycoprotein IIb/IIIa receptor antagonists reduce mortality after percutaneous coronary interventions. *J Am Coll Cardiol* 2003;41:26–32.

Kereiakas DJ, Kleiman NS, Ambrose J, et al. Randomized double-blind, placebo-controlled dose-ranging study of tirofiban (MK-383) platelet IIb/IIIa blockade in high risk patients undergoing coronary angioplasty. *J Am Coll Cardiol* 1996;27:356–542.

Kong DF, Califf RM, Miller DP, et al. Clinical outcomes of therapeutic agents that block the platelet glycoprotein IIb/IIIa integrin in ischemic heart disease. *Circulation* 1998;98:2829–2835.

Montalescot G, Barrgan P, Wittenberg O, et al. for the ADMIRAL Investigators. Platelet glycoprotein IIb/IIIa inhibition with coronary stenting for acute myocardial infarction. *N Engl J Med* 2001;344:1895–1903.

Ohman EM, Kleiman NS, Gacioch G, et al. for the IMPACT-AMI Investigators. Combined accelerated tissue-plasminogen activator and platelet glycoprotein IIb/IIIa integrin receptor blockade with integrilin in acute myocardial infarction. Results of a randomized, placebo-controlled, dose-ranging trial. *Circulation* 1997;95:846–854.

Philips DR, Scarborough RM. Clinical pharmacology of eptifibatide. *Am J Cardiol* 1997;| 80:11B–20B.

PRISM PLUS Study Investigators. Inhibition of platelet glycoprotein IIb/IIIa receptor with tirofiban in unstable angina and non-Q wave myocardial infarction. *N Engl J Med* 1998;338:1488–1497.

PRISM Study Investigators. A comparison of aspirin plus tirofiban with aspirin plus heparin for unstable angina. *N Engl J Med* 1998;338:1498–1505.

PURSUIT Trial Investigators. Inhibition of platelet glycoprotein IIb/IIIa with eptifibatide in patients with acute coronary syndromes. *N Engl J Med* 1998;339:436–443.

RESTORE Investigators. Effects of platelet glycoprotein IIb/IIIa blockade with tirofiban on adverse cardiac events in patients with unstable angina or acute myocardial infarction undergoing coronary angioplasty. *Circulation* 1997;96:1445–1453.

Roffi M, Chew DP, Mukherjee D, et al. Platelet glycoprotein IIb/IIIa inhibitors reduce mortality in diabetic patients with non-ST-segment-elevation acute coronary syndromes. *Circulation* 2001;104:2767–2771.

Topol EJ, Califf RM, Weisman HF, et al. for the EPIC Investigators. Randomized trial of coronary intervention with antibody against platelet IIb/IIIa integrin for reduction of clinical restenosis: results at six months. *Lancet* 1994;343:881–886.

Topol EJ, Ferguson JJ, Weisman HF, et al. for the EPIC Investigator Group. Long-term protection from myocardial ischemic events in randomized trial of brief integrin B_3 blockade with percutaneous coronary intervention. *JAMA* 1997;278:479–484.

Topol EJ, for the GUSTO V Investigators. Reperfusion therapy for acute MI with fibrinolytic therapy or combination reduced fibrinolytic therapy and platelet glycoprotein IIb/IIIa inhibition: The GUSTO V randomised trial. *Lancet* 2001;357:1905–1914.

Topol EJ, Moliterno DJ, Herrmann HC, et al., for the TARGET Investigators. Comparison of two platelet glycoprotein IIb/IIIa inhibitors, tirofiban and abciximab, for the prevention of ischemic events with percutaneous coronary revascularization. *N Engl J Med* 2001;344:1888–1894.

Valgimigli M, Percoco G, Barbieri D, et al. The additive value of tirofiban administered with the high-dose bolus in the prevention of ischemic complications during high-risk coronary angioplasty. The ADVANCE trial. *J Am Coll Cardiol* 2004;44:14–19.

Aggrenox and Cilostazol

10

The dipyridamole component of Aggrenox and cilostazol, both phosphodiesterase inhibitors, are used predominantly in patients with peripheral vascular and cerebrovascular disease.

Aggrenox

Aggrenox is a combination platelet antagonist that includes aspirin (25 mg) and dipyridamole (200 mg extended-release preparation). It is typically taken twice daily.

Mechanisms of Action

Aspirin's mechanism of action has been discussed previously. Dipyridamole inhibits cyclic adenosine monophosphate (cAMP)-phosphodiesterase (PDE) and cyclic-3′, 5′-guanylate monophospate (GMP)-PDE (Bunag et al., 1964).

Pharmacokinetics

The pharmacokinetic profile of aspirin has been summarized previously. Peak dipyridamole levels in plasma are achieved within several hours of oral administration (400 mg dose of Aggrenox). Extensive metabolism via conjugation with glucuronic acid occurs in the liver. There are no significant pharmacokinetic interactions between aspirin and dipyridamole coadministered as Aggrenox.

Pharmacodynamics

Dipyridamole inhibits platelet aggregation by two distinct mechanisms. First, it attenuates adenosine uptake into platelets (as well as endothelial cells and erythrocytes). The resulting increase elicits a rise in cellular adenylate cyclase concentrations, resulting in elevated cAMP levels, which inhibit platelet activation to several agonists, including adenosine diphosphate (ADP), collagen, and platelet-activating factor. Dipyridamole also inhibits PDE. The subsequent increase in cAMP elevates nitric oxide concentration, facilitating platelet inhibitory potential (Eisert, 2001).

Adverse Effects

The European Stroke Prevention Study (ESPS)-2 reported that 79.9% of patients experienced at least one on-treatment adverse event. The most common side effects were gastrointestinal complaints and headache.

Dipyridamole has vasodilatory effects and should be used with caution in patients with severe coronary artery disease in whom episodes of angina pectoris may increase. Patients receiving Aggrenox should not be given adenosine for myocardial perfusion studies.

Administration in Older Patients

Plasma concentrations of dipyridamole are approximately 40% higher in patients greater than 65 years of age compared with younger individuals.

Clinical Experience

Aggrenox has not been studied in patients with acute coronary syndrome (ACS). The ESPS-2 included 6,602 patients with ischemic stroke (76% of the total population) or transient ischemic attack who were randomized to receive Aggrenox, dipyridamole alone, aspirin alone, or placebo. Aggrenox reduced the risk of stroke by 22.1% compared with aspirin and by 24.4% compared with dipyridamole. Both differences were statistically significant ($p = .008$ and $p = .002$, respectively) (Diener et al., 1996).

Aggrenox is not considered interchangeable with its individual components, particularly aspirin, which may be required in larger doses among patients with coronary artery disease (CAD). In addition, the vasodilatory effects of dipyridamole can cause coronary "steal" and angina pectoris. Accordingly, Aggrenox should be used cautiously, if at all, in the setting of advanced CAD.

Cilostazol

Cilostazol is a quinolinone derivative that inhibits cellular phosphodiesterase.

Mechanism of Action

Cilostazol inhibits PDE III, reducing cAMP degradation. The resulting increase within platelets and endothelial cells impairs platelet aggregation and leads to vasodilation (Umekawa et al., 1984).

Pharmacokinetics

Cilostazol is well absorbed after oral administration, particularly when given with a high-fat meal. Metabolism occurs via the hepatic cytochrome enzymes, and most of the metabolites are excreted in the urine (75% of overall clearance). One of the two active metabolites is responsible for more than 50% of PDE III inhibition. The elimination half-life of cilostazol (and its metabolites) is approximately 12 hours.

Pharmacodynamics

Increasing cAMP concentrations within endothelial cells causes vasodilation, whereas elevated levels in platelets impair their ability to aggregate.

Adverse Effects

The most common adverse effect associated with cilostazol administration is headache. Other relatively frequent causes of drug discontinuation include palpitations and diarrhea.

Several PDE III inhibitors have been associated with decreased survival in patients with class III/IV congestive heart failure. Accordingly, cilostazol should *not* be administered to patients with congestive heart failure (of any severity).

Use in Older Patients

The clearance of cilostazol (and its metabolites) has not been determined in patients older than age 65.

Use in Patients with Renal Insufficiency

Moderate to severe renal impairment increases cilostazol metabolite levels and alters protein binding of the parent compound. Patients with advanced renal insufficiency have not been studied.

Clinical Experience

Cilostazol is approved for the treatment of intermittent claudication. Across eight clinical trials, the improvement in walking distance (compared with placebo) was approximately 40% to 50% (Dawson et al., 1998). Although there is experience with cilostazol after coronary arterial stenting (Kozuma, 2001), its long-term administration to patients with coronary artery disease has not been studied. Short-term coadministration with aspirin reduced ADP-mediated platelet aggregation by 30% to 40% (compared with aspirin alone). There are no randomized clinical trials of cilostazol in ACS.

Cilostazol is recommended for patients with disabling claudication, particularly when revascularization cannot be offered. Although it has platelet-inhibiting properties, cilostazol should not be considered a substitute for aspirin or clopidogrel in patients with ACS who have concomitant peripheral vascular disease. Although the data are modest in terms of randomized trials, cilostazol has been used in combination with aspirin following coronary artery stenting (Han 2005). Whether long-term beneficial effects are the result of platelet inhibition, improved lipid profiles, and/or prevention of neointimal proliferation will require further evaluation.

Summary

Aggrenox and cilostazol are phosphodiesterase inhibitors that are used in patients with ischemic stroke, transient ischemic attacks, and peripheral vascular disease causing activity-limiting claudication. They should not be considered equivalent to aspirin (in terms of benefit) among patients with CAD. Aggrenox should be avoided in patients with active CAD, while cilostazol is contraindicated among those with reduced left ventricular performance.

References

Bunag RD, Douglas CR, Imai S, Berne RM. Influence of pyrimidopyrimidine derivative on determination of adenosine by blood. *Circ Res* 1964;15:83–88.

Dawson DL, Cutler BS, Meissner MH, et al. Cilostazol has beneficial effects in treatment of intermittent claudication: results from a multicenter, randomized, prospective, double-blind trial. *Circulation* 1998;98:678–686.

Diener HC, Cunha L, Forbes C, et al. European Stroke Prevention Study-2: dipyridamole and acetylsalicylic acid in the secondary prevention of stroke. *J Neurol Sci* 1996;143:1–13.

Eisert WG. Near-field amplification of antithrombotic effects of dipyridamole through vessel wall cells. *Neurology* 2001;57(5 suppl 2):S20–S23.

Han Y, Wang S, Li Y, et al. Cilostazol improves long-term outcomes after coronary stent implantation. *Am Heart J* 2005;150:568e1–568e5.

Kozuma K. Effects of cilostazol on late lumen loss and repeat revascularization after Palmaz-Schatz coronary stent implantation. *Am Heart J* 2001;141:124–130.

Umekawa H, Tanaka T, Kimura Y, et al. Purification of cyclic adenosine monophosphate phosphodiesterase from human platelets using new-inhibitor Sepharose chromatography. *Biochem Pharmacol* 1984;33:3339–3344.

Novel Platelet Antagonists

The development of pharmacologic agents that inhibit platelet performance could not have proceeded without a fundamental knowledge of normal biology and a clear understanding of the laws that govern cellular events in the circulatory system (Table 11.1 and Figure 11.1).

Platelet Antagonists

Agents That Inhibit Platelet Adhesion

The adhesion of platelets to a site of vessel wall injury is mediated by von Willebrand factor (vWF), which binds to the platelet glycoprotein (GP) Ib/IX-V complex receptor (and the GPIIb/IIIa receptor under high shear stress conditions). Monoclonal antibodies to vWF have been developed and tested in animal models, as has aurintricarboxylic acid (Strony et al., 1990), a triphenylmethyl compound that inhibits vWF binding. To date, investigation in humans has not taken place, perhaps because of concerns regarding the potential risk for hemorrhagic complications. Nevertheless, the scientific community remains interested in vWF and its platelet surface receptor as potential pharmacology-directed targets.

Although the GPIIb/IIIa receptor antagonists are best known for their ability to inhibit platelet aggregation, under high shear stress conditions vWF can also bind the GPIIb/IIIa receptor, facilitating adhesion. As a result, GPIIb/IIIa antagonists may have an impact on both platelet adhesion and aggregation.

Agents That Inhibit Platelet Activation

As previously discussed, platelet activation is followed by a series of intracellular events that culminate in the release of calcium and substances that augment platelet aggregation and support coagulation protease binding. Thus, pharmacologic agents that inhibit initial surface receptor–mediated activation may also impair platelet aggregation.

Prostaglandin E and Prostacyclin

Several natural prostanoids (prostaglandin [PG] E_1 and PGI_2) can inhibit platelet activation and aggregation by elevating cyclic adenosine monophosphate (cAMP) levels. Although the mechanism is complex, the primary mode of inhibition is

Table 11.1 A Platelet Biology-Based Approach to Inhibition

Agents That Inhibit Platelet Adhesion
  von Willebrand factor monoclonal antibodies
  Aurintricarboxylic acid
  GPIIb/IIIa receptor antagonists (high shear stress)
Agents That Inhibit Platelet Activation
  Prostacyclin
  Prostaglandin E_1
  Prostanoid analogs (iloprost, beraprost, cicaprost, ciprostene)
  Thromboxane/endoperoxide receptor antagonists
  PAF antagonists
Agents That Inhibit Platelet Aggregation
  Nitric oxide/nitric oxide donors
  Apyrase
  GPIIb/IIIa receptor antagonists
  Aspirin
  Nonsteroidal antiinflammatory agents
  Dipyridamole
  Ticlopidine
  Clopidogrel
  Omega-3 fatty acids
  Cilostazol
  Ketanserin
  Ridogrel
Agents That Inhibit Platelet Secretion
  Calcium channel antagonists

GP, glycoprotein; PAF, platelet-activating factor.

through the activation of adenylate cyclase (with a subsequent rise in cAMP concentrations), which in turn prevents calcium mobilization. The clinical application of PGE_1 and PGI_2 has been limited by their effect on vascular tone, producing substantial systemic hypotension (Emmons et al., 1967; Terres et al., 1989), and by extensive first-pass metabolism in the lungs (70% of the active compound is rapidly cleared) (Kleiman et al., 1994).

The prostanoid analogs (i.e., iloprost, beraprost, cicaprost, and ciprostene) are more stable compounds than are PGE_1 and PGI_2; however, their development has focused primarily on potential use in patients with primary pulmonary hypertension (Okano et al., 1997).

Thromboxane/Endoperoxide Receptor Antagonists

This class of compounds is designed to prevent platelet activation in response to TXA_2 and other endoperoxides. There is limited experience with the thromboxane receptor antagonists sulotroban and SQ30741 in patients with myocardial infarction (MI) treated with streptokinase (Kopia et al., 1989) and tissue plasminogen ac-

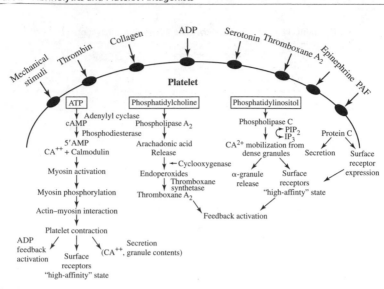

Figure 11.1 Platelet activation is triggered by a variety of biochemical and mechanical stimuli that provoke a series of internal events (signaling) following their initial binding to specific surface receptors. The phosphoinositide and phosphatidylcholine pathways provide the release of calcium and physiologic agonists that stimulate further activation and potentiate aggregation through surface receptor expression. ADP, adenosine 5' diphosphate; PAF, platelet-activating factor; ATP, adenosine 5' triphosphate; cAMP, cyclic adenosine monophosphate; PIP_2, phosphatidylinositol 4–5 biphosphate; IP_3, inositol 1,4,5-triphosphate.

tivator (tPA) (Grover et al., 1991), respectively. Ridogrel, a thromboxane synthetase antagonist that also has antagonistic effects on the thromboxane receptor, was shown to reduce recurrent ischemia compared with aspirin when used adjunctively with fibrinolytic therapy (Transchesi et al., 1992); however, further investigation on a large scale has not yet taken place.

Serotonin Receptor Antagonists

Ketanserin, a serotonin receptor antagonist, has been studied in animal models of coronary thrombosis and fibrinolysis. These models show that when administered concomitantly with a TXA_2 receptor antagonist, ketanserin improves reperfusion and decreases reocclusion following tPA administration (Golino et al., 1988).

P2Y$_{12}$ Receptor Antagonists

Adenosine triphosphate (ATP) is a competitive $P2Y_{12}$ receptor antagonist that can inhibit ADP-mediated platelet aggregation (Feolde et al., 1995); however, because

ATP functions as an agonist at other P_2 receptor sites, efforts are underway to develop selective $P2Y_{12}$ receptor antagonists (oral and intravenous) that can be used clinically in situations where platelet activation, platelet aggregation, and platelet-rich thrombosis are prevalent (e.g., acute coronary syndromes).

A novel ATP analog, FPL66096 (2-propylthio-D-B, 4-difluoromethylene ATP), produces a dose-dependent inhibition of ADP-mediated platelet aggregation with a high degree of selectivity for $P2Y_{12}$ receptors (Humphries et al., 1995). The dichloro-derivative molecule, FPL67085 is a potent ADP-mediated platelet antagonist as well, and has been shown to prevent cyclic flow variations in a Folts model. Its antithrombotic effects were similar to those of a GPIIb/IIIa antagonist but with considerably less prolongation of the bleeding time (Figure 11.2 C). When compared with ticlopidine and aspirin in an anesthetized rat model, FPL67085 was found to be a more effective inhibitor of ADP-mediated platelet aggregation.

A second novel ATP analog, AR-C69931 MX (2-methylthio-ethyl-2–3,3, 3-trifluoropropyl; adenylic acid), is a potent inhibitor of ADP-induced aggregation in human washed platelets (in vitro). It has also been shown to prevent arterial thrombosis in a canine model with minimal prolongation of the bleeding time. The latter observation has been confirmed in studies of healthy human volunteers in whom platelet aggregation in response to ADP was eventually abolished at doses that prolonged the bleeding time by approximately twofold. ADP-mediated ex vivo aggregation returned to normal within 20 minutes of terminating the infusion (Humphries, unpublished data, 1998). The metabolism of AR-C69931 MX is pre-

Figure 11.2 A–C: Comparison of the antithrombotic effect of the $P2Y_{12}$ receptor antagonist FPL67085 and two glycoprotein (GP) IIb/IIIa receptor antagonists (Ro449883 and GR144053) in a canine model of coronary thrombosis (percentage inhibition of cyclic flow reduction) (bleeding time increase ×). (From Humphries RG, Tomlinson W, Clegg JA, et al. Pharmacological profile of the novel P_{2T}-purinoceptor antagonist, FPL 37085 *in vitro* and in the anaesthetized rat *in vivo*. *Trends Pharmacol Sci* 1995;16:179–181.)

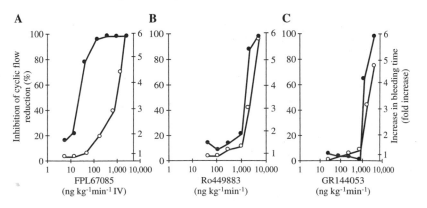

dominately via the hepatic route, with less than 10% being excreted through the kidneys. A phase 3 program with cangrelor is ongoing.

Several oral ADP ($P2Y_{12}$) receptor antagonists are under development. Prasugrel, a novel thienopyridine platelet antagonist with rapid onset of action, was evaluated in JUMBO (Joint Utilization of Medications to Block Platelets Optimally)-TIMI 26 (Wiriott 2005). A total of 904 patients undergoing elective or urgent PCI received either clopidogrel (300 mg oral oad, 75 mg daily) or prasugrel (40–60 mg load, 7.5–15.0 mg daily). Hemorrhagic events (TIMI major plus minor) were infrequent and did not differ between groups. Among prasugrel-treated patients, there were numerically lower incidences of major adverse cardiac events at 30-day follow-up.

Agents That Inhibit Platelet Aggregation

Aspirin, a platelet cyclooxygenase acetylator that impairs prostaglandin metabolism and TXA_2 synthesis, has been discussed in detail. The potent class of platelet antagonists preventing fibrinogen binding to its GPIIb/IIIa receptor (GPIIb/IIIa receptor antagonists) on the platelet surfaces has also been summarized previously.

Thromboxane Synthetase Inhibitors

Thromboxane synthetase antagonists, including dazoxiben and pirmagrel, suppress platelet thromboxane synthesis and platelet aggregation (Mullane and Foinabaio, 1988). Clinical development has been hampered by the aggregating potential of endoperoxide intermediates and by the incomplete inhibition of thromboxane synthesis by currently available compounds.

Dextran

Dextran is a polysaccharide preparation that ranges in molecular weight from 65,000 to 80,000 Da. It prolongs the bleeding time, probably by interfering with surface membrane receptor function and fibrinogen binding. Dextran also reduces plasma viscosity.

Omega-3 Fatty Acids

Omega-3 fatty acids decrease platelet membrane arachidonic acid concentration, reducing thromboxane A_2 synthesis. The competition of N-3 polyunsaturated fatty acids for cyclooxygenase also reduces platelet-aggregating capacity by facilitating the synthesis of biologically inactive prostanoids.

Nitric Oxide

Nitric oxide (NO) is a naturally occurring molecule derived from the amino acid L-arginine. It is a product of normal vascular endothelial cells that contributes to physiologic vasoreactivity and thromboresistance.

Nitric oxide prevents platelet adhesion, agonist-dependent G-protein–mediated phospholipase C activation, calcium release, P-selectin expression, and calcium-dependent conformation change in platelet surface GPIIb/IIIa. It has also been shown to potentiate platelet disaggregation by preventing the stabilization of fibrinogen–GPIIb/IIIa interactions (Gries et al., 1998). Beyond having potent platelet inhibitory effects, NO also inhibits neutrophil aggregation in vitro and prevents leukocyte adhesion to the vascular endothelium.

Although the endothelial cell is a major source of NO, it is not the only source. Platelets themselves and their precursor megakaryocytes possess NO synthase activity.

Organic nitrates and other nitrosovasodilators serve as an exogenous source of NO. Both nitroglycerine and nitroprusside have platelet inhibitory effects and promote platelet disaggregation in vitro (Mellion et al., 1981). The administration of L-arginine hydrochloride (8.4 g/day orally) to hypercholesterolemic patients reduced platelet aggregation in response to collagen. The effect lasted for 2 weeks after completion of the treatment phase (Wolf et al., 1997). L arginine has been shown to reduce human monocyte adhesion to endothelial cells and may also decrease the expression of several cellular adhesion molecules (Adams et al., 1997).

In addition to their direct effects, organic nitrates undergo denitrification with formulation of S-nitrosothiol (RSNO) intermediates. These species inhibit platelet aggregation through cyclic guanosine 3', 5'-monophosphate (cGMP) (Loscalzo, 1992). A polynitrosated RSNO, S-nitroso-BSA, administered locally following femoral artery injury in a rabbit model prevented neointimal proliferation and platelet adhesion. N-acetyl-L-cysteine enhanced the platelet inhibitory effects of nitroglycerin, and S-nitroso-N-acetyl-L-cysteine decreased platelet aggregability by reducing the expression of ligand-receptive GPIIb/IIIa. In patients with acute coronary syndromes, S-nitrosoglutathione was shown to inhibit platelet activation and GPIIb/IIIa expression (Langford et al., 1996).

NONOates

Complexes of NO with nucleophiles, NONOates, are capable of spontaneously generating NO and, as a result, may offer therapeutic benefit in the treatment of NO deficiency states. The biologic potency as well as the duration of action can be modified by altering the carrier nucleophile. For example, diethylamine (DEA)/NO possess a shorter half-life than spermine (SPER)/NO (2.1 vs. 39 minutes, respectively), resulting in an earlier peak activity (5 vs. 15 minutes) and shorter duration of action. In contrast to the acid stability of RSNOs, NONOates are alkali stable and decompose rapidly at low pH levels (Morley et al., 1993). Both possess platelet inhibitory properties.

The NONOate group can be incorporated into polymeric matrices and applied to artificial (prothrombotic) surfaces such as vascular grafts. When compared to uncoated grafts, NO-treated grafts are less thrombogenic (Smith et al., 1996).

Molsidomine and SIN-1

A novel class of nitrosovasodilators, known as sydnonimines (molsidomine and its active metabolite, SIN-1), have been evaluated in clinical trials. The European Study of Prevention of Infarct with Molsidomine (ESPRIM Investigators, 1994) trial randomized 4,017 patients with acute MI to receive either SIN-1 (1 mg/hour intravenously for 48 hours) followed by molsidomine (16 mg orally for 12 days) or placebo. There was no difference in all-cause mortality between treatment groups at either 35 days or 13 months.

An oral extended-release preparation of molsidomine was evaluated in a small randomized trial of 50 patients with ischemic heart disease and chronic stable angina to determine its effect on anginal symptoms and exercise tolerance. Exercise duration was increased and ischemic ST-segment depression was reduced up to 10 hours following drug administration. Anginal attacks and the requirement for sublingual nitroglycerine were also reduced in the treatment group (Messin et al., 1995).

Molsidomine and SIN-1, as NO donors, inhibit vascular smooth muscle cell proliferation; therefore, it has been suggested that these agents may reduce the occurrence of restenosis following percutaneous coronary intervention (PCI). The Angioplastic Coronaire Corvasal Diltiazem (ACCORD) study included 700 patients with stable coronary artery disease who were scheduled for coronary angioplasty and randomized them to receive either SIN-1 or diltiazem. The study drug was administered prior to PCI and continued for a total of 6 months afterward. Patients receiving SIN-1 demonstrated a greater luminal diameter pre- and postangioplasty as well as at 6-month angiographic follow-up. Although restenosis was reduced in the SIN-1 group, there was no difference in combined clinical events, including death and nonfatal MI (Lablanche et al., 1997).

New NO Donors

Several novel NO donors are currently under development. A compound known as FK 409 releases NO at a relatively slow rate; however, it has demonstrated potent vasorelaxation properties with a short half-life (Kita et al., 1995).

SPM-5185

The compound SPM-5185 is an effective NO donor that, when compared to nitroglycerin in an ex vivo preparation of human saphenous vein grafting and internal mammary arteries obtained at the time of bypass grafting, produced comparable relaxation in both arteries and veins and was less likely to cause vascular tolerance (Lefer et al., 1993).

Summary

A physiology-based approach to platelet antagonists provide a direct means to understand their mechanisms of action and anticipated use in clinical practice. It also fosters a rational approach to combination drug therapy, designed to inhibit several fundamental steps in platelet behavior. Novel agents have been developed; however, relatively few have progressed beyond phase II clinical trials. Future efforts will address methods to identify the most clinically relevant targets and their safe and effective inhibition.

References

Adams Mr, Jessup W, Hailstones D, et al. L-Arginine reduces human monocyte adhesion to vascular endothelium expression of cell adhesion molecules. *Circulation* 1997; 95:662–668.

Emmons PR, Hamptom JR, Harrison MJG, et al. Effect of prostaglandin E_1 on platelet behavior *in vitro* and *in vivo*. *Br Med J* 1967;2:468–472.

ESPRIM Trial. Short-term treatment of acute myocardial infarction with molsidomine. European Study of Prevention of Infarct with Molsidomine. *Lancet* 1994;344:91–97.

Feolde E, Vigne P, Breittmayer JP, et al. ATP, a partial agonist of atypical P_{2Y} purinoceptors in rat brain capillary endothelial cells. *Br J Pharmacol* 1995;115:1199–1203.

Golino P, Ashton JH, Glas-Greenwalt P, et al. Mediation of reocclusion by thromboxane A_2 and serotonin after thrombolysis with tissue-type plasminogen activator in a canine preparation of coronary thrombosis. *Circulation* 1988;77:678–684.

Gries A, Bode C, Peter K, et al. Inhaled nitric oxide inhibits human platelet aggregation, P-selectin expression, and fibrinogen binding *in vitro* and *in vivo*. *Circulation* 1998; 97:1481–1487.

Grover GJ, Parham CS, Schumacher WA. The combined antiischemic effects of the thromboxane receptor antagonist SQ 30741 and tissue-type plasminogen activator. *Am Heart J* 1991;121:426–433.

Humphries RG, Tomlinson W, Clegg JA, et al. Pharmacological profile of the novel P_{2T}-purinoceptor antagonist, FPL 37085 in vitro and in the anaesthetized rat in vivo. Br J Pharmacol 1995;115:1110–1116.

Kita Y, Ohkubo K, Hirasawa Y, et al. FR 14420, a novel, slow nitric oxide-releasing agent. Eur J Pharmacol 1995;275:125–130.

Kleiman NS, Tracy RP, Tracy RP, et al. Prostaglandin E_1 does not accelerate rTPA-induced thrombolysis in acute myocardial infarction. Am Heart J 1994;127:738–743.

Kopia GA, Kopaciewicz LJ, Ohlstein EH, et al. Combinations of the thromboxane receptor antagonist, sulotraban, with streptokinase: demonstration of thrombolytic synergy. J Pharmacol Exp Ther 1989;250:887–894.

Lablanche JM, Grollier G, Lussion JR, et al. Effect of the direct nitric oxide donors linsidomine and molsidomine on an angiographic restenosis after coronary balloon angioplasty. The ACCORD Study. Circulation 1997;95:83–89.

Langford EJ, Wainwright RJ, Martin JF. Platelet activation in acute myocardial infarction and unstable angina inhibited by nitric oxide donors. Arterioscler Thromb Vasc Biol 1996;16:51–55.

Lefer DJ, Nakanishi K, Johnston WE, et al. Antineutrophil and myocardial protection actions of a novel nitric oxide donor after acute myocardial ischemia and reperfusion of dogs. Circulation 1993;88:2337–2350.

Loscalzo J. Antiplatelet and antithrombotic effects of organic nitrates. Am J Cardiol 1992; (Suppl)70:18B–22B.

Mellion BT, Ignarro LJ, Ohlstein EH, et al. Evidence for the inhibitory role for guanosine 3', 5'-monophosphate in ADP-induced human platelet aggregation in the presence of nitric oxide and related vasodilators. Blood 1981;57:946–955.

Messin R, Boxho G, De Smedt J, et al. Acute and chronic effect of molsidomine on exercise capacity in patients with stable angina, a double-blind cross-over clinical trial versus placebo. J Cardiovasc Pharmacol 1995;25:558–563.

Morley D, Keefer LK. Nitric oxide/nucleophile complexes: a unique class of nitric oxide-based vasodilators. J Cardiovasc Pharmacol 1993;22(suppl):S3–S9.

Mullane KM, Foinabaio D. Thromboxane synthetase inhibitors reduce infarct size by a platelet dependent, aspirin-sensitive mechanism. Circ Res 1988;62:668–678.

Okano Y, Yoshioka T, Shimouchi A, et al. Orally active prostacyclin analogue in primary pulmonary hypertension. Lancet 1997;349:1365–1368.

Smith DJ, Chakravarthy D, Pulfer S, et al. Nitric oxide-releasing polymers containing the [N(O)NO]-group. J Med Chem 1996;39:1148–1156.

Strony J, Phillips M, Brands D, et al. Aurintricarboxylic acid in a canine model of coronary artery thrombosis. Circulation 1990;81:1106–1114.

Terres W, Beythien C, Kupper W, et al. Effects of aspirin and prostaglandin E_1 on in vitro thrombolysis with urokinase. Circulation 1989;79:1309–1314.

Transchesi B, Caramelli B, Bevara O, et al. Efficacy and safety of ridogrel versus aspirin in coronary thrombolysis with alteplase for myocardial infarction [Abstract]. *J Am Coll Cardiol* 1992;19:92A.

Wiriott SD, Antman EM, Wirters KJ, et al. for the JUMBO-TIMI 26 investigators. Randomized comparison of prasugrel (CS-747, LT640315), a novel thienopyridine P2T$_{12}$ antagonists, with clopidogrel in percutaneous coronary intervention. *Circulation* 2005;111:3366–3373.

Wolf A, Zalpour C, Theilmeier G, et al. Dietary L-arginine supplementation normalizes platelet aggregation in hypercholesterolemic humans. *J Am Coll Cardiol* 1997;29: 479–785.

Combination
Pharmacotherapy

12

The goal of improving coronary arterial patency, microcirculatory blood flow, and myocardial perfusion represents the essence of fibrinolytic–adjunctive therapy combinations. Because fibrinolytic resistance, patency without perfusion, and reocclusion are platelet-mediated phenomena, considerable emphasis has been placed on the development of platelet antagonists.

Platelet-Fibrin Thrombi

Coronary arterial thrombi consist of platelets and fibrin bound in a tightly packed meshwork. Platelets modify the intrinsic properties of the fibrin network, causing changes in permeability and vasoelasticity, which decrease fibrinolysis rates. The addition of aspirin and the glycoprotein (GP) IIb/IIIa receptor antagonist abciximab modulates the interaction of platelets and fibrin, improving both accessibility to fibrinolytics and the overall rates of fibrinolysis (Collet et al., 2001).

Clinical Experience

Abciximab

The Thrombolysis in Myocardial Infarction (TIMI) 14 trial (Antman et al., 1999) randomized 888 patients with ST-segment elevation myocardial infarction (MI) to receive (1) accelerated tissue plasminogen activator (tPA; ≤100 mg) plus standard dose of unfractionated heparin (UFH); (2) tPA (920 mg bolus) plus abciximab (0.25 mg/kg bolus, 7 μg/min); (3) streptokinase (800,000 to 1.5 million units) and low-dose UFH; or (4) abciximab plus low-dose UFH. TIMI 3 flow rates 90 minutes from treatment initiation were 52%, 53%, 42%, and 32%, respectively. In subsequent dose/strategy studies, a combination of tPA (35 mg) plus abciximab and tPA (15 mg bolus, 31 mg over 60 minutes) plus abciximab revealed 63% and 73% TIMI 3 flow rates, respectively. Rates of major hemorrhage were similar in all tPA treatment groups.

The Strategies for Patency Enhancement in the Emergency Department (SPEED) trial (SPEED Group, 2000) included two phases. Phase A (*n* = 241) randomized patients to receive either abciximab (bolus plus infusion) alone or combined with 5 U, 7.5 U, 10 U, 5 U + 2.5 U, or 5U + 5 U of reteplase. Phase B tested the best strategy from phase A (abciximab plus 5 U + 5 U of reteplase) against 10 U + 10 U of reteplase. In phase A, 62% of the abciximab–reteplase 5 U + 5 U patient group had TIMI 3 flow rates at 60 to 90 minutes vs. 27% of those given abciximab alone ($p = .001$).

In phase B, 54% of the abciximab–reteplase 5 U + 5 U group had TIMI 3 flow rates compared to 47% of the reteplase-alone patients ($p = .32$). Major bleeding rates were increased with combination therapy.

Despite encouraging findings in two phase II clinical trials, the Global Use of Strategies to Open Occluded Arteries (GUSTO) V trial (Topol and the GUSTO V Investigators, 2001) demonstrated similar 30-day mortality rates in patients receiving either standard-dose reteplase or half-dose reteplase combined with abciximab (5.9% and 5.6%, respectively). Reinfarction and urgent revascularization occurred less frequently with combination therapy.

The Assessment and Safety and Efficacy of a New Thrombolytic Agent (ASSENT)-3 trial (ASSENT-3 Investigators, 2001) evaluated combination therapy from a broadened perspective with a third-generation fibrinolytic agent. A total of 6,095 patients with ST-segment elevation MI were randomly assigned to one of three regimens: full-dose tenecteplase (30–50 mg) plus enoxaparin (30 mg IV, 1 mg/kg SC every 12 hours); ½ dose tenecteplase (15–25 mg) plus weight-adjusted UFH (40 U/kg bolus; 7 U/kg/h) and a 12-hour infusion of abciximab; or full-dose tenecteplase with weight-adjusted UFH. The primary endpoints were the composite of 30-day mortality, in-hospital reinfarction, or in-hospital refractory ischemia (efficacy endpoint) and the efficacy endpoint plus in-hospital intracranial hemorrhage or major bleeding (efficacy plus safety endpoints). There were significantly fewer efficacy endpoints in the enoxaparin (7.40%) and abciximab (11.1%) groups than in the UFH group (15.4%). The same was true for the efficacy plus safety endpoint: 13.7%, 14.2%, and 17%, respectively (Figure 12.1). Vital status at 1 year was available for 5,942 patients enrolled in the ASSENT-3 trial (Sinnaeve et al., 2004). Mortality at 1 year was 7.9% in the UFH group, 8.1% in the enoxaparin group, and 9.3% in the abciximab group (no statistically significant differences).

The ASSENT-3 PLUS randomized trial (Wallentin et al., 2003) included 1,639 patients with MI who received either tenecteplase plus enoxaparin (30 mg IV bolus, 1.0 mg/kg SC q12h) or tenecteplase plus UFH in the prehospital setting. Although enoxaparin tended to reduce the composite of 30-day mortality, reinfarction, and refractory ischemia compared to UFH (17.4% vs. 14.2%; $p = .08$), intracranial hemorrhage rates were significantly higher with enoxaparin treatment (2.20% vs. 0.97%; $p = .047$). The increase was observed in patients greater than 75 years of age (Figure 12.2).

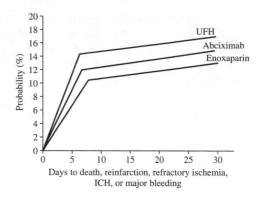

Figure 12.1 Combined safety plus efficacy endpoint (Kaplan-Meir curve) in ASSENT-3. Enoxaparin in combination with tenecteplase yielded the most favorable results. ICH, intracerebral hemorrhage; UFH, unfractionated heparin. (From ASSENT-3 Investigators. Efficacy and safety of tenecteplase in combination with enoxaparin, abciximab or unfractionated heparin. The ASSENT-3 randomized trial in acute myocardial infarction. *Lancet* 2001;358:605–613.)

The combined administration of tenecteplase, enoxaparin, and abciximab was investigated in the ENTIRE (Enoxaparin and Tenecteplase Tissue Plasminogen Activator with or without GPIIb/IIa Inhibitor as the Reperfusion Strategy in the STEMI trial)-TIMI 23 trial (Antman et al., 2002). A total of 483 patients received full-dose tenecteplase and either UFH (bolus 60 U/kg; infusion 12 U/kg/h) or enoxaparin, or half-dose tenecteplase plus abciximab and either UFH (bolus 40 U/kg; infusion 7 U/kg/h) or enoxaparin (0.3 to 0.75 mg/kg SC q12h ± 30 mg initial IV bolus). The TIMI 3 flow rates at 60 minutes were 52%, 50%, 48%, and 52%, respectively. The 30-day death/recurrent MI rates were 15.9%, 4.4%, 6.5%, and 5.5%, respectively. The rates of major hemorrhage were 2.4%, 1.9%, 5.2% and 8.5%, respectively.

Considered collectively, and in the absence of a phase III clinical trial investigating the combination of the tenecteplase, enoxaparin, and abciximab, the available data do not support the routine combination of tPA-based fibrinolytic therapy and abciximab in the treatment of ST-segment elevation MI.

Integrilin

The Integrilin to Minimize Platelet Aggregation and Coronary Thrombosis-After Myocardial Infarction (IMPACT-AMI) study (Ohman et al., 1997) determined the potential impact of combination therapy with alteplase and Integrilin among 132 patients with MI. The Integrilin doses ranged from 36 to 180 U/kg (bolus) and 0.2 to 0.75 μg/kg/min infusion. The alteplase strategy was a standard full dose. A dose-response for Integrilin and TIMI 3 flow rates were observed.

The INTEGRITI (Integrin and Tenecteplase in Acute Myocardial Infarction) angiographic trial (Giugliano et al., 2003) included 438 patients. In the dose-finding study, 189 patients were randomized to receive different doses of double-bolus In-

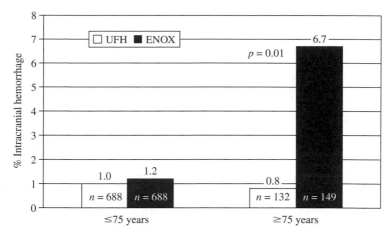

Figure 12.2 Intracranial hemorrhage in patients greater than or less than 75 years of age in the ASSENT-3 PLUS Study. ENOX, enoxaparin; UFH, unfractionated heparin. (From Wallentin L, Goldstein P, Armstrong PW, et al. Efficacy and safety of tenecteplase in combination with the low-molecular-weight heparin enoxaparin or unfractionated heparin in the prehospital setting: the assessment of the safety and efficacy of a new thrombolytic regimen (ASSENT)-3 PLUS randomized trial in acute myocardial infarction. *Circulation* 2003;108:135–142)

tegrilin and reduced-dose tenecteplase. In the dose-confirmation phase, 249 patients received eptifibatide 180 µg/kg bolus, 2 µg/kg/min infusion, and 180 µg/kg bolus 10 minutes later plus half-dose (0.53 µg/kg) tenecteplase monotherapy. All patients received UFH (60 U/kg bolus; 7 U/kg/h [combination], 12 U/kg/h [monotherapy]). The TIMI 3 flow rates at 60 minutes (dose-confirmation phase) were 59% and 49%, respectively ($p = .15$). Major hemorrhage and transfusion requirements were greater with combination therapy.

Summary

The pathobiology of arterial thrombosis and existing limitations of fibrinolytic therapy support platelet-based (and factor Xa-directed) adjunctive therapies. The available information from clinical trials does not support the routine use of GPIIb/IIIa receptor antagonists with either second- or third-generation fibrinolytics. The combination of tenecteplase and enoxaparin is particularly attractive; however, dosing modifications will be required in older patients. Aspirin will remain a mainstay of therapy, while aspirin–clopidogrel combinations will likely become an important treatment option (see Chapter 18).

References

Antman EM, Giugliano RP, Gibson CM, et al., for the TIMI 14 Investigators. Abciximab facilitates the rate and extend of thrombolysis: results of the TIMI 14 trial. *Circulation* 1999;99:2720–2732.

Antman EM, Louwerenburg HW, Baars HF, et al. Enoxaparin as adjunctive antithrombin therapy for ST-elevation myocardial infarction: results of the ENTIRE-Thrombolysis in Myocardial Infarction (TIMI) 23 trial. *Circulation* 2002;105:1642–1649.

ASSENT-3 Investigators. Efficacy and safety of tenecteplase in combination with enoxaparin, abciximab or unfractionated heparin. The ASSENT-3 randomized trial in acute myocardial infarction. *Lancet* 2001;358:605–613.

Collet JP, Montalescot G, Lesty C, et al. Disaggregation *in vitro* preformed platelet-rich clots by abciximab increased fibrin exposure and promotes fibrinolysis. *Arterioscler Thromb Vasc Biol* 2001;21:142–148.

Giugliano RP, Roe MT, Harrington RA, et al. Combination reperfusion therapy with eptifibatide and reduced-dose tenecteplase for ST-elevation myocardial infarction: results of the Integrilin and tenecteplase in acute myocardial infarction (INTEGRITI) phase II angiographic trial. *J Am Coll Cardiol* 2003;41:1251–1260.

Ohman EM, Kleiman NS, Gacioch G for the IMPACT-MI Investigators. Combined accelerated tPA and platelet GPIIb/IIIa integrin receptor blockade with Integrilin in acute myocardial infarction: results of a randomized placebo-controlled dose-ranging trial. *Circulation* 1997;95:846–854.

Sinnaeve PR, Alexander JA, Bogaerts K, et al. Efficacy of tenecteplase in combination with enoxaparin, abciximab, or unfractionated heparin: one-year follow-up results of the Assessment of the Safety of a New Thrombolytic-3 (ASSENT-3) randomized trial in acute myocardial infarction. *Am Heart J* 2004;147:993–998.

SPEED Group. Trial of abciximab with and without low-dose reteplase for acute myocardial infarction. *Circulation* 2000;101:2788–2794.

Topol EJ, for the GUSTO V Investigators. Nonperfusion therapy for acute myocardial infarction with fibrinolytic therapy or combination reduced fibrinolytic therapy and platelet GPIIb/IIIa inhibitor: the GUSTO V randomized trial. *Lancet* 2001;357:1905–1914.

Wallentin L, Goldstein P, Armstrong PW, et al. Efficacy and safety of tenecteplase in combination with the low-molecular-weight heparin enoxaparin or unfractionated heparin in the prehospital setting: the assessment of the safety and efficacy of a new thrombolytic regimen (ASSENT)-3 PLUS randomized trial in acute myocardial infarction. *Circulation* 2003;108:135–142.

Facilitated Percutaneous
Coronary Intervention

The failure of fibrinolytic therapy to restore physiologic myocardial perfusion in upward of 40% of patients supports the development of strategies to improve response rates to percutaneous coronary intervention (PCI) in those requiring early procedures. The construct of facilitated PCI (pharmacoinvasive therapy) provides a platform for utilizing the strengths of existing therapies and treatment modalities.

The Heparin in Early Patency (HEAP) trial (Zijlstra et al., 2002) included 1,702 patients treated with primary PCI for myocardial infarction (MI); 860 patients received aspirin (500 mg IV) and UFH ($\geq$5,000 U IV) before being transported to the hospital and 842 patients received the same antithrombotic therapy in the hospital. TIMI 2 or 3 flow rates were higher in the pretreated group (31% vs. 20%; p = .001), and patients with TIMI 2 or 3 flow initially had a higher PCI success rate (94% vs. 89%; p <.001) and a lower 30-day mortality (1.6% vs. 3.4%; p = .04).

The Plasminogen Activator Angioplasty Compatibility Trial (PACT) randomized 606 patients to receive a 50-mg bolus of alteplase or placebo, followed by immediate angiography and angioplasty if needed (Ross et al., 1999). TIMI flow rates on arrival to the catheterization laboratory were 33% and 15%, respectively. Facilitated PCI and primary PCI restored TIMI 3 flow in occluded vessels equally (77% and 79%, respectively). There were no differences in major bleeding. Left ventricular ejection fraction was highest in those with TIMI 3 flow on arrival to the catheterization laboratory or following PCI within 1 hour of alteplase administration.

Full-dose fibrinolytic therapy with alteplase or reteplase followed by coronary angiography and PCI (if no clinical evidence of reperfusion) was evaluated retrospectively in the Global Use of Strategies to Open Occluded Arteries (GUSTO) III trial (Miller et al., 1999). Among those undergoing PCI (n = 392), 87 patients received in-laboratory abciximab. A trend toward reduced mortality was observed in abciximab-treated patients, but at a higher cost of hemorrhagic complications.

In the Strategies for Patency Enhancement in the Emergency Department (SPEED) trial (Herrmann et al., 2000), 323 patients who underwent PCI had an 88% procedural success rate and a 30-day composite of death, reinfarction, or revascularization of 5.6%. Early PCI was required less often in patients receiving combination therapy with reteplase and abciximab. They were also more likely to have TIMI flow at the time of initial coronary angiography. Post-PCI TIMI 3 flow rates were approximately 90%.

The benefit derived from PCI following fibrinolytic therapy as a standard strategy for ST-segment elevation MI, although anticipated (and frequently entertained in clinical practice), has not been confirmed in randomized trials. Two trials, Facilitated INtervention and Enhanced Reperfusion Speed to Stop Events (FINESSE) and Assessment and Safety and Efficacy of a New Thrombolytic Agent (ASSENT)-4 PCI, will provide key data to clarify the risks and benefits of pharmacoinvasive therapy. In FINESSE, pre-PCI treatment with half-dose reteplase plus abciximab or abciximab alone were compared with primary angioplasty plus procedural abciximab. In ASSENT-4 PCI, patients were given full-dose tenecteplase (TNK-tPA) before PCI and compared with patients undergoing primary angioplasty (glycoprotein [GP] IIb/IIIa receptor antagonist use will be up to the primary operator). The trial was terminated early because of high event rates in the combined treatment modality (pharmacoinvasive) group.

Summary

Pharmacologic strategies designed to improve clinical outcomes following PCI for ST-segment elevation MI have not shown a consistent benefit and there may be added risk with regard to hemorrhagic complications (particularly with GPIIb/IIIa receptor antagonists). Ongoing clinical trials with clopidogrel and the low-molecular-weight heparin enoxaparin may shed additional light on the important area.

References

Herrmann HC, Moliterno DJ, Ohman EM, et al. Facilitation of early percutaneous coronary intervention after reteplase with or without abciximab in acute myocardial infarction. *J Am Coll Cardiol* 2000;36:1489–1496.

Miller JM, Smalling R, Ohman EM, et al. Effectiveness of early coronary angioplasty and abciximab for failed thrombolysis (reteplase or alteplase) during acute myocardial infarction (results from the GUSTO-III trial). Global Use of Strategies To Open occluded coronary arteries. *Am J Cardiol* 1999;84:779–784.

Ross AM, Coyne KS, Reiner JS, et al. A randomized trial comparing primary angioplasty with a strategy of short-acting thrombolysis and immediate planned rescue angioplasty in acute myocardial infarction: the PACT trial. *J Am Coll Cardiol* 1999;34: 1954–1962.

Zijlstra F, Ernst N, de Boer MJ, et al. Prehospital aspirin and heparin in acute MI. *J Am Coll Cardiol* 2002;39:1733–1737.

Part III
Anticoagulants

Thrombin-Directed Therapy

14

Anticoagulant therapy in general is designed to prevent either the generation or activity of thrombin; however, a cell-based model of coagulation provides a physiologic view of individual phases of the process, allowing more specific targets for attenuating the initiation, priming, or propagation of thrombus formation. Future categorization schemes will consider individual coagulation factors, individual sites on a given coagulation factor, and specific phases of coagulation to better identify an agent's biochemical and physiologic activity.

Unfractionated Heparin

Unfractionated heparin (UFH) is a heterogeneous, negatively charged mucopolysaccharide consisting of approximately 18 to 50 saccharide units (molecular weight 5000–30,000 Da) (Figure 14.1). Antithrombin (AT), required for the interaction (and subsequent neutralization) of UFH with thrombin and coagulation proteases including factors Xa, IXa, XIa, and XIIa, is bound by one third of administered drug (only molecules containing the critical pentasaccharide sequence can bind AT).

Following IV administration, UFH binds to a variety of plasma proteins, endothelial cells, and macrophages, explaining, in part, the wide variability in anticoagulant effects for a given dose. It is cleared from the circulation through both a rapid saturable mechanism and a slower first-order mechanism. As a result, there is a dose-dependent half-life ranging from 60 minutes after a dose of 100 U/kg to 180 minutes for a dose of 400 U/kg (Beguin et al., 1988; Lam et al., 1976).

Heparin-induced thrombocytopenia and hemorrhage are the most feared complications of UFH administration (see Chapter 29). Other adverse effects include osteopenia (with long-term administration).

Low-Molecular-Weight Heparin

Low-molecular-weight heparin (LMWH) is prepared by the depolymerization of porcine UFH. A variety of processes are used, giving distinctive products whose molecular weights range from 4,000 to 6,500 Da (Hirsh and Levine, 1992) (Table 14.1). Like UFH, approximately one third of LMWH polysaccharide chains contain the pentasaccharide binding site for antithrombin. The LMWH–antithrombin

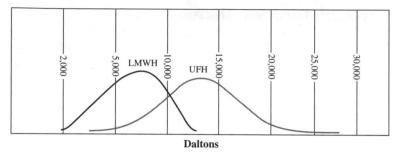

Figure 14.1 Comparative molecular weight distributions for unfractionated heparin (UFH) and low-molecular-weight heparin (LMWH).

complex (consisting of a predominance of shorter chain polysaccharides) has relatively weak antithrombin activity but retains the ability to inactivate factor Xa (Figure 14.2). The ratio of anti-Xa activity to anti-IIa (antithrombin) activity varies from 2:1 to 4:1. Similar to UFH, LMWH is not able to inhibit thrombin bound to fibrin (Weitz, 1997).

When LMWH is given in either fixed or weight-adjusted doses by the subcutaneous route, greater than 90% of the dose is absorbed. In contrast to UFH, LMWH has minimal binding to cells or plasma proteins, resulting in persistence of free drug in the circulation and a longer half-life of activity. While the half-life of UFH averages about 90 minutes, the half-life of LMWH averages about 180 minutes (the half-lives of three LMWHs range from 90 to 260 minutes).

Thrombocytopenia is infrequently associated with LMWH administration, but antibodies directed against complexes of LMWH and platelet factor have been detected in some patients. On rare occasions, the full-blown syndrome of heparin-induced thrombocytopenia (HIT) occurs. Equally rare is necrosis at the site of skin injections with LMWH, which may represent an early feature of HIT.

Warfarin

Coumarins inhibit the enzymatic reduction of vitamin K epoxide. Vitamin K (in the reduced state) is the coenzyme responsible for the carboxylation of glutamic acid and resides on factors II, VII, IX, and X and proteins C, S, and Z. Carboxylation is essential for calcium binding. The noncarboxylated forms of these coagulation proteases can be detected in the circulation of treated patients, but do not exert coagulant activity.

Several coumarins have been developed for clinical use: Acenocoumarol is available in Europe but is not used in the United States, where warfarin is the most

Table 14.1 Low-Molecular-Weight Heparins

International Nonproprietary Name	Molecular Weight (daltons)	Method of Preparation	Chemical Modification	Anti-Xa:Anti-IIa
Enoxaparin	4,371	Benzoylation followed by alkaline hydrolysis	Introduction of double bond at the end group	2.7:1
Dalteparin	5,819	Controlled nitrous acid depolymerization	Formation of anhydromannose (5-member ring)	2.1:1
Fraxiparine	4,855	Fractionated, optimized nitrous acid depolymerization	Formation of anhydromannose (5-member ring)	3.2:1
Tinzaparin		Heparinase digestion	Introduction of double bond at the end groups	3.5:1
Reviparin		Nitrous acid digestion	Formation of anhydromannose (5-member ring)	3.6:1

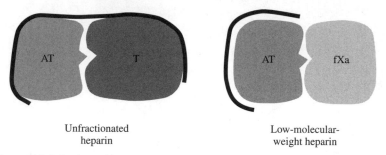

Unfractionated
heparin

Low-molecular-
weight heparin

Figure 14.2 Unfractionated heparin, containing chains mostly in excess of 18 saccharide units, interacts with antithrombin (AT) and thrombin (T), forming a ternary complex. In contrast, low-molecular-weight heparin preparations consist of a greater proportion of short chains (<18 saccharide units), allowing binding of factor Xa (fXa) (to a relatively greater degree than thrombin).

commonly used vitamin K antagonist. Warfarin is rapidly absorbed from the gastro-intestinal tract and has a half-life ranging from 36 to 72 hours. After an oral dose, the synthesis of carboxylated factors ceases, but the overall effects on coagulation will depend on the disappearance of carboxylated factors formed prior to warfarin exposure. The disappearance of these factors, in turn, is a function of their half-lives (factor VII and protein C: 6 to 7 hours; factors IX and X: 24 hours; prothrombin: 90 hours). Thus, following a dose of warfarin, factor VII and protein C will be 20% of normal at 48 hours, but prothrombin will not be reduced to this extent for 5 to 7 days. Since effective anticoagulation requires a decrease in clotting factors to 20% of normal, warfarin is considered a slow-acting anticoagulant (Hirsh, 1991).

Warfarin binds to plasma proteins (predominantly albumin) and is metabolized by the cytochrome P450 (CYP) system of the liver. Persons with genetic polymorphisms of the CYP 2C9 enzyme (CYP 2C9*2 and CYP 2C9*3) may have impaired metabolism of warfarin (specifically the S enantiomer) and may require lower doses for anticoagulation than those with the wild-type enzyme (Taube et al., 2000). Drugs that alter protein binding or affect the liver may potentiate or inhibit the activity of warfarin (Table 14.2) (Wells et al., 1994). Herbal remedies such as ginkgo and ginseng, as well as numerous others, may alter warfarin metabolism. Other factors that affect warfarin response are dietary content of vitamin K, the ability to absorb vitamin K (altered by diarrheal disease), and advanced malignancy. High-fat, low-carbohydrate meals impair warfarin's anticoagulant effect.

An important adverse reaction to warfarin therapy is tissue necrosis due to rapidly decreased levels of protein C or S. This complication occurs most often in the setting of acute thrombosis and is characterized by microvascular thrombosis involving the postcapillary venules in patients with inherited or acquired (transient

Table 14.2 Drug Interactions with Warfarin

Interaction	Antibiotics	Cardiac	Anti-inflammatory	CNS	GI
Potentiate	Cotrimoxazole Erythromycin Fluconazole Isoniazid Metronidazole	Amiodarone Clofibrate Propafenone Propranolol Sulfinpyrazone	Phenylbutazone Piroxicam	Alcohol (with liver disease)	Cimetidine Omeprazole
Inhibit	Griseofulvin Nafcillin Rifampin	Cholestyramine		Barbiturates Carbamazepine Chlordiazepoxide	Sucralfate
No effect	Enoxacin	Atenolol Bumetanide Felodipine Metoprolol	Diflunisal Ketoralac Naproxen	Alcohol Fluoxetine Nitrazepam	Antacids Famotidine

CNS, central nervous system; GI, gastrointestinal

Wells PS, Holbrook AM, Crowther NR, Hirsh J. Interactions of warfarin with drugs and food. Ann Intern Med 1994;121;676–683.

as an acute phase response and/or following large doses of warfarin) protein C or S deficiency. The sudden decline in proteins C and S leads to thrombus formation in venules with extensive skin and subcutaneous fat necrosis. Even more profound thrombosis, producing limb gangrene, occurs with warfarin given to patients with HIT. The mechanism appears to be similar—an underlying deficiency in protein C that is exacerbated by the administration of warfarin (Warkentin et al., 1997).

Other adverse effects attributed to warfarin are fetal embryopathy, especially with exposure to the drug between the sixth and twelfth week of gestation, and "purple toes" related to embolization of cholesterol-rich material from atheromatous aortic plaques.

A prolonged prothrombin time due to warfarin declines within 24 to 48 hours of drug discontinuation if the patient is eating. Vitamin K represents a widely available antidote.

Anticoagulants Currently Under Development

A wide variety of intravenous and oral compounds are currently under development; these include inhibitors of factors IIa, VIIa, IXa, Xa, and XIIIa. Several have embarked upon phase II and III clinical trials.

References

Beguin S, Lindhout t, Hemker HC. The mode of action of heparin in plasma. Thromb Haemost 1988;60:457–462.

Hirsh J. Oral anticoagulant drugs. N Engl J Med 1991;324:1865–1875.

Hirsh J, Levine MN. Low molecular weight heparin. Blood 1992;79:1–17.

Lam LH, Silbert JE, Rosenberg RD. The separation of active and active forms of heparins. Biochem Biophys Res Commun 1976;69:570–577.

Taube J, Halsall D, Baglin T. Influence of cytochrome P-450 CYP2C9 polymorphisms on warfarin sensitivity and risk of over-anticoagulation in patients on long-term treatment. Blood 2000;96:1816–1819.

Warkentin TE, Elavathil LJ, Hayward CP, Johnston MA, Russett JI, Kelton JG. The pathogenesis of venous limb gangrene associated with heparin-induced thrombocytopenia. Ann Intern Med 1997;127:804–812.

Weitz JI. Low-molecular-weight heparins. N Engl J Med 1997;337:688–968.

Wells PS, Holbrook AM, Crowther NR, Hirsh J. Interactions of warfarin with drugs and food. Ann Intern Med 1994;121:676–683.

Factor Xa Inhibitors

15

The importance of factor Xa in the initiation and propagation of coagulation, as well as its pluripotential cellular properties, has been discussed previously. Considered collectively, the effects exhibited by this particular protease make it an attractive target for pharmacologic inhibition.

Classification

Factor Xa inhibition can be classified and subcategorized as follows: indirect (antithrombin [AT]-dependent), nonselective (e.g., unfractionated heparin); indirect, semi-selective (e.g., low-molecular-weight heparin); indirect, selective (e.g., fondaparinux); and direct, selective (e.g., DX-9065a [in early stage of development]) (Table 15.1) Oral factor Xa inhibitors are in phase II testing.

Fondaparinux

Fondaparinux (Arixtra) is a synthetic pentasaccharide that requires AT for selective fXa binding (Petitou et al., 1991). Unlike heparin compounds, fondaparinux does not inhibit thrombin directly nor does it interact with platelets (or platelet-derived proteins). After subcutaneous administration in healthy volunteers, fondaparinux was nearly 100% bioavailable, and absorption was rapid (C_{max} within 2 hours) (Donat et al., 2002). Clearance is through renal mechanisms with a terminal half-life of 17 ± 3 hours (slightly longer in elderly volunteers). Overall, drug clearance is 25% lower in patients with mild renal impairment (creatinine clearance [CrCl] 50–80 mL/min), approximately 40% lower in patients with moderate renal impairment (CrCl 30–50 mL/min), and 55% lower in patients with severe renal impairment (CrCl <30 mL/min).

Table 15.1 Proposed Classification for Factor Xa Inhibitors

Category	Compound
Indirect, nonselective	Unfractionated heparin
Indirect, semiselective	Low-molecular-weight heparin
Indirect, selective	Synthetic pentasaccharide (fondaparinux)
Direct, selective	DX-9065a, apixaban

Fondaparinux in Acute Coronary Syndromes

OASIS-5, the largest trial performed to date in non-ST segment elevation acute coronary syndromes (ACS), randomized 20,078 patients to fondaparinux (2.5 mg subcuaneous once daily) or enoxaparin (1 mg/kg twice daily) for 2 to 8 days. The primary outcome (composite of death, MI, and refractory ischemia on day 9) was 5.9% and 5.8%, respectively. Major bleeding rates were 2.1% and 4.0%, respectively (hazard ratio 0.53; $p < .001$). By 6-month follow-up, the endpoints of death, death/MI, stroke, and composite of death/MI/stroke were significantly reduced in those receiving fondaparinux. Catheter thrombosis (during PCI) was 3-fold higher in fondaparinux-treated patients compared to those receiving enoxaparin (1.3% vs. 0.5%, respectively) (European Society of Cardiology presentation, September 2005). The clinical use of fondaparinux for venous thromboembolism prophylaxis will be discussed in Chapter 22.

References

Donat F, Duret JP, Santoni A, et al. The pharmacokinetics of fondaparinux sodium in healthy volunteers. *Clin Pharmacokinet* 2002;41(Suppl 2):1–9.

Petitou M, Lormeau JC, Choay J. Chemical synthesis of glycosaminoglycans: a new approach to antithrombotic drugs. *Nature* 1991;350(Suppl):30–33.

Direct Thrombin Inhibitors

16

The pivotal role of thrombin in all phases of coagulation, cellular proliferation, and cellular interactions involved centrally in inflammatory processes provides an attractive target for pharmacologic inhibition. The development of direct thrombin inhibitors has evolved rapidly to include both intravenous and oral preparations.

Intravenous Direct Thrombin Inhibitors

Hirudin

Hirudin is extracted from the parapharyngeal gland of the medicinal leech *Hirudo medicinalis*. Several derivatives and recombinant preparations have been developed, including the most widely used agent lepirudin (Refludan).

Hirudin binds to both the catalytic and fibrinogen-binding sites of thrombin and thus is considered a bivalent inhibitor.

The plasma half-life of hirudin is 50 to 65 minutes, with a biologic half-life of 2 hours (Verstraete et al., 1993). The properties of heparin, hirudin, and bivalirudin are highlighted in Table 16.1. The predominant renal clearance of hirudin must be emphasized for safe clinical use (Table 16.2).

Hirudin forms a tight complex with thrombin, inhibiting the conversion of fibrinogen to fibrin as well as thrombin-induced platelet aggregation (Verstraete, 1997). These actions are independent of the presence of antithrombin, and also affect thrombin bound to fibrin. On the downside, the ability of thrombin to complex with thrombomodulin, activating protein C, is also inhibited. Hirudin does not bind to platelet factor , nor does it elicit antibodies that induce platelet and endothelial cell activation; thus, it can be safely administered to patients with heparin-induced thrombocytopenia (HIT). Hirudin does have weak immunogenicity, so diminished (or rarely increased) responsiveness after repeated dosing is possible (Table 16.3). The use of hirudin in the management of heparin-induced thrombocytopenia is discussed in Chapter 29.

Table 16.1 Properties of Heparin, Bivalirudin, and Hirudin

Property	Heparins	Bivalirudin and Hirudin
Thrombin inhibition	Require AT	Directly inhibit
Clot-bound thrombin	Not inhibited	Inhibited
Thrombocytopenia	Yes	No
Immunogenicity	Yes	Rare
Effect on aPTT	Yes (modest with LMWH)	Yes
Effect on PT	Minimal	Moderate+
Metabolism	Liver, kidney	Kidney
Antidote	Protamine*	None

*60% reversal of LMWH.
+Greater effect with bivalirudin.
APTT, activated partial thromboplastin time; AT, antithrombin; LMWH, low-molecular-weight heparin; PT, prothrombin time.

Table 16.2 Hirudin Dosing in Patients with Impaired Renal Function

Creatinine Clearance (mL/min)	Serum Creatinine (mg/dL)	Adjusted Infusion Rate	
		% of Standard Initial Infusion	mg/kg/h
45–60	1.6–2.0	50%	0.075
30–44	2.1–3.0	30%	0.045
15–29	3.1–6.0	15%	0.0245
Below 15*	Above 6.0*	—	

*Among patients with acute renal failure or hemodialysis-dependent renal failure, hirudin should be avoided or discontinued.

Table 16.3 Comparative Pharmacologic Characteristics of Hirudin, Bivalirudin, and Argatroban

	Hirudin	Bivalirudin	Argatroban
Molecular weight (d)	7,000	1,980	527
Mechanism of thrombin inhibition	Bivalent	Bivalent	Univalent
Clearance	Renal	Renal	Hepatic
Plasma half-life (min)	60	25	45
FDA-approved indication	HIT	PCI in ACS HIT in PCI	HIT HIT (or at risk for HIT in PCI)

Bivalent: Catalytic site and anion-binding exosite
Univalent: Catalytic site
ACS, acute coronary syndromes; FDA, Food and Drug Administration; HIT, heparin-induced thrombocytopenia; PCI, percutaneous coronary intervention.

References

Verstraete M, Nurmohamed M, Klenast J, et al. Biologic effects of recombinant hirudin (CGP 39.9.) in human volunteers. European Hirudin in Thrombosis Group. *J Am Coll Cardiol* 1993;22:1080–1088.

Verstraete M. Direct thrombin inhibitors. Approval of the antithrombotic/hemorrhagic balance. *Thromb Haemost* 1997;78:357–363.

Novel Anticoagulants

17

While all anticoagulants have, to a certain extent, novel properties, the development of agents that inhibit specific coagulation proteases through structural affinity and can be inhibited themselves by the concomitant production of antidotes (drug–antidote pair construct) has the potential to revolutionize the field.

Protein-Binding Oligonucleotides

With the evolution of our thinking toward hemostasis and thrombosis has come new pharmacologic constructs for safe and effective treatment. Aptamers are single-stranded nucleic acids that inhibit a protein's function by folding into a specific three-dimensional structure that defines high-affinity binding to the target protein (White et al., 2000). The term *aptamer* (from the Latin *aptus,* "to fit") was coined by Ellington and Szostak (1990) following their pioneering work published originally in *Nature.* Based on iterative selection techniques, aptamers that bind essentially any protein or small molecule can be generated. A high-affinity, specific inhibitor that interacts with functional groups (on both the nucleic acid and the protein) can be constructed if a small amount of pure target is available.

The initiation point for aptamer development is a combinatorial library composed of single-stranded nucleic acids (RNA, DNA, or modified RNA), typically containing 20 to 40 randomized positions (10^{24} different sequences). Isolation of high-affinity nucleic acid ligands involves a process known as SELEX (systemic evolution of ligands by exponential enrichment). The starting library is incubated with the protein of interest. Nucleic acid molecules that adopt conformations that allow target protein binding are subsequently partitioned from other sequences (that do not bind the protein). The bound sequences are removed and amplified by reverse transcription and polymerase chain reaction (PCR) (for RNA-based libraries) or PCR alone (for DNA-based libraries). After repeating the process several times, the selected ligands are secured and evaluated for binding affinity and ability to inhibit activity (of the target protein) (Figure 17.1). Postselection optimization steps typically include (1) reduction in aptamer length (from a starting molecule of 80–100 nucleotides to 40 nucleotides); (2) enhanced stability in biologic systems (achieved by substitution of ribonucleotides with 2-amino, 2′-fluoro, or 2′-0-alkyl nucleotides and protection from exonuclease digestion by 3′ end capping); and (3) reduced renal clearance (achieved by increasing the molecules' mo-

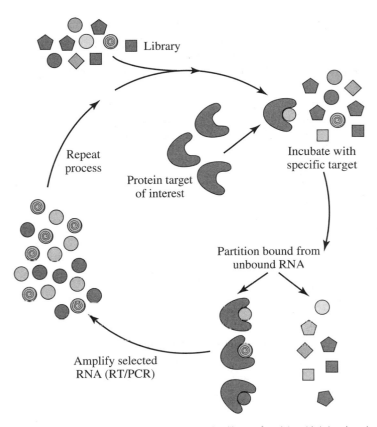

Figure 17.1   An overview of the SELEX process. A starting library of nucleic acids is incubated with the protein target of interest. Molecules that bind to the target protein are then partitioned from other sequences in the library. The bound sequences are then amplified to generate a library enriched in sequences that bind to the target protein. PCR, polymerase chain reaction; RT, reverse transcriptase. (From White RR, Sullenger BA, Rusconi CP. Developing aptamers into therapeutics [Perspective Series]. *J Clin Invest* 2000;106:929–934.)

lecular weight through site-specific addition of polyethylene glycol moieties or other hydrophobic groups.

A 15-nucleotide DNA aptamer developed to thrombin inhibited fibrin clot formation in vitro using either purified fibrinogen or human plasma (Bock et al., 1992). A combinatorial library was used to isolate a high-affinity, nuclease-resistant RNA ligand that bound specifically to factor VIIa, preventing its complexing with tissue factor. The factor VIIa aptamer prolonged tissue factor–induced clotting times of human plasma in a concentration-dependent manner and was stable (in plasma) with a half-life in excess of 15 hours (Rusconi et al., 2000).

An aptamer against factor IXa exhibiting greater than 5,000-fold specificity to this protein vs. the structurally similar coagulation proteases VIIa, Xa, and XIa and activated protein C inhibited the activation of factor Xa (by the preassembled factor IX–factor VIII complex) on a liposome surface and prolonged the clotting time (activated partial thromboplastin time) in human plasma (Rusconi et al., 2000). An oligonucleotide complex to the aptamer, which altered its shape (from an active to an inactive conformation), completely attenuated the anticoagulant effect (drug–antidote pair construct) in vitro and in plasma derived from patients with heparin-induced thrombocytopenia.

The ability to concomitantly design inhibitors to specific coagulation proteases and their antidotes provides an opportunity to ensure patient-specific and regulated therapeutics.

References

Bock LC, Griffin LC, Latham JA, Vermaas EH, Toole JJ. Selection of single-stranded DNA molecules that bind and inhibit human thrombin. *Nature* 1992;355:564–567.

Ellington AD, Szostak JW. In vitro selection of RNA molecules that bind specific ligands. *Nature* 1990;346:818–819.

Rusconi CP, Yeh A, Lyerly HK, Lawson JH, Sullenger BA. Blocking the initiation of coagulation by RNA aptamers to factor VIIa. *Thromb Haemost* 2000;84(5):841–848.

White RR, Sullenger BA, Rusconi CP. Developing aptamers into therapeutics [Perspective Series]. *J Clin Invest* 2000;106:929–934.

Part IV
Management of Arterial Thrombotic Disorders

The 20th century witnessed dynamic international changes in cardiovascular disease mortality, including death and disability from coronary heart disease, stroke, and peripheral vascular disease. Although many western countries, including the United States, have experienced a reduction in events following a peak in the 1960s and 1970s, cardiovascular disease represents the leading cause of death in most industrialized nations, with an alarming increase in both incidence and health care costs world wide. Future efforts will continue to focus on prevention, health care awareness, and quality of care derived from existing and emerging therapies.

Acute Coronary Syndromes

For over a century astute clinicians have recognized that prodromal symptoms often precede acute myocardial infarction (MI). The evolution of symptoms was subsequently found to correlate with changes in atherosclerotic plaque composition, morphology, and thrombogenicity, leading to the classification of symptoms that are currently categorized to better delineate diagnostic and management strategies (Table 18.1).

Acute coronary syndromes (ACSs) are traditionally divided into two separate categories—ST-segment elevation and non–ST-segment elevation ACS—based on the presenting electrocardiogram. The latter category is then subdivided into unstable angina and non–ST-segment elevation MI, based on the absence or presence of elevated cardiac biomarkers, respectively.

This chapter considers ST-segment elevation MI and non–ST-segment elevation ACS based on pharmacologic and clinical (diagnostics and routine management) constructs.

ST-Segment Elevation MI

ST-segment elevation MI (STEMI), in a vast majority of cases, is caused by occlusive thrombosis at a site of plaque rupture. In others, particularly when the stimulus for thrombosis is strong, occlusion may follow minor disruption of the plaque surface (erosion) or occur in areas of endothelial cell injury (activation with inflammatory features and concomitantly impaired vascular thromboresistance). Coronary arterial spasm, in the absence of intrinsic vascular disease (as may be seen with cocaine use), can also impair restrictive blood flow to the myocardium, resulting in cellular death.

Pharmacology-Based Construct

The goal of pharmacology-based therapy (and mechanical intervention) is to restore myocardial blood flow as quickly and completely as possible. The "open vessel hypotheses" predicts that rapid, complete, and sustained myocardial perfusion through the prompt restoration of physiologic blood flow will minimize (salvage) myocardium, promote ventricular performance, and reduce mortality.

Table 18.1 Past Contributions in the Diagnosis and Management of Acute Coronary Syndromes

Past 50 Years

Clinical recognition of the presence of a premonitory syndrome to acute myocardial infarction

Development of blood tests to predict and/or quantify myocardial necrosis (serum CK, CK-MB, troponin I and T, myoglobin)

Development of myocardial perfusion and functional imaging using nuclear, echocardiographic, and MRI techniques

Insights into the pathogenesis of ACS and recognition of the importance of inflammation and thrombosis

Emphasis on identifying increases in serum C-reactive protein, fibrinogen, troponin T and/or I, and serum amyloid-like protein as markers of a difficult future prognosis

Development of coronary bypass surgery

Development of percutaneous interventional procedures, including angioplasty, stents

Development and application of the statins

Recognition of the importance of aspirin and of other potent antiplatelet and antithrombotic medications (including heparins and other thrombin antagonists, ADP antagonists, and inhibitors of platelet GPIIb/IIIa receptors)

Development, refinement, and application of fibrinolytic agents

Development of left ventricular assist devices and cardiac transplantation

Development of pacemakers and defibrillators, including implantable defibrillators

---

ACS, acute coronary syndrome; ADP, adenosine 5'-diphosphate; CK, creatine kinase; GP, glycoprotein; MRI, magnetic resonance imaging.

Theroux P, Willerson JT, Armstrong PW. Progress in the treatment of acute coronary syndromes. Circulation 2000; 102:IV2–IV3.

Open-Vessel Hypothesis

Strong support for the open-vessel hypothesis can be traced to the Thrombolysis and Myocardial Infarction (TIMI) trial performed in the 1980s (Dalen et al., 1988; TIMI Study Group, 1985). Patients with patent infarct-related coronary arteries 90 minutes after the initiation of fibrinolytic therapy had an 8.1% mortality at 1 year, compared to a 14.8% mortality among those with an occluded vessel. Since that time, several large-scale clinical trials have confirmed the importance of an open infarct-related coronary artery for early, intermediate, and long-term outcome. The TIMI angiographic grading system and, more recently, the TIMI Frame Count have shed additional light by showing that normal, brisk flow (TIMI grade 3) is associated with the lowest mortality (Anderson et al., 1996; Cannon and Braunwald, 1994; Vogt et al., 1993). The Global Use of Strategies to Open Occluded Arteries (GUSTO)-1 angiographic study (GUSTO Angiographic Investigators, 1993; Simes et al., 1995), representing the largest prospective trial to examine the relationship between coronary blood flow and patient outcome, provided incontrovertible proof in support of the open-vessel hypothesis, providing a quantitative "gold standard" for developing new fibrinolytic and adjunctive treatment strategies for patients with ST-segment elevation/bundle-branch block MI. The benefit of early and complete reperfusion (TIMI grade 3 flow) is sustained beyond the initial 30 days (Ross et al., 1998) and most evident among patients with preserved left ventricular performance (ejection fraction >40%) (Goodman et al., 1998).

Time to Treatment

The benefit of coronary fibrinolysis and other reperfusion modalities is based on the early establishment of physiologic blood flow and myocardial perfusion. In the Gruppo Italiano per lo Studio della Streptochinasi nell'Infarcto Miocardico (GISSI)-1 trial (GISSI, 1987), patients treated within 1 hour of symptom onset had a 50% reduction in mortality, representing a twofold reduction when compared with the overall patient group treated with fibrinolytics (time treatment up to 12 hours). This striking observation has subsequently been confirmed by several investigators (Newby et al., 1996), including the Myocardial Infarction Triage Investigation (MITI) Study Group, which demonstrated a 1.2% mortality in patients treated within 70 minutes from symptom onset (in the field or in the hospital), compared with 8.7% for those treated between 70 minutes and 3 hours (Weaver et al., 1993). In the TIMI 2 trial (TIMI Study Group, 1989), a 1% absolute decrease in mortality was observed for each hour of decreasing time to treatment. Despite the clear benefits of early reestablishment of coronary arterial blood flow, achieving an open vessel even after the period of potential myocardial salvage may yield benefit as well (Table 18.2).

Clinical Trials of Fibrinolytic and Adjunctive Antithrombotic Therapy

The development of fibrinolytic therapy as a definitive treatment for STEMI has progressed steadily "from bench to bedside." Each fibrinolytic agent has been tested rigorously as a means to define, as clearly as possible, its respective efficacy and safety profile. Beyond the unique characteristics of individual agents has been the challenge of determining the optimal dosing and best adjunctive antithrombotic strategies (Tables 18.3–18.8).

Table 18.2 Benefits of Achieving an Open Vessel

Time-dependent effects ↓ Early restoration of coronary flow	Time-independent effects ↓ Restoration of coronary flow
Myocardial salvage Reduced infarct size Preserved ventricular performance	Improved electrical stability Decreased infarct expansion Decreased remodeling Improved collateral blood supply

Table 18.3 Angiographic Patency: Streptokinase

Study Investigator	n	Dose (mU)	Time to Treatment	Time to Coronary Angiography	Patency (%) (TIMI 2/3)
GUSTO-1 (1993)					
(SC heparin)	260	1.5	<6 h	90 min	54 (140/260)
(IV heparin)	261	1.5	<6 h	90 min	59 (153/261)
Total	**1,310**				**53 (704/1320)**
60 min					
Cribier et al. (1986)	21	1.5	115 min	74 min	52 (11/21)
PRIMI (1989)	203	1.5	140 min	61 min	48 (82/171)
Total	**224**				**48 (93/192)**
90 min					
Lopez-Sendon et al. (1988)	25	1.5	<6 h	90 min	60 (15/25)
Charbonnier et al. (1989)	58	1.5	168 min	93 min	51 (27/53)
Hogg et al. (1990)	63	1.5	209 min	90 min	53 (31/58)
ECSG-2 (1985)	65	1.0	156 min	75–90 min	55 (34/62)
TIMI-1 (1985)	159	1.5	286 min	90 min	43 (63/146)
PRIMI (1989)	203	1.5	140 min	91 min	64 (124/194)
Stack (1988b)	216	1.5	180 min	90 min	44 (95/216)
120–180 min					
Monnier (1987)	11	1.5	135 min	150 min	64 (7/11)
Vogt et al. (1994)	31	1.5	138 min	176 min	72 (21/30)
Six et al. (1990)	56	1.5	150 min	168 min	60 (32/53)
TEAM-2 (1991)	182	1.5	158 min	126 min	73 (129/176)
Total	**280**				**70 (189/270)**

Table 18.4 Angiographic Patency: Anistreplase

Study Investigator	n	Dose (U)	Time to Treatment	Time to Coronary Angiography	Patency (%) (TIMI 2/3)
60 min					
Kasper (1986)	50	30	151 min	64 min	64 (32/50)
TAPS (1991)	210	30	<6 h	60 min	60 (122/204)
Total	**260**				**61 (154/254)**
90 min					
Lopez-Sendon et al. (1988)	22	30	<6 h	90 min	86 (19/22)
Charbonnier et al. (1989)	58	30	162 min	95 min	72 (38/54)
Hogg et al (1990)	65	30	199 min	90 min	55 (32/60)
Relik-van Wely (1991)	156	30	106 min	96 min	73 (106/145)
TAPS (1991)	210	30	<6 h	90 min	70 (142/202)
Total	**511**				**70 (337/483)**

Table 18.5 Angiographic Patency: Tissue Plasminogen Activator, Accelerated Infusion

Study Investigator	n	Dose (mg)	Time to Treatment	Time to Coronary Angiography	Patency (%) (TIMI 2/3)
60 min					
Gemmell et al. (1991)	33	70 mg/h	208 min	49 min	77 (23/30)
Purvis et al. (1991)	60	70–100 mg/60 min	130 min	60 min	80 (35/44)
Neuhaus et al. (1989)	80	100 mg/90 min	<6 h	60 min	74 (54/73)
Smalling et al. (1990)	84	1.2 mg/kg/60 min	216 min	56 min	65 (51/79)
RAAMI (1990)	143	100 mg/90 min	<6 h	60 min	76 (66/87)
TAPS (1991)	210	100 mg/90 min	<6 h	60 min	73 (145/199)
Total	**610**				**74 (401/545)**
90 min					
Gemmell et al. (1991)	33	70 mg/h	208 min	90 min	87 (26/30)
Purvis et al. (1991)	60	70–100 mg/60 min	130 min	60 min	81 (48/59)
TAMI-7 (1990)	61	1.25 mg/kg/90 min	151 h	90 min	84 (51/61)
Neuhaus et al. (1989)	80	100 mg/90 min	<6 h	90 min	91 (67/74)
Smalling et al. (1990)	84	1.2 mg/kg/ 90 min	216 h	56 min	84 (68/81)
RAAMI (1990)	143	100 mg/90 min	<6 h	90 min	82 (105/128)
TAPS (1991)	210	100 mg/90 min	<6 h	90 min	84 (168/199)
GUSTO-Angiographic Investigators (1993)	272	100 mg/90 min	<6 h	90 min	81 (220/272)
Total	**943**				**83 (753/904)**

Fibrinolytic Therapy

All of the available fibrinolytic agents activate single-chain plasma plasminogen via a direct or indirect enzymatic reaction to the active fibrinolytic agent, double-chain plasmin. Characteristics of the currently available agents, streptokinase (SK), anistreplase, alteplase, reteplase (rPA), and tenecteplase (TNK-tPA) are summarized in Table 18.9.

Benefits of Fibrinolytic Therapy

Observations from experimental animal models and clinical studies performed in humans demonstrated that prompt recanalization of the infarct artery salvaged myocardium, preserved left ventricular performance, and improved outcome in a time-dependent fashion.

Comparative Clinical Trials

Several randomized clinical trials have compared the most widely used fibrinolytic agents, streptokinase and tissue plasminogen activator (tPA): GISSI-2 (GISSI-2, 1990),

Table 18.6 Angiographic Patency Tissue Plasminogen Activator Bolus Dosing

Study Investigator	n	Dose	Time to Coronary Angiography	Angiographic Patency (%) (TIMI 2/3)
Tebbe et al. (1989)	20	50-mg bolus	60 min	75 (15/20)
Verstraete et al. (1985b)	29	50-mg bolus	60 min	45 (13/29)
	28	60-mg bolus		32 (9/28)
	25	70-mg bolus		72 (18/25)
Tranchesi et al. (1991)	60	70-mg bolus	60 min	55 (33/60)
			90 min	48 (29/60)
Gemmell et al. (1991)	33	35-mg bolus	90 min	87 (29/33)
		Wait 30 min		
		35-mg bolus	24 h	83 (24/29)
Purvis et al. (1994)	84	50-mg bolus	60 min	91 (58/64)
		Wait 30 min	90 min	93 (78/84)
		50-mg bolus	18–48 h	96 (66/69)
Total	**279**			**74 (372/501)**

ISIS-3 (International Study of Infarct Survival; ISIS-3 Collaborative Group, 1992), and GUSTO-1 (GUSTO Angiographic Investigators, 1993) (Table 18.10). The largest trial, GUSTO-1, randomized 41,000 patients with ST-segment elevation to one of four treatment strategies. Accelerated "front-loaded" tPA with IV unfractionated heparin reduced 30-day mortality by 15% compared with SK with IV or subcutaneous unfractionated heparin. This benefit was maintained at 1 year (Figure 18.1). Although hemorrhagic stroke occurred more often with tPA (0.7%) than with SK (0.4%), a net clinical benefit was still achieved with tPA, as evidenced by nine fewer deaths or disabling strokes per 1,000 patients treated.

Reteplase, a deletion mutant of tPA, and tenecteplase, a single-bolus mutant of tPA, were both found to be similar in outcome and efficacy compared with tPA in the GUSTO-3 (GUSTO III Investigators, 1997) and Assessment of the Safety and Efficacy of a New Thrombolytic (ASSENT)-2 (ASSENT-2 Investigators, 1999) trials.

Heparin Preparations

Heparin is a naturally occurring inhibitor of thrombin, requiring formation of a ternary complex with antithrombin for an inhibitory effect. A composite of trials performed in the pre-reperfusion era demonstrated a 17% mortality reduction and a 22% reduction in risk of reinfarction with unfractionated heparin (MacMahon et al., 1988).

These "historical" data, as well as the reduction in the incidence of venous thromboemboli, provided support for the use of IV unfractionated heparin (UFH) or SC UFH in patients with MI.

Table 18.7 Angiographic Patency: Third-Generation Fibrinolytic Agents

Study Investigator	Agent	n	Dose (mg)	Time to Treatment Angiography	Time to Coronary (TIMI 2/3)	Patency (%)
GRECO I	rPA	42	10-mU bolus	2.9 h	60 min	73 (30/41)
					90 min	66 (28/42)
					24–48 h	92 (39/42)
GRECO II	rPA	51	10-mU bolus		60 min	72 (36/50)
			Wait 30 min	<6 h	90 min	78 (39/50)
			5-mU bolus		24–48 h	94 (47/50)
GRECO I	rPA	100	15-mU bolus	2.9 h	60 min	74 (73/99)
					90 min	75 (74/99)
					24–48 h	92 (87/95)
RAPID - 1	rPA	137	10-mU bolus Wait 30 min 5-mU bolus	2.7 h	90 min	66.2 (93/41)
RAPID - 1	rPA	141	10-mU bolus Wait 30 min 5-mU bolus	2.7 h	90 min	66.2 (93/41)
RAPID - 1	rPA	142	15-mU bolus	2.7 h	90 min	65 (92/142)
RAPID - 2	rPA	165	10-mU bolus Wait 30 min 10-U bolus	3.2 h	60 min	80 (132/165)
TIMI 10A	TNK tPA	113	30-mg bolus	<12 h	60 min	82 (23/28)
					75 min	87 (28/32)
					90 min	88 (36/41)
			50-mg bolus		60 min	79 (11/14)
					75 min	82 (14/17)
					90 min	86 (19/22)
TIMI 10B	TNK-tPA	526	30-mg bolus	<12 h	90 min	77 (234/304)
			40-mg bolus			79 (115/146)
			50-mg bolus			80 (67/176)
TIMI 10B	nPA	602	15 kU/kg		90 min	54.1 (66/122)
			30 kU/kg			62.4 (67/108)
			60 kU/kg			72.5 (89/122)
			120 kU/kg			83.0 (101/122)
Total		**2019**				**82 (1871/2276)**

nPA, novel plasminogen activator; rPA, reteplase; TNK-tPA, tenecteplase.

Patients experiencing an anterior infarction with akinesis or dyskinesis, significant left ventricular dysfunction, left ventricular aneurysm, congestive heart failure, thrombus in the left ventricle documented by echocardiography, a history of a previous embolic event, and atrial fibrillation are at a high risk for systemic embolization. Although randomized trial data are sparse, there is evidence that the risk of systemic emboli can be reduced by early initiation of heparin therapy. Therefore, independent of the fibrinolytic agent choice, heparin is recommended for patients at high risk for systemic embolism. Unless a contraindication exists, oral

Table 18.8 Angiographic Patency: Fibrinolytic/GPIIb/IIIa Receptor Antagonist Combined Pharmacotherapy

Study Investigator	n	Fibrinolytic	Dose	GPIIb/IIIa Antagonist Dose	Time to Coronary Angiography	Patency (%) (TIMI 2/3)
IMPACT-AMI		tPA	≤100 mg	Eptifibatide	90min	
	18			36 µg/kg B, 0.2 µg/kg/min		78 (14/18)
	14			72 µg/kg B, 0.4 µg/kg/min		69 (10/14)
	12			108 µg/kg B, 0.6 µg/kg/min		75 (9/12)
	15			135 µg/kg B, 0.75 µg/kg/min		79 (12/15)
	15			180 µg/kg B, 0.75 µg/kg/min		86 (13/15)
	16			180 µg/kg B, 0.75 µg/kg/min		93 (15/16)
TIMI 14	36	tPA	20 mg (bolus)	Abciximab (0.25 mg/kg bolus) 0.125 µg/kg/min × 12 h	90 min	53 (19/36)[a]
	40		35 mg (bolus)	Abciximab (0.25 mg/kg bolus)		38 (15/40)[a]
	50		35 mg (30 min infusion)	Abciximab (0.25 mg/kg bolus)		62 (31/50)[a]
	28		50 mg (bolus)	Abciximab (0.25 mg/kg bolus) 0.125 µg/kg/min × 12 h		54 (15/28)[a]
	46		50 mg (30-min infusion)	Abciximab (0.25 mg/kg bolus) 0.125 µg/kg/min × 12 h		61 (28/46)[a]
	34		50 mg (15 mg b1 35 mg) infusion × 60 min	Abciximab (0.25 mg/kg bolus) 0.125 µg/kg/min × 12 h		79 (27/34)[a]
SPEED	36	tPA	5 U	Abciximab (0.25 mg/kg bolus) 0.125 µg/kg/min × 12 h	90 min	52 (19/36)[a]
	35		7.5 U	Abciximab (0.25 mg/kg bolus) 0.125 µg/kg/min × 12 h		46 (16/35)[a]
	48		10 U	Abciximab (0.25 mg/kg bolus) 0.125 µg/kg/min × 12 h		48 (23/48)[a]
	70		5 U/5 U	Abciximab (0.25 mg/kg bolus) 0.125 µg/kg/min × 12 h		67 (47/70)[a]
Total	**477**					**72 (393/493)**

[a]TIMI 3 flow.
GP, glycoprotein; tPA, tissue plasminogen activator.

Table 18.9 Pharmacologic Features of Fibrinolytic Agents

Feature of Agent	Streptokinase	Anistreplase	Alteplase	Reteplase	Tenecteplase
Dose	1.5 MU in 30–60 min	30 mg in 5 min	100 mg in 90 min	10 U × 2 over 30 min	0.55 mg/kg over 5–10 sec
Bolus administration	No	Yes	No	Yes	Yes
Antigenic	Yes	Yes	No	No	No
Allergic reactions (hypotension most common)	Possible	Possible	No	No	No
Systemic fibrinogen depletion	Marked	Marked	Mild	Moderate	Mild
90-min patency rates (%)	~50	~65	~75	~75	~75
TIMI grade 3 flow (%)	32	43	54	60	~60
Average mortality rate in comparative trials (%)	7.3	10.5	7.2	6.0	6.0
Cost per dose	+			++	++	++

+, relatively low; ++, relatively high.
From ACC/AHA Joint Guidelines Statement.

anticoagulant therapy with warfarin (target international normalized ratio [INR] 2.5) may be continued for several months.

Patients receiving fibrin-selective agents tPA, rPA, or TNK-tPA should receive weight-adjusted IV UFH (target activated partial thromboplastin time [aPTT] 50–70 seconds) for 48 hours (Ryan et al., 1999). The dosing strategy is as follows: a 60 U/kg bolus at initiation of fibrinolytic therapy, followed by an initial maintenance dose of 12 U/kg/h (maximum bolus of 4,000 U and 1,000 U/h infusion in patients weighing >70 kg). If non–fibrin-selective fibrinolytics are used, such as SK or anistreplase, patients at low risk for thromboemboli can receive subcutaneous heparin, 7,500 to 10,000 U every 12 hours, until ambulatory.

Low-Molecular-Weight Heparin and Direct-Acting Antithrombins

Low–molecular-weight heparins provide several potential advantages over conventional UFH, owing to their improved bioavailability, enhanced antithrombotic effects mediated by "upstream" inhibition of the coagulation cascade, and ease of use.

Table 18.10 Mortality Rates in Comparative Trials of Fibrinolytic Therapy

Study	No. of Patients	Agents, Dose	Time (h)	Follow-up	Mortality		RRR (%)/ ARR (%)	p Value
					Therapy (%)	Control (%)		
GISSI-2	12,490	SK 1.5 MU, 0.5–1 h vs. tPA 100 mg, 3 h; heparin SC vs. control	<6	Hospital	SK, 8.6	tPA, 9.0	—	Not significant
International Study Group	20,891	SK 1.5 MU, 0.5–1 h vs. tPA 100 mg, 3 h; heparin SC vs. control	<6	Hospital	SK, 8.5	tPA, 8.9	—	Not significant
ISIS-3	41,291	SK 1.5 MU, 1 h; APSAC 30 U, 3–5 min; duteplase 0.6 MU/kg; heparin SC vs. control	<24	35 d	SK, 10.5	APSAC, 10.6; tPA, 10.3	—	Not significant
INJECT	6,010	SK 1.5 MU, 1 h; rPA 10 U, repeated after 30 min; heparin IV to all	<12	35 d	SK, 9.53	rPA, 9.02	0.51	Not significant
GUSTO-1	41,021	SK 1.5 MU, 1 h + heparin SC or IV or SK 1.0 MU, 1 h + tPA 1.0 mg/kg, 1 h + heparin, or tPA up to 100 mg, 1.5 h + heparin	<6	30 d	SK SC heparin, 7.2; SK IV 7.4	SK, 7.0; tPA, 6.3; rtPA, 6.3	Accelerated tPA, vs. SK 14/1.0	0.001
GUSTO-III	15,059	tPA up to 100 mg, 1.5 h or rPA 10 U, repeated after 30 min; heparin IV to all	<6	30 d	tPA, 7.24	rPA, 7.47	0.23	0.54
COBALT	7,169	tPA up to 100 mg, 1.5 h rtPA 50-mg bolus, repeated (50 or 40 mg) after 30 min; heparin IV to all	<6	30 d	tPA accelerated, 7.53	tPA 2 bolus, 7.98	0.45	Not significant

APSAC, anisoylated plasminogen-streptokinase activator complex; ARR, absolute risk reduction; rPA, reteplase; RRR, relative risk reduction; rtPA, recombinant tissue plasminogen activator; SK, streptokinase; tPA, tissue plasminogen activator.

Cairns JA, Theroux P, Lewis HD Jr, Ezekowitz M, Meade TW. Antithrombotic agents in coronary artery disease. Chest 1998;114(Suppl):636S.

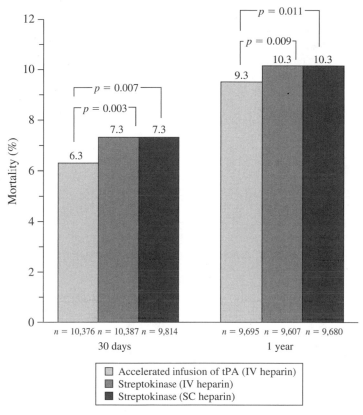

Figure 18.1 In the GUSTO-1 study, the combination of alteplase, IV unfractionated heparin, and aspirin was associated with the lowest 30-day and 1-year mortality rates. tPA, tissue plasminogen activator.

The ASSENT-3 trial provided encouraging results for the combination of enoxaparin and TNK-tPA (ASSENT-3 Investigators, 2001), but bleeding was a concern, particularly in older patients in whom enoxaparin dose modifications may be required.

Low-Molecular-Weight Heparin

A total of 400 patients with ST-segment elevation MI participating in the Heparin and Aspirin Reperfusion Therapy (HART) II study who received alteplase were randomized to receive either UFH or enoxaparin (30 mg IV bolus, 1 mg/kg every 12 hours) for 3 days. The 90-minute patency rates were similar at 75.1% and 80.1%, respectively, while reocclusion rates were lower with enoxaparin (9.1% vs. 3.1%;

161

$p = .02$). Clinical endpoints including 30-day mortality and major hemorrhage were low in both groups (Ross et al., 2001).

Baird and colleagues (2002) randomized 300 patients who had received fibrinolytic therapy (anistreplase, streptokinase, or tPA) to either UFH or enoxaparin (40 mg IV bolus, 40 mg SC every 8 hours) for a total of 4 days. The triple endpoint of death, nonfatal reinfarction, or readmission for unstable angina occurred more frequently in patients receiving UFH (36% vs. 26%; $p = .04$). Major hemorrhage was reported in 9% and 3% of patients, respectively.

Bivalirudin

Bivalirudin may be utilized with streptokinase instead of UFH in patients with suspected or known heparin-induced thrombocytopenia (HIT) as well as among patients considered to be at high risk for reinfarction. A dose of 0.25 mg/kg bolus, followed by an infusion of 0.5 mg/kg/h (for up to 36 hours), is recommended. The infusion rate should be reduced if the aPTT exceeds 75 seconds within the first 12 hours.

Warfarin

The evolution of oral anticoagulants (vitamin-K antagonists) for the management of ACSs has taken a circuitous path; however, much insight has been achieved along the way. The Warfarin Aspirin Reinfarction Study (WARIS-1) (Smith et al., 1990) included 1,219 patients with MI who received either warfarin (INR 2.8–4.8) or placebo. Although major hemorrhage was increased twofold by warfarin treatment, mortality and reinfarction were reduced by 24% and 34%, respectively.

Interest in oral anticoagulants waned over the following decade because of two large-scale trials, the Coumadin-Aspirin Reinfarction Study (CARS) ($n = 8,803$; median INR 1.3) (Fuster, 1997) and the Combination Hemotherapy and Mortality Prevention (CHAMP) study ($n = 5,059$; median INR 1.8) (Fiore et al., 2002), both of which found no reduction in mortality, reinfarction, or stroke with warfarin (alone or in combination with aspirin) as compared with aspirin monotherapy.

The favorable results observed in WARIS-1, coupled with the disappointing findings of CARS and CHAMP, not only established the need for a definitive trial of anticoagulant therapy in ACSs, but also raised the very important possibility of a "threshold" effect for benefit (as previously observed for venous thromboembolic disorders and atrial fibrillation). Indeed, WARIS-II (Hurlen et al., 2002), the Antithrombotics in the Secondary Prevention of Events in Coronary Thrombosis (ASPECT)-2 study (Van Es et al., 2002), and the Antithrombotics in the Prevention of ReOcclusion in Coronary Thrombolysis (APRICOT)-2 trial (Brouwer et al., 2002) support a target level of anticoagulation (INR) approaching 3.0 (range 2.5–3.5) for anticoagulation monotherapy and 2.5 (range 2.0–3.0) for combination therapy with aspirin. Thus, the available data, based on nearly 20,000 patients participating in randomized clinical trials, are strong and show that oral anticoagulants, when given in adequate doses, reduce reinfarction and thromboembolic stroke, but at a cost of increased hemorrhagic events.

Maximizing benefit while minimizing the risk associated with oral anticoagulant therapy is linked closely to management strategies designed to achieve and maintain a target level of inhibition. Because coumarin compounds exhibit complex pharmacokinetic and pharmacodynamic properties and are among the most challenging drugs to regulate, coordinated anticoagulation clinics may represent the preferred means to provide safe and effective care. Accumulating data show a 50% reduction in thromboembolism, major hemorrhage, and emergency medical visits using this strategy, and the use of portable, point-of-care coagulation monitors, by providing a mechanism for frequent testing, could improve outcomes further (Burken and Whyte, 2002). Even under ideal circumstances, the complexities of coumarin therapy create real obstacles for clinicians and their patients. In WARIS-II, approximately one third of the patients were below the target INR range; one third discontinued warfarin treatment at some point during the 80-month study period; 5% to 7% were withdrawn from treatment because of hemorrhagic complication; and 2% to 3% were deemed noncompliant. The exclusion of patients greater than 75 years of age undoubtedly reduced the warfarin-associated hemorrhagic risk.

Aspirin and Antiplatelet Therapy

ISIS-2 (ISIS-2 Collaborative Group, 1988) was a randomized, placebo-controlled, double-blind trial of short-term therapy with IV SK, oral aspirin (160 mg daily for 1 month), both, or neither among 17,187 patients with suspected acute MI. In addition to the 23% risk reduction in the 5-week vascular mortality rate among patients receiving SK, there was a 21% reduction among those receiving aspirin and a 40% reduction among those receiving a combination of SK and aspirin, which are all highly significant reductions. The early reduction in mortality with aspirin persisted when the patients were observed for a mean of 15 months. Aspirin reduced the risk of nonfatal reinfarction by 49% and nonfatal stroke by 46%.

The Antiplatelet Trialists' Collaboration update (Antiplatelet Trialists' Collaboration, 2002) included 287 studies involving 135,640 high-risk (acute or previous vascular disease or another predisposing condition) patients in comparisons of antiplatelet therapy vs. control and 77,000 in comparisons of different antiplatelet regimes. The analysis extended the direct evidence of benefit from antiplatelet therapy to a much wider range of patients at high risk of occlusive vascular disease.

Among 18,788 patients with a history of MI, allocation to a mean duration of antiplatelet therapy of 27 months resulted in 36 fewer serious vascular events per 1,000 patients (25% odds reduction; $p < .001$). This benefit reflects large and highly significant reductions in nonfatal MI (18 fewer per 1,000; $p < .0006$), as well as a smaller, but still significant, reduction in nonfatal stroke (5 fewer per 1,000; $p < .002$). The overall benefits were larger than the excess risk of major extracerebral hemorrhage (3 per 1,000 or 1 per 1,000 patients per year).

Data were available on 19,288 patients with suspected acute MI. Allocation to a mean treatment duration of 1 month of antiplatelet therapy led to a 30% odds reduction in vascular events (38 fewer serious vascular events per 1,000 patients treated) ($p < .001$). This reflects a large and highly significant reduction in nonfatal reinfarction (13 fewer per 1,000; $p < .001$) and in vascular death (23 fewer per 1,000; $p = .02$). The risk of major extracranial bleeding was approximated at 1 to 2 per 1,000 patients treated.

The updated meta-analysis also provided additional information on the effects of different doses of aspirin. Overall, among 3,570 patients in three trials directly comparing aspirin ($\geq$75 mg daily vs. <75 mg daily), there were significant differences in vascular events (two trials compared 72–325 mg aspirin daily vs. <75 mg daily and one trial compared 500–1,500 mg aspirin daily vs. 75 mg daily). Considering both direct and indirect comparisons of aspirin dose, the proportional reduction in vascular events was 19% with 500 to 1,500 mg daily, 26% with 160 to 325 mg daily, and 32% with 75 to 150 mg daily. Whether the greater reductions observed with decreasing doses are clinically meaningful will require a large-scale, randomized trial in patients with coronary heart disease. Similarly, the relative benefits for patients with non–ST-segment elevation ACS compared to other subsets must be more clearly defined through large-scale studies. Regardless of the chosen dose, aspirin should be administered unless contraindications (rare) exist (Burns et al., 1999).

The effect of antiplatelet drugs other than aspirin (vs. control) was assessed in 166 trials including 81,731 patients. Indirect comparisons provided no clear evidence of differences in reducing serious vascular events (χ^2 for heterogenicity between any aspirin regimen and other antiplatelet drugs = 10.8; ns). Most direct comparisons assessed the effects of replacing aspirin with another antiplatelet agent. In the Clopidogrel versus Aspirin in Patients at Risk for Ischaemic Events (CAPRIE) trial (CAPRIE Steering Committee, 1996), which included 19,185 patients with a history of MI, stroke, or peripheral vascular disease, clopidogrel reduced serious vascular events by 10% compared with aspirin ($p = .03$).

The effect of adding another antiplatelet drug to aspirin (vs. aspirin alone) has been assessed in 43 trials including 39,205 patients. Overall, a 15% reduction in serious vascular events was observed ($p = .0001$). The benefits of adding an intravenous glycoprotein (GP) IIb/IIIa receptor antagonist to aspirin were particularly evident among patients undergoing percutaneous coronary intervention (PCI).

Summary

Acute thrombotic occlusion of an epicardial coronary artery, the most common cause of ST-segment elevation MI, is the end result of platelet activation and aggregation, followed by activation of the extrinsic and intrinsic pathways of coagulation. The clinician's antithrombotic armamentarium includes:

- Fibrinolytics used alone or as part of a facilitated (PCI) strategy
- Mechanical techniques, such as immediate angioplasty and/or stenting, to restore perfusion and maintain patency
- Antiplatelet agents that inhibit platelet activation as well as aggregation through blockade of the GPIIb/IIIa receptor
- Antithrombotic compounds that prevent propagation of thrombus, particularly after successful reperfusion therapy

Current research efforts are directed toward defining the safest and most efficacious pharmacologic and mechanical treatments that achieve rapid and sustained patency of the infarct vessel and limit subsequent atherothrombotic events.

ST-Segment Elevation MI: Clinical Construct

The classic symptom profile of patients experiencing MI includes burning, pressing, aching, or "viselike" retrosternal pain lasting from 30 minutes to several hours and not relieved by nitrates. The pain typically radiates to the neck, jaw, shoulder, or arms and is often accompanied by nausea, diaphoresis, and indigestion. Patients with a prior history of angina may describe recent worsening or "acceleration" of symptoms. Because patients with aortic dissection, pulmonary embolism, and pericarditis can also experience severe and protracted chest pain, it is crucial to elicit a complete history and perform a careful physical examination to exclude these diagnoses. Because 20% of patients with MI present to the hospital with atypical symptoms (Bayer et al., 1986), a high index of suspicion is required. Of importance, elderly and diabetic patients as well as individuals with hypertension are more likely to suffer silent infarctions.

Patients without Chest Pain

A total of 434,877 patients enrolled in the NRMI (National Registry of Myocardial Infarction)-2 were assessed for their presenting signs and symptoms upon hospital presentation. Of all patients diagnosed with an MI, 142,445 (33%) did not have chest pain at the time of arrival. These patients (compared to those with chest pain) tended to be older, more often had diabetes mellitus, had a longer delay (nearly 8 hours), were less likely to receive fibrinolytic therapy or undergo PCI, and experienced a 23.3% in-hospital mortality (Canto et al., 2000).

Electrocardiographic Features

The initial electrocardiogram (ECG) is of considerable diagnostic importance, and up to 60% of patients will have abnormalities compatible with myocardial injury (Figure 18.2). However, the presenting ECG is completely normal in 5% to 10% of patients. The evolution of ECG changes in MI is outlined in Figure 18.3.

The ECG will typically reveal ST-segment elevation (injury pattern); however, ST-segment depression in leads V_1 to V_3 is observed in true posterior wall infarctions (Gau, 1987). Localization of infarction can be achieved by recognizing the ECG–anatomic relationships. Leads V_1 and V_2 represent the septal region, V_3 and V_4 the midanterior wall, V_5 and V_6 the low lateral or apical aspect of the left ventricle, I and aV_L the high lateral wall of the left ventricle, and V_7, V_8, and V_9 the posterior aspect of the left ventricle. The association between coronary anatomy (involved coronary artery) and site of myocardial damage is outlined in Table 18.11. A new

Figure 18.2a Component parts of the surface electrocardiogram (ECG).

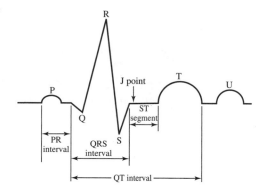

Figure 18.2b Electrocardiographic features of an acute injury pattern with convex upward ST-segment elevation.

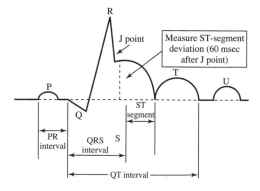

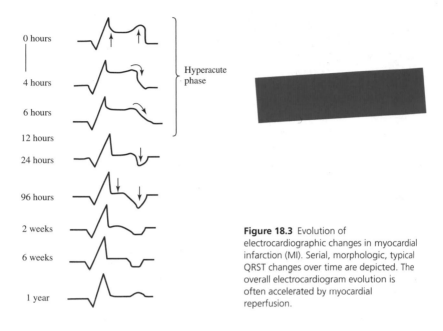

Figure 18.3 Evolution of electrocardiographic changes in myocardial infarction (MI). Serial, morphologic, typical QRST changes over time are depicted. The overall electrocardiogram evolution is often accelerated by myocardial reperfusion.

left bundle-branch block (LBBB) or an old LBBB with pronounced ST-segment elevation may represent a pattern of infarction. The presence of ST-segment elevation in V_{4R} is a specific finding for right ventricular infarction. A new right bundle-branch block (RBBB) or an old RBBB with ST-segment elevation and/or reversal of reciprocal ST changes (pseudonormalization) may also represent acute injury. In the appropriate clinical context (but without diagnostic ECG changes), noninvasive

Table 18.11 Association of ECG Lead Changes of Injury with the Most Commonly Involved Coronary Artery and Site of Myocardial Damage

Leads with ECG Changes	Injury/Infarct Artery	Area of Damage
V_1–V_2	LCA: LAD–septal branch	Septum; bundle of His; bundle branches
V_3–V_4	LCA: LAD–diagonal branch	Anterior wall LV
V_5–V_6 plus I and a VL	LCA–circumflex branch	High lateral wall LV
V_{4R} (II, III, aVF)	RCA–proximal branches	RV: inferior wall LV; posterior wall LV
V_1–V_4 (ST depression)	Either LCA–circumflex or RCA–posterior descending branch	Posterior wall LV

ECG, electrocardiogram; LCA, left coronary artery; LAD, left anterior descending artery; RCA, right coronary artery; LV, left ventricle; RV, right ventricle.

imaging modalities may show focal wall motion abnormalities or abnormal perfusion (American College of Cardiology [ACC]/American Heart Association [AHA] Guidelines, 1999; Hilton et al., 1994). Sgarbossa and colleagues (1996a) described a scoring system for diagnosis of acute infarction in the setting of LBBB:

ST-segment elevation ≥ 1 mm concordant with the QRS (Score 5)
ST-segment depression ≥ 1 mm in lead V_1 or V_3 (Score 3)
ST-segment elevation ≥ 5 mm discordant with the QRS (Score 2)

A score greater than or equal to 3 was associated with a 90% specificity for infarction. If the score was greater to or equal than 5, a sensitivity of 73% was achieved (Sgarbossa et al., 1996a).

Current Approach to Myocardial Infarction and Its Management

Patient Selection

Given its proven beneficial effects, fibrinolytic therapy has become the global standard of care for patients threatened with MI. Appropriate patient selection is the key to safe and effective care and requires a thorough assessment prior to initiating treatment. An overview of inclusion and exclusion criteria is presented in Table 18.12a and b.

In general, patients expected to derive the greatest overall benefit from fibrinolytic therapy (and other forms of reperfusion) include those with large areas of jeopardized myocardium who receive treatment soon after symptom onset (Rawles, 1997).

Patient Subgroups

Older Patients

Myocardial infarction is the leading cause of morbidity and mortality among individuals greater than 80 years of age. As the world's population continues to age, the prevalence of "at-risk" patients will rise steadily as well. Greater than 60% of all randomized clinical trials for fibrinolytic therapy have excluded patients greater than 75 years of age. This serves as the basis for a class IIa recommendation for fibrinolytic therapy in patients 70 to 75 years of age and a class IIb recommendation for those greater than 75.

Hospital mortality among patients older than 70 years of age approaches 25%, nearly four times that for younger individuals (Lesnefsky et al., 1996). This high

Table 18.12a Patient Selection for Fibrinolytic Therapy

Indication(s) for Treatment
  Patient history consistent with acute MI
  Ischemic myocardial pain
    >30 min duration
    <12 h from symptom onset
    Unrelieved by sublingual nitroglycerin
  ECG changes consistent with transmural infarction[a]
    >0.1 mV ST-segment elevation in:
      Two or more inferior leads (II, III, aV_f)
      Two or more contiguous precordial leads $(V_1 - V_6)$
      I and aVL
Potential Exclusion(s) from Treatment
  Absolute
    Bleeding diathesis
    History of cerebrovascular accident or transient ischemic attack
      (particularly within the past 6 mo)
    Active internal bleeding
    Intracranial neoplasm, arteriovenous malformation, or aneurysm
    Recent intracranial/intraspinal surgery or trauma (within 2 mo)
    Significant trauma (within 2 mo)
    Recent major surgery (within 4 wk)
    Pregnancy
    Recent puncture of noncompressible vessel (within 10 days)
    Previous intracranial hemorrhage (any cause)
  Relative
    Active peptic ulcer disease (within 6 mo)
    Recent obstetric delivery or organ biopsy
    Acute pericarditis
    High likelihood of left-heart thrombus
    Subacute bacterial endocarditis
    Significant liver dysfunction
  Hypertension
    Severe hypertension (systolic blood pressure >180 mmHg,
      diastolic blood pressure >110 mmHg)
    Long-standing, poorly controlled hypertension
  Current oral anticoagulation therapy
  Knitted Dacron graft (placed within 6 mo)
  Prosthetic device
    Mechanical valve
    Caval filter (placed within 3 mo)

---

[a]*Presence of Q-waves does not preclude treatment.*
ECG, electrocardiogram; MI, myocardial infarction.

mortality reflects an inherently high-risk subset of patients with existing comorbid conditions, including hypertension, diabetes mellitus, and prior MI; however, data also show that elderly patients delay seeking medical attention, and once hospitalized, they experience further delay in receiving treatment (Tresch et al., 1996). This undoubtedly adds to their already high mortality rate. In addition, elderly patients

Table 18.12b Approach to Patients with ST-Segment Elevation MI

Presentation within 3 h of symptom onset
No delay for primary angioplasty
No absolute contraindication for fibrinolytic therapy

Fibrinolysis Generally Preferred	Invasive Strategy Generally Preferred
Early presentation and delay to invasive strategy	Skilled PCI laboratory available
Invasive strategy not an option	Door-to-balloon time <90 min
Catheterization laboratory not available	High risk
Vascular access limitations	Cardiogenic shock
PCI operator experience limited	Killip class ≥3
Delay to invasive strategy	Relative contraindications for fibrinolytic therapy
Prolonged transport	Symptom onset >3 h
Door-to-balloon time >90 min	Diagnosis of STEMI in question

MI, myocaridal infarction; PCI, percutaneous coronary intervention; STEMI, ST-segment elevation myocardial infarction.

Antman EM, Anbe DT, Armstrong PW et al. ACC/AHA Guidelines for the management of pateints with ST-segment elevation MI. J Am Coll Cardiol 2004;44:671–719.

have a greater decrease in left ventricular performance after MI than do younger patients, even in the presence of a patent infarct-related coronary artery.

There is little question that elderly patients are at increased risk for hemorrhagic complications following fibrinolytic therapy, adjunctive antithrombotic agents, and invasive procedures. It is likely that existing concerns regarding bleeding risk have contributed greatly to the comparatively low fibrinolytic administration rates among elderly patients (Krumholz et al., 1997); however, the potential benefits of treatment outweigh the risks (Gurwitz et al., 1991, 1996).

In NRMI-1, fibrinolytic therapy use was inversely related to patient age even when adjusted for sex, diagnosis by initial ECG, and time from symptom onset to hospital presentation; however, the relative increase in fibrinolytic therapy use since the mid-1990s has been greater in older patients (Fibrinolytic Therapy Trialists' [FTT] Collaborative Group, 1994).

Patients with Diabetes Mellitus

The relationship between diabetes mellitus and vascular events, including MI and cardiac death, is well established. In addition, diabetic patients have a higher mortality than do nondiabetic patients following MI, due at least in part to more advanced coronary artery disease and their increased sensitivity to catecholamine stimulation. Oral hypoglycemic agents may also contribute to this higher mortality by attenuating the protective effect of preconditioning and increasing the propensity toward malignant ventricular arrhythmias (Tomai et al., 1994).

Despite experiencing relatively poor outcomes following MI, diabetic patients respond well to reperfusion therapy and have a greater absolute risk reduction of death than do nondiabetic patients (Woodfield et al., 1996).

Late Treatment

Animal models provided the initial supportive basis for late perfusion, including (1) improved infarct healing, (2) limited myocardial wall thinning, (3) reduced aneurysm formation, and (4) improved electrical stability (Jeremy et al., 1987; Kersschot et al., 1986). The important hypothesis that required confirmation was that establishing infarct-related coronary arterial patency beyond a point capable of salvaging myocardium could still provide benefit. In addition, the potential for relatively late treatment to occasionally limit infarct size (depending on the precise time of complete coronary occlusion) should not be overlooked.

Several clinical trials have supported the use of fibrinolytic therapy up to 12 hours from symptom onset. In the Late Assessment of Thrombolytic Efficacy (LATE) trial (LATE Study Group, 1993), 5,711 patients with symptoms and ECG findings of MI were randomized, between 6 and 24 hours from symptom onset, to receive either tPA (100 mg IV over 3 hours) or placebo. Mortality at 35 days was 8.8% and 10.3%, respectively (14% reduction mortality favoring tPA). Patients treated within 12 hours had mortality rates of 8.9% and 11.9%, respectively (25.6% relative reduction). Although modest support for late treatment with streptokinase was derived from Estudio Multicéntrico Estreptoquinasa Repúblicas de América del Sur (EMERAS) (EMERAS Collaborative Group, 1993), an overview of nine clinical trials, including more than 58,000 patients with ST-segment elevation or bundle-branch block MI treated within 12 hours from symptom onset, revealed a mortality reduction of 20 per 1,000 treated patients; 10 lives were saved for every 1,000 patients treated between 13 and 18 hours (Kersschot et al., 1986).

Despite the proven benefit of fibrinolytic therapy achieved beyond 6 hours from symptom onset, many clinicians still choose to restrict treatment to a 6-hour time window. One explanation may be the perceived increased risk of cardiac rupture. Data derived from the LATE study, however, suggested that rupture is not increased with treatment beyond 12 hours (Becker et al., 1995a).

Q Waves on Presenting Electrocardiogram

The presence of Q waves is a marker of myocardial necrosis, leading clinicians to perceive that patients with this abnormality have little myocardium to salvage. Data from the Western Washington Study and MITI trial revealed that more than 50%

of patients presenting to the hospital within 1 hour of symptom onset already had Q waves on their initial ECG. Although infarct size was larger in these patients, benefit was still seen (Raitt et al., 1995).

Bundle-Branch Block on Presenting Electrocardiogram

The presence of bundle-branch block, particularly complete LBBB, tends to conceal the ECG ST-segment changes of acute MI. As a result, therapy may be delayed or not given at all. The GUSTO investigators established criteria for diagnosing acute MI in the presence of a LBBB (Sgarbossa et al., 1996a). These criteria can also be used in the presence of a paced ventricular rhythm (Sgarbossa et al., 1996b).

An overview of randomized studies compiled by the FTT Group (1994) showed convincingly that patients with ST-segment elevation—or new (presumably new) bundle-branch block—benefit from fibrinolytics, irrespective of age, sex, blood pressure, heart rate, and history of prior MI or diabetes mellitus. The greatest benefit was derived from early treatment (within 6 hours of symptoms onset), amounting to 30 lives per 1,000 patients treated.

Smokers

Trials of fibrinolytic therapy have revealed a favorable prognosis for "current" smokers (Barbash et al., 1995). In the TAMI (Thrombolysis and Agioplasty in Myocardial Infarction) trial, smokers were more likely to have TIMI 3 coronary arterial blood flow at 90 minutes following treatment initiation than were nonsmokers (41.1% vs. 34.6%) (Grines et al., 1995). Other studies have revealed similar findings (de Chillou et al., 1996). The presence of a procoagulant state in smokers supported higher fibrinogen levels and baseline hematocrits. Thus, it had been hypothesized that thrombus burden is greater in smokers (with less underlying atherosclerotic disease and smaller plaque dimensions), improving the response to fibrinolysis.

Women

Data from several large epidemiologic and clinical studies have suggested that the prognosis after MI is worse for women than for men (Becker et al., 1994a). In the TIMI II study, 597 women received fibrinolytic therapy and either invasive (18–48 hours percutaneous transluminal coronary angioplasty [PTCA] when feasible) or conservative management. The 6-week mortality was greater among women than among men (9.0% vs. 4.0%; adjusted relative risk 1.54). The combined endpoint of death or MI was also higher (15.9% vs. 9.5%; adjusted relative risk 1.37). Older age and a higher incidence of diabetes mellitus accounted for part but not all of the observed differences in outcome. Data from the NRMI-1 support these conclusions and raise concerns over a selection bias for invasive procedures among women (Becker et al., 1995b). Of further concern, NRMI-1 and NRMI-2 both show a tendency for women, already being treated with decreased frequency, to receive fibrinolytics later than do men. On further analysis, women delay seeking treatment longer than do men, and once hospitalized, they experience further delay. As previously discussed, there is an increasing use of fibrinolytics in women, including elderly women; however, the overall rate of treatment still lags considerably behind men.

In an overview of hemorrhagic complications among patients participating in the TAMI trials, female gender was shown to be an independent risk factor, as were advanced age, reduced body weight, and history of cerebrovascular disease. Similar observations have emerged from the TIMI experience (Becker et al., 1994a). Female gender may also be a risk factor for intracranial hemorrhage (White et al., 1993), independent of age. This area warrants further investigation. Finally, cardiac rupture has been observed more frequently among women receiving fibrinolytics, particularly women greater than 70 years of age. This may explain the higher mortality rate among older women compared with men.

Body Weight

In epidemiologic studies, excessive body weight, independent of other risk factors, portends a poor prognosis after MI. Questions of dosing (underdosing) have been considered in the reperfusion era given similar observations; however, the greatest concern is among patients with low body weight. In the NRMI-1 study (Becker et al., 1995b), patients weighing less than 70 kg were older, received treatment later, and were less likely to undergo invasive procedures than were patients of greater weight. In fact, low body weight was independently associated with hemorrhagic complications and in-hospital mortality (Figure 18.4). Despite receiving a lower dose of tPA per kg body weight, high-weight patients (>85 kg) experienced a low incidence of cardiogenic shock, recurrent MI, and death.

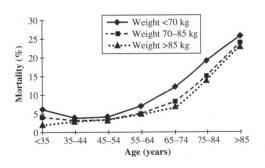

Figure 18.4 Low body weight is associated with higher mortality at all age strata, particularly in the elderly.

Menstruation

Although anecdotal case reports have suggested that fibrinolytic therapy is safe for most women during menstruation, the potential risk is poorly defined. In the GUSTO study (Karnash et al., 1995), 12 actively menstruating women received fibrinolytic therapy for acute MI. Three women had moderate bleeding (vaginal in two patients) that required transfusion. None of the women died or experienced severe bleeding. Thus, the potential benefit appears to outweigh the risk.

Cardiogenic Shock

Shock, as currently defined, is a syndrome (i.e., a recognizable collection of symptoms, signs, and laboratory abnormalities) characterized by (1) hypotension and (2) hypoperfusion associated with widespread cellular and vital organ dysfunction.

Cardiogenic shock is associated with an in-hospital mortality approaching 80%. Clinical experience in trials of coronary fibrinolysis indicates that 2% to 3% of patients with MI are in shock on hospital arrival, whereas an additional 3% to 4% develop this complication after initial treatment. A large proportion of patients who develop cardiogenic shock are initially classified as Killip class I or II, suggesting that subsequent events (recurrent ischemia, infarct extension, early infarct expansion) contribute. Predictors of poor outcomes in patients sustaining acute MI include advanced age, prior infarction, anterior site of infarction, ejection fraction less than 35%, and diabetes mellitus (Hands et al., 1989).

The in-hospital mortality among patients with cardiogenic shock treated with fibrinolytic therapy has remained high, paralleling Killip's experience in the prefibrinolytic era (Killip and Kimbal, 1967). The fact remains that cardiogenic shock is the strongest independent predictor or mortality after acute MI.

It is clear from clinical trials that the beneficial effects of coronary fibrinolysis are determined by prompt and complete restoration of coronary arterial blood flow. There is evidence that successful reperfusion is also a pivotal factor in the setting of cardiogenic shock. This observation is supported by the findings of retrospective studies in patients with shock undergoing coronary angioplasty. A consecutive series of 500 patients with MI complicated by cardiogenic shock in the Duke database identified patency of the infarct-related coronary artery among the most important predictors of in-hospital mortality (Kennedy et al., 1985; Mathey et al., 1981). Of major concern, however, are the low patency rates experienced by patients with cardiogenic shock after fibrinolytic therapy. Experimental data obtained by magnetic resonance imaging (MRI) and by photographing clot dissolution in vitro have shown that clots dissolve two orders of magnitude faster when fibrinolytic agents are introduced by pressure-induced permeation instead of by diffusion (Blinc et al., 1990). When coronary perfusion pressure is low, the velocity of fibrinolysis is limited by the diffusion constraints of the plasminogen activator itself and by plasmin (the active enzyme). As the concentration profile of diffusing molecules falls exponentially with distance, even high concentrations of fibrinolytics would not be expected to fully compensate for slowed transport into a thrombus.

Intraluminal pressure is of particular importance in areas of dynamic coronary arterial stenosis (soft plaque) because it represents the opposing force to both vasoconstriction and passive collapse. Perfusion pressure is decreased in patients with cardiogenic shock, favoring passive collapse of compliant areas and potentially influencing fibrinolytic response (Freedman et al., 1982; Li et al., 1989; Sabol et al., 1994).

Metabolic factors may also have an impact on the ability of fibrinolytic agents to dissolve an occlusive thrombus. Increased plasma fibrinogen and local thrombin concentrations, common among patients with acute coronary artery disease, are associated with formation of thin fibrin strands. In turn, a thrombus composed of thin, tightly packed fibrin strands restricts the transport of plasminogen, plasmin, and plasminogen activators. Furthermore, metabolic acidemia may impair the conversion of plasminogen to plasmin by increasing the Michaelis constant and lowering the catalytic rate. Thus, an "unfriendly" metabolic environment may limit fibrinolysis even if coronary perfusion pressure is increased.

Coronary Revascularization in Patients with Cardiogenic Shock

Despite significant advances in the treatment of cardiogenic shock, including coronary care unit monitoring, vasopressor and inotropic agents, and circulatory support measures, mortality rates remain unacceptably high. Several studies (Gacioch et al., 1992; Hibbard et al., 1992; Lee et al., 1988; Moosvi et al., 1992; Stack et al., 1988a) examined in-hospital and long-term mortality rates in patients who have undergone mechanical revascularization. Survival to hospital discharge ranged from 50% to 71%. A factor common to all studies that have indicated a benefit is successful reperfusion of the infarct-related artery. Bengston et al. (1992) found a mortality rate of 33% in patients with patent infarct-related arteries compared with 75% in patients with an occluded vessel and 84% in patients whose patency status was unknown.

Long-term clinical outcome from prior retrospective studies also suggests a significant improvement in survival rates for patients who underwent successful PCI compared with patients who had unsuccessful PCI or when intervention was not attempted. Stack et al. (1988a) initially reported a 4% mortality rate at 6- and 12-month follow-up in 25 survivors of cardiogenic shock who had successful PCI and survived to hospital discharge. Other studies have reported mortality rates after hospitalization of 11% to 20% (Gacioch et al., 1992; Lee et al., 1991; Moosvi et al., 1992). Therefore, on the basis of clinical observations, it appears that establishing coronary arterial reperfusion in patients with single-vessel coronary disease, acute MI, and cardiogenic shock improves both short- and long-term survival.

The clinical outcome among patients with cardiogenic shock and multivessel disease who undergo PCI may not be as promising. Lee et al. (1988) reported an 83% mortality rate in patients with multivessel disease, despite successful PCI of the infarct-related coronary artery. However, in a study by Hibbard et al. (1992), 9 of 12 patients with three-vessel coronary disease survived to hospital discharge, and 47% were alive at 6-month follow-up.

Although successful PCI appears to improve survival in patients who have suffered cardiogenic shock even up to 24 hours previously, among patients with multivessel disease, reperfusion fewer than 6 hours from the onset of symptoms may be an important variable that significantly influences outcome.

The use of PCI in patients with prior coronary artery bypass grafting (CABG) and cardiogenic shock was investigated by Kahn et al. (1990). In-hospital survival for 9 to 11 patients in shock who underwent successful PCI was 64%, suggesting that coronary angioplasty should be considered in carefully selected patients.

Patients with cardiogenic shock resulting from ischemic papillary muscle dysfunction have also been treated successfully with PCI. A significant reduction in mitral regurgitation was achieved, enabling resolution of cardiogenic shock and avoiding both valve replacement and long-term anticoagulation.

In the SHOCK (Should We Emergently Revasuclarize Occluded Coronary Arteries in Cardiogenic Shock) trial (Hochman, 1999), patients receiving aggressive medical therapy (fibrinolytics and intraaortic balloon pumps) experienced a 56% mortality at 30 days compared with 47% in those who underwent revascularization (PCI or bypass surgery). Although the early outcomes did not differ by 6 months, patients less than 75 years of age undergoing immediate revascularization had lower mortality rates (48% vs. 69%).

Risk Stratification Models

A TIMI risk score was developed as a readily available means to predict 30-day mortality. The baseline variables accounted for 97% of the predictive capacity of multivariate modeling (Table 18.13). This risk score showed a greater than 40-fold graded increase in mortality, with scores ranging from 0 to greater than 8 (Morrow et al., 2000) (Figure 18.5).

Prehospital Destination Protocols

Based on available data, the ACC/AHA Guidelines for the Management of Patients with ST-Segment Elevation MI (Antman et al., 2004) recommend that each com-

Table 18.13 TIMI Risk Score for Predicting Mortality in Patients with ST-Segment Elevation MI

Age 65–74 yr . . . . 2 points
Age >75 yr . . . . 3 points
Systolic blood pressure <100 mmHg . . . . 2 points
Killip class II–IV . . . . 2 points
Anterior site of infarction or left bundle branch block . . . . 1 point
Diabetes, history of angina, or history of hypertension . . . . 1 point
Weight <67 kg . . . . 1 point
Time to treatment . . . . 1 point
  >4 hours . . . . 1 point
Risk score . . . . 0–14 possible points

MI, myocardial infarction.

munity develop a written protocol designed to guide EMS systemic personnel in rapidly triaging persons with suspected or confirmed MI.

Class I recommendations are as follows:

1.   Patients with STEMI who have cardiogenic shock and are <75 years of age should be brought immediately or secondarily transferred to facilities capable of cardiac catheterization and rapid revascularization (PCI or CABG) if it can be performed within 18 hours of shock onset.

2.   Patients with STEMI who have contraindications to fibrinolytic therapy should be brought immediately or secondarily transferred promptly (within 30 minutes) to a facility capable of cardiac catheterization and rapid revascularization.

Class IIa recommendations are as follows:

1.   Patients with cardiogenic shock who are >75 years of age should be considered for immediate or prompt secondary transfer to facilities capable of cardiac catheterization and rapid revascularization.

2.   Patients with a high risk profile, including those with severe congestive heart failure, should be considered for immediate or prompt secondary transfer (within 30 minutes) to facilities capable of cardiac catheterization and rapid revascularization.

Defining Hemorrhagic Risk for Patients Treated with Fibrinolytic and Antithrombotic Agents

One of the great challenges in clinical practice is the administration of agents that are designed to prevent or, in the case of fibrinolytic agents, remove pathologic ar-

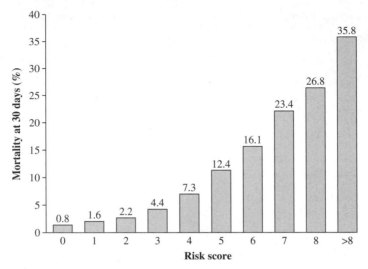

Figure 18.5 TIMI risk score for predicting 30-day mortality. (From Morrow DA, Antman EM, Charlesworth A, et al. TIMI risk score for ST-elevation myocardial infarction: a convenient, bedside, clinical score for risk assessment at presentation: an Intravenous nPA for Treatment of Infarcting Myocardium Early II trial substudy. *Circulation* 2000;102:2031–2037.)

terial thrombi without causing a profound perturbation of the hemostatic mechanism that can predispose to serious bleeding. Over the years, randomized clinical trials, large-scale registries, and widespread experience has helped define patient, clinical, and laboratory predictors of hemorrhagic risk that can be applied directly to decision making and everyday patient care.

Patient Characteristics

Patients with recognized bleeding diatheses are at increased risk for bleeding, as are those patients who have had recent surgery, major trauma invasive procedures, and existing pathology within the gastrointestinal tract (malignancy, atrioventricular [AV] malformations, polyps, peptic ulcer disease). A careful history should be obtained from all patients being considered for treatment with a fibrinolytic and/or antithrombotic agent. Interviewing family members can also be useful.

The risk of bleeding, in general, increases with patient age, and particularly with fibrinolytic therapy. Hypertension, low body weight, renal insufficiency, hepatic insufficiency, and female gender have also been associated with increased bleeding risk.

Fibrinolytic Therapy

Fibrinolytic agents, through the production of plasmin, a nonspecific protease, impair hemostasis at several specific sites. As a result, the potential for bleeding complications is increased in all patients; however, an ever-increasing lytic dose and elevated aPTT are independent risk factors (Bovill et al., 1991). Thrombocytopenia and hypofibrinogenemia also increase the likelihood of hemorrhage. Intracranial hemorrhage, the most feared and devastating bleeding complication, is associated with age greater than 65 (odds ratio 2.2), body weight less than 70 kg (odds ratio 2.1), hypertension (systolic >140 mmHg, diastolic >100 mmHg; odds ratio 2.0), and high-dose fibrin-specific fibrinolytic agents (odds ratio 1.6) (Simoons et al., 1993). Other risk factors include female gender, Black ethnicity, history of stroke, and tPA dose greater than 1.5 mg/kg (Gurwitz et al., 1998) (Table 18.14).

A major risk factor for bleeding following fibrinolytic therapy is the performance of invasive procedures, particularly coronary bypass surgery (TIMI Research Group, 1988). Although the vast majority of events occur at vascular access sites, some are sufficiently severe to require transfusions and surgical interventions.

Safety of Third-Generation Fibrinolytics

While the administration of fibrinolytic drugs (and concomitant antithrombotic agents) is associated with hemorrhagic risk, it is important to assess new drugs and strategies as they emerge. In the ASSENT-2 trial, 4.66% of patients in the tenecteplase group experienced major noncerebral bleeding, in comparison with 5.94% in the alteplase group ($p = .0002$). Independent risk factors for bleeding were older age, female sex, and lower body weight (van de Werf, 2001). Female patients greater than 75 years of age weighing less than 67 kg were at greater risk for intracranial hemorrhage; however, the overall risk was less with the tenecteplase than with alteplase treatment (1.14% vs. 3.02%).

Table 18.14 Risk Factors for Intracranial Hemorrhage with Fibrinolytic Therapy

Older age
Higher systolic blood pressure (>140 mmHg)
Higher diastolic blood pressure (>100 mmHg)
Lower body weight
Prior stroke or transient ischemic attack
Fibrin-specific fibrinolytic agent
Higher dose of fibrin-specific agent

Anticoagulants

There is an association between the intensity of anticoagulation and hemorrhagic risk in the presence or absence of concomitant fibrinolytic therapy. The relationship, as determined by the aPTT, is most clear with UFH (Granger et al., 1996) (Figure 18.6), in which values in excess of 70 seconds (at any time) are associated with the greatest overall risk (1% increased risk for every 10-second increase in aPTT). An elevated aPTT also predicts hemorrhagic risk with direct thrombin antagonists as well (Antman et al., 1994; GUSTO IIa Investigators, 1994; Neuhaus et al., 1994). The experience gained from TIMI 9A, GUSTO IIa, and HIT-3 also show that impaired renal function (with slowed clearance of hirudin) increase the risk of major hemorrhage. Point-of-care determination of the aPTT may be particularly useful, as it provides a means to rapidly identify elevated aPTT values prompting dose titration (Becker et al., 1994b). In GUSTO-1, point-of-care coagulation monitoring was associated with a reduced incidence of moderate or severe bleeding compared with central laboratory aPTT monitoring (Zabel et al., 1998).

Because low-molecular-weight heparins (LMWHs) do not prolong the aPTT to any meaningful degree, it has been difficult to establish a laboratory-based pa-

Figure 18.6 The probability of intracranial hemorrhage as a function of activated partial thromboplastin time (aPTT) in the GUSTO-1 trial. A: The risk of intracranial hemorrhage increases significantly at 12 hours after fibrinolytic therapy if the aPTT exceeds 70 seconds. B: The overall probability of intracranial hemorrhage is modestly increased 24 hours after fibrinolytic therapy, and the relationship between aPTT and its occurrence, although still present, is less robust. (From Granger CB, Hirsh J, Califf RM, et al. for the GUSTO-1 Investigators. Activated partial thromboplastin time and outcome after thrombolytic therapy for acute myocardial infarction. Results from the GUSTO-1 trial. *Circulation* 1996;93:870–878.)

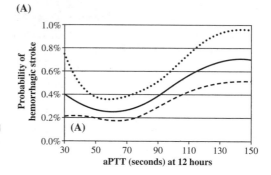

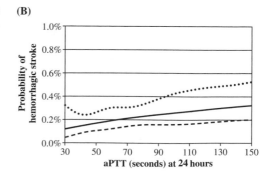

rameter that can be used to predict hemorrhagic risk. A heparin assay (Xa method) can be used to determine the intensity of anticoagulation, and levels greater than 1.5 anti-Xa U/mL have been associated with an increased risk of hemorrhage, particularly at instrumented sites (TIMI IIA Trial Investigators, 1997). In most patients, a dose of 100 anti-Xa units per kilogram of body weight yields a safe and effective level of anticoagulation; however, patients with renal insufficiency and patients of lower body weight (<60 kg) may achieve higher levels of systemic anticoagulation with standard dosing, and therefore must be observed closely. Alternatively, heparin levels can be followed with a target of 1.0 to 1.5 anti-Xa U/mL (peak level obtained 4 hours after dosing). A steady-state level of approximately 0.5 anti-Xa U/mL is considered safe and effective.

Warfarin

The intensity of anticoagulation, as determined by the INR, is strongly associated with hemorrhagic risk in warfarin-treated patients. In general, INR values greater than 4.0 increase the risk for major bleeding, particularly among patients over 65 years of age. The relationship between high-intensity anticoagulation and hemorrhage is seen in patients with a variety of thrombotic disorders, including atrial fibrillation, venous thromboembolism, and mechanical heart valve replacement.

In general, the combination of platelet antagonists and warfarin increases the risk of hemorrhage; however, this is predominantly seen with intermediate to high doses. For example, the addition of low-dose aspirin (≤100 mg) to moderate-intensity warfarin (INR 2.0–3.0) increases the risk slightly, whereas more intense treatment (higher doses of aspirin or high-intensity warfarin) is associated with much greater risk.

Platelet Antagonists

Aspirin, when given alone in doses ranging from 162 to 325 mg daily, has an acceptable safety profile with a relatively low incidence of major hemorrhagic events. A possible exception is primary prevention, in which aspirin has been associated with an increased risk of hemorrhagic stroke (relative risk 2.14; $p = .06$). Aspirin used in conjunction with fibrinolytic therapy increases the risk of minor hemorrhage and, as discussed previously, increases the risk of major hemorrhage when combined (in a dose >100 mg) with warfarin (moderate- to high-intensity anticoagulation) (Steering Committee of the Physicians' Health Study Research Group, 1989).

Ticlopidine/Clopidogrel

Ticlopidine and clopidogrel have overall safety profiles that are similar to aspirin with an increased risk of minor hemorrhage expected at currently recommended doses. Major bleeding may be encountered in the presence of profound thrombocytopenia. Ongoing clinical trails will better define the risk of combination oral platelet antagonists.

Glycoprotein IIb/IIIa Antagonists

The currently available GPIIb/IIIa antagonists (IV preparations) cause substantial platelet inhibition and, therefore, increase the risk of bleeding. With time and experience, it has become clear that bleeding risk is closely associated with heparin dose and sheath care for patients undergoing PCI. A target activated clotting time (ACT) between 200 and 250 seconds (rather than >300) reduces bleeding risk, as does early sheath removal (<12 hours) (Aguirre et al., 1995). Although the benefit of combination fibrinolytic–GPIIb/IIIa receptor antagonists therapy has not been established, the potential risk for hemorrhagic complications has been recognized (see Chapter 28).

Primary PCI for ST-Segment Elevation MI

Since 1990, coronary angioplasty has been used increasingly in the treatment of patients with acute myocardial infarction (MI). Because interventional capabilities are *not* immediately available in most hospitals, it is important to review the indications as determined by the results of large-scale registries and, more important, randomized clinical trials. Rather then being viewed as adversaries, coronary angioplasty and fibrinolysis should be considered treatment alternatives to be used as indicated to optimize patient care (see Table 18.12b).

Registry Data

The pooled data from two MI registries—the Maximal Individual TheRapy in Acute myocardial infarction (MITRA) study and the Myocardial Infarction Registry (MIR)—included 8,579 patients treated with thrombolytics and 1,327 patients who underwent primary PCI (both ≤12 hours from symptom onset). Mechanical reperfusion was associated with a 42% relative risk reduction in mortality compared with pharmacologic reperfusion (6.4% vs. 11.3%). This observation was consistent across all major risk groups and there was a significant correlation between mortality and absolute risk reduction with primary PCI (Figure 18.7) (Zahn et al., 2001).

Meta-Analysis of Randomized Trials

A total of 23 randomized trials comparing primary PCI ($n = 3,872$) and fibrinolytic therapy ($n = 3,867$) in the setting of acute ST-segment elevation MI were col-

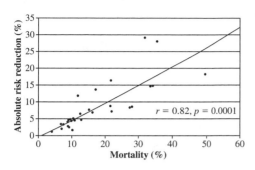

Figure 18.7 Relationship between overall mortality and absolute risk reduction of dying by treatment with primary angioplasty compared with thrombolysis in the subgroups analyzed. (From Zahn R, Schneider S, Gitt AK, et al. Primary angioplasty versus intravenous thrombolysis in acute myocardial infarction: can we define subgroups of patients benefiting most from primary angioplasty? Results from the pooled data of the maximal individual therapy in Acute Myocardial Infarction Registry and the Myocardial Infarction Registry. *J Am Coll Cardiol* 2001;37:1827–1835.)

lectively analyzed by Keeley and colleagues (2003). Primary PCI (often with coronary stenting) was more effective than fibrinolytic therapy at reducing short-term mortality (3% vs. 7%, $p = <.0001$), stroke (1% vs. 2%; $p = .0004$), and the combined endpoint of death, nonfatal reinfarction, and stroke (80% vs. 14%, $p < .0001$) (Figure 18.8a and b). Similar results were seen whether or not the patient was transferred for primary PCI.

Reperfusion Strategies in Clinical Practice

The benefit of primary angioplasty for managing patients with ST-segment elevation MI is recognized widely; however, reperfusion strategies used in clinical practice must consider the available resources and expertise, as well as opportunities to deliver optimal care.

In a meta-analysis of six clinical trials (3,750 patients) comparing immediate fibrinolysis and hospital transfer for primary angioplasty, death, reinfarction, and stroke (combined outcome) were reduced by 42%, favoring transfer-primary angioplasty. The transfer time was always less than 3 hours (Dalby et al., 2003).

Given the observations with primary angioplasty, many clinicians have questioned whether mechanical reperfusion should be offered in community hospitals (which may lack cardiac surgery programs). In the PAMI (Primary Angioplasty in Myocardial Infarction)-No SOS (Surgery on Site) study (Wharton et al., 2004), 500 patients underwent primary angioplasty at hospitals without SOS and were compared with 71 patients enrolled in the Air PAMI study (transfer for primary angioplasty).

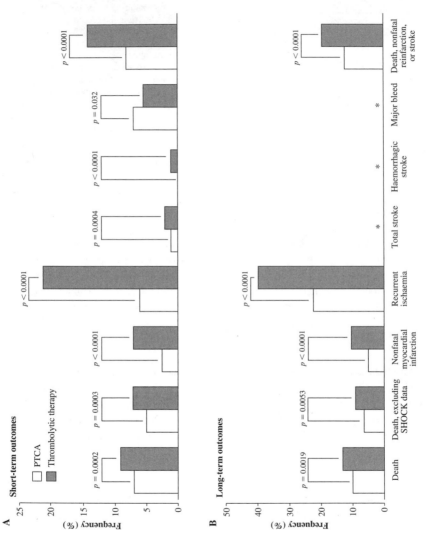

Figure 18.8 Meta-analysis of 23 randomized trials of primary percutaneous coronary intervention (PCI) vs. thrombolysis including short- (A) and long-term (B) outcomes. CVA, cerebrovascular accident. (From Keeley EC, Boura JA, Grines CL. Primary angioplasty intravenous thrombolytic therapy for acute myocardial infarction: a quantitative review of 23 randomised trials. *Lancet* 2003;361:13–20.)

Patients transferred had a longer time to treatment (187 vs. 120 minutes; $p < .0001$), lower TIMI 3 flow rates (86% vs. 96%; $p = .004$), and higher composite event rate (30-day death, reinfarction, and disabling stroke) (8.5% vs. 5%; $p = .27$) than those who underwent angioplasty on-site.

The importance of time to treatment for reperfusion strategies was investigated in the Comparison of Angioplasty and Prehospital Thrombolysis in Acute MI (CAPTIM) trial (Steg et al., 2003). A total of 834 patients were randomized to either prehospital tPA or primary angioplasty. Patients randomized within 2 hours of symptom onset had strong trends toward lower 30-day mortality with prehospital thrombolysis compared with those who underwent primary angioplasty (2.2% vs. 5.7%; $p = .058$). Prehospital treatment with reteplase (double bolus) is also a consideration (Lamfers et al., 2003).

A large-scale registry of 443 intensive care units in France, which tracked patient outcomes following ST-segment elevation MI, identified prehospital fibrinolysis as a predictor of a very high 1-year survival rate (0.52 relative risk of death compared to in-hospital fibrinolysis or primary PCI) (Danchin et al., 2004).

The overriding importance of time to reperfusion can not be overstated. Fibrinolytic therapy administered to patients less than 75 years of age and at low risk for major hemorrhagic complications within 2 hours of symptom onset is effective. Beyond 2 hours, primary angioplasty should be considered strongly, even if hospital transfer is required (assuming that the intervention can be performed within the next 120 minutes) (Tables 18.5 and 18.6).

From clinical data and expert consensus, the ACC/AHA Task Force on Practice Guidelines (Antman et al., 2004) considers primary PCI without surgical backup a class IIb recommendation to be undertaken only by experienced operators at facilities with a proven plan for rapid (and effective) PCI and rapid access to cardiac surgery at a nearby hospital.

Table 18.15 ST-Segment Elevation Myocardial Infarction (STEMI): Site-, Specialty-, and Spectrum-of-Care Strategies for Outcome-Effective Management CATH Panel SOS-ACS Guidelines and Recommendations

---

ACS CARE LEVEL: A SITE
Interventional cardiology services are available, percutaneous coronary intervention (PCI) is the dominant strategy for patients with STEMI, and coronary artery bypass graft (CABG) is available: ACS Care Level A institutions maintain cardiac catheterization facilities and skilled interventional operators capable of performing cardiac angiography and (PCI), as well as facilities for performing CABG. As a result, interventional strategies will dominate management of STEMI patients at these sites, and pharmacologic antithrombotic therapy should be consistent with this approach.

(continued)

Table 18.15 (*continued*)

Level A Site:
Emergency Department
    At ACS Care Level A site, STEMI patients should be managed with PCI as the dominant strategy. Pharmacologic stabilization and antithrombotic therapy prior to PCI should include:
- **Aspirin 162–325 mg PO**
- **UFH or enoxaparin**

If patient is to be transferred directly from the emergency department to the cardiac catheterization laboratory to undergo coronary angiography and possible PCI, the emergency physician, in consultation with the interventional cardiologist, may initiate antiplatelet therapy with the GPIIb/IIIa inhibitor abciximab in addition to the core regimen above:
- **Abciximab (0.25 mg/kg bolus IV, followed by 0.125 μcg/kg/min [max 10 μcg/min] infusion for 12 h)**

As dictated by clinical presentation and need to implement appropriate measures for acute medical management of ischemic chest pain, pulmonary edema, hypertension, and other hemodynamic abnormalities in the emergency department, the following agents may be initiated according to clinical protocols:
- Nitroglycerin IV/SC/TC/SL
- Morphine sulfate IV
- Lopressor 5 mg q5min × 3 doses

Cardiac Catheterization Laboratory/PCI
    STEMI patients should undergo invasive assessment of their coronary anatomy with the intention for PCI in cardiac catheterization laboratory. The pharmacological foundation regimen in these patients should include the following:
- **Abciximab (0.25 mg/kg bolus IV, followed by 0.125 μcg/kg/min [max 10 μcg/min] infusion for 12 h)** if not already started in the emergency department (alternative GPIIb/IIIa inhibitor for primary PCI: eptifibatide, 180 μcg/kg IV bolus × 2, 10 min apart, followed by 2.0 μcg/kg/min infusion for 18–24 hr)[1] **Plus**
- **Clopidogrel 300 mg loading dose (if stent placed)**
- **Aspirin 162–325 mg PO**
- **UFH or enoxaparin**

As dictated by clinical presentation and need to implement appropriate measures for acute management of ischemic chest pain, pulmonary edema, hypertension, and/or other hemodynamic abnormalities, adjunctive pharmacology should be employed per standard protocols.

Inpatient Care (Step-Down Unit/Coronary Care Unit/Medical Intensive Care Unit)
    After coronary angiography/PCI, the following pharmacologic agents should be continued and initiated in the coronary care unit or other inpatient setting prior to discharge:
- **Aspirin 162 mg PO QD**
- **Abciximab (continue infusion for 12 h)** (alternative GPIIb/IIIa inhibitor for primary PCI: eptifibatide, 180 μcg/kg IV bolus × 2, 10 min apart, followed by 2.0 μcg/kg/min infusion for 18–24 hr)
- **Clopidogrel 75 mg PO QD** (if coronary stent placed)

As dictated by presentation, and based on the presence of ischemic symptoms, abnormal hemodynamic parameters, cardiac risk factors, hypertension, diabetes, and/or left ventricular dysfunction, the following agents, it not continued for cardioprotection and/or management of symptoms following discharge:
- Statin therapy (within 96 h of acute ischemic event)
- Beta-blockers
- ACE inhibitors
- Maintenance nitrate therapy

ACS, acute coronary syndrome; GP, glycoprotein; UFH, unfractionated heparin.

Interventional Cardiology Consensus Reports 2003.

Table 18.16 ST-Segment Elevation Myocardial Infarction (STEMI): Site-, Specialty-, and Spectrum-of-Care Strategies for Outcome-Effective Management (*continued*) CATH Panel SOS-ACS Guidelines and Recommendations

ACS CARE LEVEL: B SITE
Medical management is the dominant strategy at ACS Care Level B site, although rapid patient transfer is possible. Level B institution or site of care has no facilities for performing percutaneous coronary intervention (PCI), although transfer of STEMI patients to an institution capable of PCI is possible or likely.

Level B Site:
Emergency Department
Medical management (fibrinolysis is dominant strategy at ACS Care Level B Site):
- **Aspirin 162–325 mg PO**
- **Enoxaparin 30 mg IV bolus followed by 1 mg/kg SC q12h** (maximum dose 100 mg SC 12 h for first 24 h)
- **Full-dose tenecteplase (TNK), weight-based dosing per package insert**
- **Alternative first-line fibrinolytic regimes:** tPA in combination with either of the following anticoagulant regimens: enoxaparin 30 mg IV bolus followed by 1 mg/kg SC 1 12 h, or unfractionated heparin (UFH) (60 U/kg bolus, followed by 12 U/gk/hr); OR rPA in combination with UFH.

As dictated by clinical presentation and need to implement appropriate measures for acute medical management of ischemic chest pain, pulmonary edema, hypertension, and other hemodynamic abnormalities in the emergency department, the following agents may be initiated according to clinical protocols:
- Nitroglycerin IV/SC/TC/SL
- Morphine sulfate IV

Inpatient Care (Step-Down Unit/Coronary Care Unit/Medical Intensive Care Unit)
If STEMI patient is not transferred to level A site, medical/fibrinolytic/antithrombotic management should be continued as follows:
- **Aspirin 162 mg PO**
- **Enoxaparin 1 mg/kg SC q12h × 7 d**
- **Consider clopidogrel therapy**

As dictated by presentation, and based on the presence of ischemic symptoms, abnormal hemodynamic parameters, cardiac risk factors, hypertension, diabetes, and/or left ventricular dysfunction, the following agents, if not contraindicated, should be considered for administration during acute hospitalization, and when indicated, these agents should be continued for cardioprotection and/or management of symptoms following discharge:
- Nitroglycerin IV/SC/TC/SL
- Morphine sulfate IV
- Statin therapy (within 96 hours of acute ischemic event)
- Beta-blockers
- ACE inhibitors

Inpatient Care (Step-Down Unit/Coronary Care Unit/Medical Intensive Care Unit)
Because ACS Level B sites do not maintain invasive cardiology capabilities, transfer of STEMI patients to an ACS Care Level A site is strongly recommended. The decision to (a) initiate immediate fibrinolysis for STEMI patients at a Level B site and then transfer or (b) facilitate immediate transfer to Level A site for catheterization/PCI without lysis will depend on timing considerations, which will vary among institutions. Although there will be exceptions, the Panel recommends that STEMI patients in whom the time from door to arrival at the B Level hospital to anticipated cath lab needle time at the Level A hospital is likely to *exceed 90 minutes*, undergo immediate fibrinolysis per protocol above at the Level B site prior to transfer.

ACS, acute coronary syndrome; rPA, reteplase; tPA, tissue plasminogen activator.

Interventional Cardiology Consensus Reports 2003.

The ACC/AHA Task Force also considers pharmacoinvasive therapy (facilitated PCI) a class IIb recommendation to be considered in high-risk patients when PCI is not immediately available and bleeding risk is low.

Process of Care Initiatives

The optimal treatment of patients with acute MI requires the frequent use of evidence-based management strategies. The national focus has evolved to include not only key indicators, but also processes of care and tool use initiatives. An ACC GAP (Guidelines Applied in Practice) project, a multifaceted intervention including kick-off presentation, customization, and implementation of care tools, local leadership, a project leader at each hospital, and grand-round site visits, was associated with MI standing orders, ACS standing orders, clinical pathway development, and MI-specific discharge form utilization, which, in turn, lead to a higher adherence to quality indicators (aspirin, angiotensin-converting enzyme inhibitors, smoking cessation, and dietary counseling) (Mehta et al., 2004).

Consideration of system-wide changes for treating patients with acute ST -segment elevation MI that adopts a strategy of community-based transfer protocols has followed several reports of improved outcomes associated with primary PCI. Despite these promising findings, several obstacles currently stand in the way of wide-scale implementation, including greater distance between community and tertiary care hospitals, an absence of integrated emergency medical services, and the medical community's limited experience with centralized acute MI care networks. The development of standardized approaches, nomenclature, and performance indicators, followed by large-scale research efforts, will be required before management can be redefined in the United States.

Summary

The available evidence suggests that, in experienced hands and medical centers, primary PCI is the safest and most effective reperfusion modality. Routine transfer to a primary angioplasty center in fibrinolytic-eligible patients is not warranted, particularly if a system to achieve an open vessel within 90 minutes is not in place. In contrast, high-risk patients may derive the greatest overall benefit from early coronary angiography and mechanical intervention. Prehospital fibrinolysis remains an area worthy of investigation. Nations, states, and communities should individually assess their resources and means to educate and provide optimal care for patients with MI. Perhaps most important, individual medical centers should have established management algorithms to facilitate safe and efficient care.

Non–ST-Segment Elevation Acute Coronary Syndromes

Patients experiencing non–ST-segment elevation ACS typically have advanced coronary artery disease (CAD) with vulnerable plaques in varying stages of development. Platelet-rich thrombi with a propensity to embolize distally to involve the coronary microvascular bed are characteristic of the disorder.

Pharmacology-Based Construct

Unfractionated Heparin

Clinical trials comparing the benefits of UFH and aspirin among patients with unstable angina and non–ST-segment elevation MI have been conducted. The first trial, performed by Théroux and colleagues (1988), compared aspirin (325 mg twice daily), UFH (5000 U bolus, 1,000 U/hr by intravenous infusion), or their combination in 479 patients. It is the only study that compared UFH (alone) and aspirin (alone) as well as combination therapy. Refractory angina occurred in 8.5%, 16.5%, and 10.7% of patients, respectively (0.47 relative risk for UFH compared with aspirin [95% confidence interval (CI), 0.21, 1 05; p = .06]). Myocardial infarction occurred in 0.9%, 3.3%, and 1.6% of patients, respectively (0.25 relative risk [95% CI, 0.03, 2.271; p = .18]), while any event was observed in 9.3%, 16.5%, and 11.5% of patients, respectively (0.52 relative risk [95% CI 0.24, 1.14; p = .10]). Serious bleeding defined as a fall in hemoglobin of 2 g or more or the need for a transfusion occurred in 1.7%, 1.7%, and 3.3% of patients, respectively. A majority of events were associated with the performance of cardiac catheterization.

The remaining trials investigated potential advantages of combination therapy (UFH plus aspirin) over aspirin monotherapy. Although not statistically different, there were consistent trends observed across each study favoring combined pharmacotherapy and its ability to reduce death or MI (combined endpoint). A pooled analysis of the ATACS (Antithrombotic Therapy in Acute Coronary Syndromes), RISC (Research Group on Instability in Coronary Artery Disease), and Théroux et al. studies yielded a relative risk of 0.44 (95% CI 021, 0.93) for death/MI, favoring combination therapy (Allison et al., 1996; Cohen et al., 1990; Cohen et al., 1994; Holdright et al., 1994; RISC Group, 1990).

Therapeutic Levels of Anticoagulation

While the pathobiology of non–ST-segment ACS is fundamentally understood, the required level of anticoagulation remains poorly defined. The challenge is multifactorial, but likely relates to inherent complexities in the pharmacokinetics and pharmacodynamics of UFH, the dynamic nature of coronary arterial thrombosis, and the use of coagulation tests designed primarily to assess hemostatic potential. In essence, current laboratory-based tests are oriented more toward the drug (and its potential to cause bleeding) than the disease.

The available evidence supports a weight-adjusted dosing regimen with UFH as a means to provide a more predictable and constant level of systemic anticoagulation. An initial bolus of 60 to 70 U/kg (maximum of 5,000 U) and initial infusion of 12–15 U/kg/hr (maximum 1,000 U/hr) titrated to a target aPTT of 50 to 75 seconds is recommended (Becker et al., 1999; Braunwald et al., 2002; Hassan et al., 1995).

A "weaning" schedule at the time of treatment completion may reduce the occurrence of rebound thrombin generation and ischemic/thrombotic events.

Low-Molecular-Weight Heparin

The original experience with LMWH (Gurfinkel et al., 1995) included 205 patients with unstable angina who were randomized to either aspirin (200 mg daily); aspirin (200 mg daily) plus UFH (5000 U bolus, 400 U/kg/day infusion); or high-dose nadroparin (214 IU/kg twice daily by SC injection) plus aspirin (200 mg daily). Patients underwent continuous ST-segment monitoring during the first 48 hours of treatment. Overall, 73% of patients receiving LMWH were free from ischemic events, compared with 39% of those receiving UFH and 40% of those given aspirin alone. There were fewer silent ischemic events in the LMWH group (18%) compared with those receiving UFH (29%) or aspirin alone (34%). Recurrent angina occurred in 9%, 26%, and 19% of patients, respectively, and MIs were not observed in LMWH-treated patients (compared with 1% in the UFH and 6% in the aspirin-alone groups). Major bleeding occurred infrequently in all treatment groups (Table 18.17).

A larger study, FRagmin during InStability in Coronary artery disease (FRISC)-1 (FRISC Study Group, 1996), included 1,506 patients with unstable angina and non–ST-segment elevation MI who were randomized to LMWH (dalteparin, 120 IU/kg body weight SC [maximum 10,000 IU] twice daily for 6 days, then 7,500 IU once daily for 35–45 days) or placebo. All patients received aspirin (300 mg first dose, 75 mg daily thereafter). Accordingly, FRISC-1 investigated the combination of LMWH plus aspirin vs. aspirin alone. The risk of death or MI was reduced by 63% at day 6. The probability of death, MI, and need for revascularization remained lower in the LMWH-treated patients at 40 days; however, little difference between groups was observed beyond the treatment period.

In the Fragmin In unstable Coronary artery disease (FRIC) study (Klein et al., 1997) 1,482 patients with unstable angina and non–ST-segment elevation MI were assigned either twice-daily weight-adjusted SC injections of LMWH (dalteparin 120 IU/kg) or dose-adjusted (target aPTT 1.5 times the control) IV UFH for 6 days (acute treatment phase). Patients randomized to UFH received a continuous infu-

Table 18.17 Trials Comparing LMWH and UFH in Patients with Non–ST-Segment Elevation Acute Coronary Syndromes

Study	No. of Patients	Study Drug	Time of Endpoints	Death / MI / Ischemic Event				Death / MI			
				LMWH, %	UFH, %	RRR%	p Value	LMWH, %	UFH, %	RRR, %	p Value
FRISC	1,482	Dalteparin	Day 6	9.3	7.6	(22)	0.25	3.9	3.6	(9)	0.76
			Days 6–45	12.3	12.3	(0)	0.99	4.3	4.7	8	0.76
ESSENCE	3,171	Enoxaparin	Day 14	16.6	19.8	16	0.02	4.9	6.1	19	0.15
			Day 30	19.8	23.3	15	0.02	6.2	6.7	19	0.108
TIMI 11B	3,910	Enoxaparin	Day 14	14.2	16.7	15	0.03	5.7	6.9	18	0.11
			Day 43	17.3	19.7	12	0.051	7.9	8.9	11	0.28
FRAXIS	2,357	Nadroparin	Day 14	17.8	18.1	1	0.88	5.3	4.5	(18)	0.37
			Day 90	26.2	22.2	(18)	0.028	8.6	7.9	(10)	0.5
All trials											
Test of heterogeneity			Early[†]	15.0	16.6	10	0.02	5.1	5.7	10	0.21
							0.135				0.298
Test of heterogeneity			Late[‡]	19.5	20.5	5	0.18	7.2	7.8	9	0.21
							0.006				0.453

*Numbers in bracket indicate an increase in relative risk.
†Early endpoints: death/MI/ischemic event 95% CI, 2–17; death/MI 95% CI, (6) to 23.
‡Late endpoints: death/MI/ischemic event 95% CI, (2) to 12; death/MI 95% CI, (5) to 20.
CI, confidence interval; LMWH, low-molecular-weight heparin; MI, myocardial infarction; RRR, relative risk reduction; UFH, unfractionated heparin.

sion for at least 48 hours and were given the option of either continuing the infusion or changing to an SC regimen (12,500 U every 12 hours). In the double-blind comparison that took place from days 6 to 45 (prolonged treatment phase), patients received either LMWH (dalteparin, 7500 IU SC once daily) or placebo. Aspirin (75–165 mg/day) was started in all patients as early as possible after hospital admission and continued throughout the study. During the first 6 days, the rate of death, recurrent angina, and MI was 7.6% in the UFH-treated patients and 9.3% in the LMWH-treated patients (relative risk 1.18; 95% CI 0.84–1.66). Revascularization was required in 5.3% and 4.8%, respectively (CI 0.57–1.35). Between days 6 and 45, the composite endpoint was reached in 12.3% of patients in both the LMWH and placebo groups.

The Efficacy and Safety of subcutaneous Enoxaparin in Non-Q Wave Coronary Events (ESSENCE) trial (Cohen et al., 1997) randomly assigned 3,171 patients with angina at rest or non–ST-segment elevation MI to either LMWH (enoxaparin, 1 mg/kg SC twice daily) or IV UFH (target aPTT 55–85 seconds). Therapy was continued for a minimum of 48 hours (maximum 8 days). All patients received aspirin (100–325 mg daily). The median duration of therapy for both groups was 2.6 days. At 14 days the risk of death, recurrent angina, or MI was 16.6% among patients receiving LMWH and 19.8% for patients given UFH (16% risk reduction). A similar risk reduction (15.0%) for the composite outcome was observed at 30 days. The benefit of LMWH treatment was maintained at 1 year (Antman et al., 2002).

The TIMI 11B study compared enoxaparin and UFH in 3,910 patients with unstable angina and non–ST-segment elevation MI (Antman and the TIMI 11B Investigators, 1999). The trial design had several unique features compared with ESSENCE. First, enoxaparin therapy was initiated with a 30-mg IV bolus, followed by 1.0 mg/kg SC twice daily. Second, UFH treatment was given according to a weight-adjusted dosing strategy (70 U/kg bolus, followed by 15 U/kg/hr infusion to a target aPTT 1.5–2.5 times control). Lastly, there was an out-of-hospital treatment phase comparing enoxaparin and placebo for approximately 6 weeks (patients ≥65 kg received <60 mg SC bid; those <65 kg received 45 mg SC bid for a total of 43 days). Treatment with enoxaparin was associated with a significant reduction in the composite outcome of death, MI, or urgent revascularization compared with UFH at day 14 (14.2% vs. 16.7%; relative risk reduction 15%; $p = .03$). Continued treatment beyond the initial hospital phase did not provide added benefit (17.3% vs. 19.7%; relative risk reduction 12%; $p = .051$).

A meta-analyses of the ESSENCE and TIMI 11B trials, totaling 7,081 patients with non–ST-segment elevation ACS, revealed a 20% reduction in the risk of any ischemic event (Antman et al., 1999) favoring enoxaparin over UFH. The differences were statistically significant at 48 hours and 43 days. The combined endpoint of death or MI was reduced by 20% at 48 hours ($p = .02$) and 18% at 43 days ($p = .02$).

A significant treatment benefit for enoxaparin on the rate of death, nonfatal MI, or urgent revascularization was observed at 1 year (hazard ratio 0.88; $p = .008$; absolute difference 2.5%). A progressively greater treatment benefit was observed as the level of patient risk at baseline increased.

Combined Pharmacology and Interventional Strategies

The FRISC II study (FRISC II Investigators, 1999) included 2,267 patients with unstable coronary disease who received 5 days of dalteparin (120 IU/kg SC q12h) and were then randomized to either an invasive or conservative treatment strategy. In a separate randomization, patients received either dalteparin (5,000 to 7,500 IU SC q12h) or placebo injections for 3 months. By 30 days there was a significant reduction in death or MI favoring dalteparin-treated patients (3.1% vs. 5.9%; $p = .002$). The benefit declined over the next 2 months. An invasive strategy (coronary angiography and revascularization) was associated with a significant reduction in death or MI at 6 months compared with ischemia-driven revascularization (9.4% vs. 12.1%; $p = .03$). The mortality rates were 1.9% and 2.9%, respectively (FRISC II Investigators, 1999). At 24-month follow-up, there were reductions in mortality (3.7% vs. 12.7%; risk ratio 0.72; $p = .005$) and the composite endpoint of death or MI (12.1% vs. 16.3%; risk ratio 0.74; $p = .003$) in the invasive compared with the noninvasive group. The need for repeat hospitalizations and late revascularization procedures was lower with an early invasive strategy as well (Lagreqvist et al., 2002).

The Randomized Intervention Trial of unstable Angina (RITA) study randomized 1,810 patients with non–ST-segment elevation ACS who received enoxaparin (1 mg/kg SC twice daily for 2 to 8 days) and aspirin to either an early intervention or conservative strategy (Fox et al., 2002). At 4 months, 9.6% of patients randomized to early intervention had either died, experienced an MI, or experienced refractory angina compared with 14.5% in the conservative group (risk ratio 0.66; 95% CI 0.51, 0.85; $p = .001$). Death or MI was similar in both treatment groups at 1 year (7.6% vs. 8.3%, respectively; risk ratio 0.91; 95% CI 0.67, 1.25; $p = .58$). Fewer patients undergoing early intervention experienced symptoms of angina or required antianginal medications.

In the Superior Yield of the New Strategy of Enoxaparin, Revascularization and Glycoprotein IIb/IIIa Inhibitors (SYNERGY) trial (Ferguson et al., 2004), 10,027 high-risk patients were randomized to UFH or enoxaparin. Overall, 92% of patients underwent coronary angiography, 47% had PCI (in-hospital), and 57% received GPIIb/IIIa antagonists. The primary endpoint of death or nonfatal MI at 30 days occurred in 14.5% of patients assigned to UFH and 14.0% of those given enoxaparin (odds ratio [OR] 0.956; 95% CI 0.869–1.063), fulfilling the noninferiority criteria. There were no differences in ischemic events during PCI between the antithrombins. Major bleeding was modestly increased with enoxaparin; however, transfusion rates did not differ and there was a relationship between advancing age, reduced creatinine clearance, and risk of hemorrhage.

The SYNERGY trial supports enoxaparin as an alternative to UFH in high-risk patients managed aggressively. The impact of age and renal insufficiency on bleeding risk is important and should stimulate further investigation of preferred dosing strategies.

LMWH and Platelet GPIIb/IIIa Receptor Antagonist Combination Therapy

A summary of clinical trials investigating combination therapy with a LMWH preparation and GPIIb/IIIa receptor antagonist appears in Table 18.18a and 18.18b (Cohen et al., 2002; Ferguson et al., 2003; Goodman et al., 2003; GUSTO IV Investigators, 2002; Mukherjee et al., 2002).

The effective level of factor Xa inhibition has not been determined for patients with ACS receiving LMWH. The available information, derived from clinical trials of PCI, shows that anti-Xa activity greater than 0.5 IU/mL is associated with a low incidence of ischemic/thrombotic and hemorrhagic events (Collet et al., 2001; TIMI 11A Investigators, 1997). Coagulation tests, including traditional aPTT and ACT assays, may provide some insight for LMWH preparations characterized by low anti-Xa–anti-IIa activity (Marmur et al., 2003).

The potential benefit of enoxaparin (1 mg/kg every 12 hours) and the platelet GPIIb/IIIa receptor antagonist tirofiban (10 mg/kg bolus, 0.1 mg/kg/min for a minimum of 48 hours), compared with weight-adjusted UFH and tirofiban, was investigated in the A to Z trial (Blazing et al., 2004)—a prospective, open-label, randomized study of 3,987 patients with non–ST-segment elevation ACS. Death, recurrent MI, or refractory ischemia at 7 days occurred in 8.4% of enoxaparin-treated patients and 9.4% of those receiving UFH (hazard ratio 0.88) (criteria for noninferiority satisfied). The risk reductions were of larger magnitude (favoring enoxaparin) among patients at highest risk and those treated conservatively.

Major bleeding was more common in patients receiving enoxaparin (0.9% vs. 0.4% with UFH; one excess major hemorrhagic event for every 200 patients treated); however, transfusion rates were low overall (0.9%) and did not differ between groups.

A systematic evaluation of clinical trials comparing enoxaparin and UFH for the treatment of ACS was conducted by Petersen and colleagues (2004). A total of six trials including 21,946 patients was analyzed and revealed a statistically significant reduction in the combined 30-day endpoint of death or MI, favoring enoxaparin (10.1% vs. 11.0%; OR 0.91). Patients receiving no pretreatment antithrombin therapy were found to have a particularly robust benefit from enoxaparin (8.0%

vs. 9.4%; OR 0.81). Major hemorrhage and blood transfusion rates did not differ between treatment groups.

Influence of Renal Function

Factor Xa inhibition pharmacokinetics were studied in 445 patients receiving enoxaparin (1.0–1.25 mg/kg SC q12h) (Becker et al., 2002). The mean apparent clearance, distribution volume, and plasma half-life were 0.733 L/hr, 5.24 L, and 5 hours, respectively. Creatinine clearance (CrCl) emerged as the most important factor affecting apparent clearance, area under the curve, and anti-Xa activity. Clearance was reduced by 22% in patients with CrCl less than or equal to 40 mL/min (compared to patients with normal renal performance [CrCl >80 mL/min]). These patients had higher peak and trough anti-Xa activity and were also more likely to experience major hemorrhagic events. Renal performance may not influence pharmacokinetics following single-dose intravenous administration of enoxaparin. Studies evaluating appropriate dosing and possible dose titration in patients with end-stage renal disease must be undertaken to provide guidance in achieving optimal (safe and effective) patient care.

Indirect, Selective Factor Xa Inhibitors

Synthetic Pentasaccharide

Fondaparinux is currently approved by the Food and Drug Administration (FDA) for prophylaxis of deep vein thrombosis (DVT) (which may lead to pulmonary embolism) in patients undergoing hip fracture surgery, hip replacement surgery, or knee replacement surgery. Its use in patients with non–ST-segment elevation ACS has been investigated in a phase II study. In the PENTasaccharide in Unstable Angina (PENTUA) study (Simoons et al., 2004), 1,147 patients were randomized to receive either enoxaparin (1 mg/kg SC bid) or fondaparinux (2.5 mg, 4 mg, 8 mg, or 12 mg SC daily) for 3 to 7 days. The primary efficacy endpoint was a composite of death, MI, or recurrent ischemia at 9 days. The composite endpoint was reached in 35.7%, 27.9%, 35.9%, 34.7%, and 30.3%, respectively ($p = $ ns), and major and minor bleeding (day 30) occurred in 3.9%, 5.4%, 5.4%, 4.6%, and 4.8% of patients, respectively. The lowest event rates were observed in the 2.5-mg fondaparinux group. A large phase 3 study (OASIS [Organization to Assess Strategies for Ischemic Syndromes]-5) showed that fondaparinux (2.5 mg) was not inferior to enoxaparin and caused less major hemorrhage (European Society of Cardiology, Stockholm, September 2005).

Table 18.18a Trials Investigating the Combined Administration of Low-Molecular-Weight Heparin and a Platelet GPIIb/IIIa Receptor Antagonist for Treatment of Non–ST-Segment Elevation Acute Coronary Syndromes

Trial*	LMWH Group			Control Group			Duration of Therapy	Primary Efficacy Outcome
	No. of Subjects	Drug	Dose	No. of Subjects	Drug	GPIIb/IIIa		
ACUTE II	315	Enoxaparin	SC 1 mg/kg twice daily	210	UFH	Tirofiban	24–96 h	Death/MI urgent revascularization
NICE 3	671	Enoxaparin	SC 1 mg/kg twice daily	...	...	Tirofiban Abciximab Eptifibatide	24–h	Death/MI urgent revascularization
GUSTO IV Dalteparin Substudy	646†	Dalteparin	SC 120 IU/kg twice daily	4,556‡	UFH	Abciximab	5–7 d	Death/ MI
INTERACT	380	Enoxaparin	SC 1 mg/kg twice daily	366	UFH	Integrilin	≥48 h	Death/MI
PARAGON-B	411	LMWH§	Not specified	2,205	UFH	Lamifiban	≥3 d	Death/MI urgent revascularization

*Major bleeding definitions were TIMI Major for all trials, except PARAGON-B, which used intracranial hemorrhage or bleeding that caused hemodynamic compromise and required intervention.

†Of this number, 315 patients received abciximab for 24 h and 331 patients received abciximab for 48 h.

‡Of this number, 2,275 patients received abciximab for 24 h and 2,281 patients received abciximab for 48 h.

§The type of LMWH was not mandated by protocol.

GP, glycoprotein; LMWH, low-molecular-weight heparin; MI, myocardial infarction; UFH, unfractionated heparin; ellipses indicate no control group.

Table 18.18b Clinical Efficacy and Major Non-CABG Bleeding in Trials Combining Low-Molecular-Weight Heparin and GPIIb/IIIa Inhibitor Combination for the Treatment of Unstable Angina/Non–ST-Segment Elevation MI

	Treatment Effect (%)				Major Non-CABG Bleeding (%)			
Trial*	Timing of Efficacy Outcome	LMWH	Control	Absolute Risk Difference	Timing of Efficacy Outcome	LMWH	Control	Absolute Risk Difference
ACUTE II	In hospital	9.2	9.0	0.2	30 d	0.3	1.0	-0.7
NICE 3	30 d	11.6[†]	...	...	30 d	1.9*	...	...
GUSTO IV	30 d	9.6	8.5	1.1	7 d	1.2	0.7	0.5
Dalteparin Substudy[‡]								
INTERACT	30 d	10.1	11.8	-1.7	96 h	1.8	4.6	-2.8 ($p = 0.03$)
PARAGON B	30 d	10.2	12.1	-1.9	30 d	1.5	1.6	-0.1

*The LMWH values for major non-CABG bleeding are: 0.8 for abciximab; 2.6 for eptifibatide; and 1.7 for tirofiban.

[†]Analysis of all patients who completed treatment with enoxaparin and any glycoprotein IIb/IIIa inhibitor.

[‡]Analysis performed with the abciximab 24-h and 48-h groups combined.

CABG, coronary artery bypass graft; GP, glycoprotein; LMWH, low-molecular-weight heparin; MI, myocardial infarction; ellipses indicate no control group.

In a pilot trial (Vullemenot et al., 1999), 61 patients undergoing PCI received a single, 5-minute intravenous infusion of 12 mg of pentasaccharide. Two patients (3.28%, 95% CI 0.4%, 11.4%) experienced abrupt vessel closure. ACT and aPTT measurements remained within the normal range; however, thrombin–antithrombin complex, prothrombin fragment 1.2, and factor VIIa levels decreased by 50% to 60% from baseline to 2 hours following injection of the test drug. There were no major hemorrhagic events.

Direct Thrombin Inhibitors

Direct thrombin inhibitors were developed to overcome several limitations of heparin compounds, which include platelet-activating properties, complex pharmacokinetics (with UFH), and an inability of the heparin–antithrombin complex to inactivate fibrin-bound thrombin.

Hirudin (Lepirudin)

In the GUSTO IIB trial (GUSTO IIB Investigators, 1996), patients with non–ST-segment elevation ACS received either UFH or hirudin (0.1 mg/kg IV bolus, 0.1 mg/kg/hr infusion). At 24 hours the risk of death or nonfatal MI was reduced in hirudin-treated patients (1.3% vs. 2.1%; $p = .001$). The primary endpoint of death or nonfatal MI at 30 days was reached in 8.9% and 9.8% of patients, respectively (odds ratio 0.89; $p = .006$). The risk of moderate bleeding was increased with hirudin treatment (8.8% vs. 7.7%; $p = .03$).

The OASIS-1 study (OASIS Investigators, 1997) included 909 patients with unstable angina or suspected MI without ST-segment elevation who were randomized to receive UFH (5,000-U bolus, 1,000–1,200 U/hr infusion), low-dose hirudin (0.2 mg/kg bolus, 0.1 mg/kg/hr infusion), or moderate-dose hirudin (0.4 mg/kg bolus, 0.15 mg/kg/hr infusion). Doses of UFH and hirudin were titrated to a target aPTT of 60 to 100 seconds. Hirudin, compared with UFH, reduced the composite incidence of cardiovascular death, MI, or refractory angina at 7 days (OR 0.57; 95% CI 0.32, 1.02) and a composite of death, MI, or refractory/severe angina requiring revascularization at 7 days (OR 0.49; 95% CI 0.27, 0.86). Overall event rates were lowest in the moderate-dose hirudin group.

The favorable results in OASIS-1 prompted a large phase III trial, OASIS-2 (OASIS-2 Investigators, 1999), which randomized 10,141 patients with non–ST-segment elevation ACS to a 72-hour infusion of either moderate-dose hirudin (as defined in OASIS-1) or UFH. The primary outcome (composite of death or MI at

7 and 35 days) was reported in 3.6% and 4.2% of patients (OR 0.87; 95% CI 0.75, 1.01), respectively. Although statistically significant differences between groups were not observed, the combined OASIS-1 and OASIS-2 experience revealed a significant reduction in the likelihood of death or MI at 35 days among hirudin-treated patients (OR 0.86; 95% CI 0.74–0.99).

Hirudin is almost exclusively excreted through the kidneys and, as a result, renal function must be considered carefully prior to administration. A majority of clinical trials excluded patients with a creatine of 2.0 mg/dL or greater. It is important to acknowledge that even in the setting of mild renal impairment (CrCl 50–80 mL/min) excessive levels of systemic anticoagulation (and accompanying risk for hemorrhage) can occur with nonmodified dosing. If hirudin is administered to patients with renal insufficiency, frequent aPTT monitoring is highly recommended.

Bivalirudin

Bivalirudin is FDA approved for use in patients with non–ST-segment elevation ACS undergoing PCI. The basis for approval stems from several large-scale clinical trials, the largest performed by Bittl et al. (1995). Among 4,312 patients with new-onset, severe, accelerating, or rest angina undergoing PCI, a 22% reduction in death, MI, or urgent revascularization at 7 days was observed in those given bivalirudin compared with UFH (6.2 vs. 7.9%, $p = .03$). The absolute and relative differences were maintained at 90 days. A marked reduction (62%) in bleeding complications among bivalirudin-treated patients was also reported.

In the Randomized Evaluation in Percutaneous coronary intervention Linking Angiomax to reduced Clinical Events (REPLACE)-1 trial (Lincoff et al., 2002), 1,020 patients received either bivalirudin (0.75 mg/kg bolus, 1.75 mg/kg/hr infusion) or UFH. Prior treatment with aspirin and a thienopyridine was encouraged in anticipation of stenting. A platelet GPIIb/IIIa receptor antagonist was administered to 71% of patients. Bivalirudin was associated with a 19% reduction in the clinical endpoint of death, MI, urgent revascularization, and bleeding complications (minor, major, transfusions) at 48 hours.

REPLACE-2 (Lincoff et al., 2003) randomized 6,010 patients undergoing urgent or elective PCI to bivalirudin plus provisional GPIIb/IIIa receptor antagonist (abciximab or eptifibatide) administration or UFH plus a GPIIb/IIIa receptor antagonist. Aspirin and clopidogrel pre-treatment were recommended. Approximately 45% of patients had either unstable angina or MI (within the prior 7 days). The composite of death, MI, and urgent revascularization at 30 days occurred in 7.1% of heparin- and 7.6% of bivalirudin-treated patients (OR 0.917, 95% CI 0.772, 1.089; $p = .32$). Major bleeding was documented in 4.1% and 2.4% of patients, respectively ($p = .001$). Minor bleeding (25.7% vs. 13.4%; $p = .001$) and thrombocytopenia ($<$1000,000/mm^3) (1.7% vs. 0.7%, p $<$.001) were also less common with bivalirudin treatment. GPIIb/IIIa receptor antagonist therapy was given to 7.2% of bivalirudin-treated patients.

Impact of Renal Insufficiency

Patients with moderate and severe renal impairment have reductions in bivalirudin clearance of 45% and 68%, respectively. An analysis of data derived from 4,312 patients with unstable angina showed increased bleeding risk for both bivalirudin- and UFH-treated patients with progressive degrees of renal insufficiency. The incidence of major bleeding was, however, consistently less for bivalirudin than UFH at all levels of renal impairment (Bittl et al., 1995).

The overall data suggest that a bivalirudin dose adjustment is indicated for patients with moderate or severe renal impairment. The encouraging results from REPLACE-2 may provide an opportunity for reducing hemorrhagic risk in patients with renal insufficiency by virtue of the short infusion length for bivalirudin administration and provisional use of GPIIb/IIIa receptor antagonists (which may themselves increase the risk of hemorrhage in this high-risk patient subset).

Argatroban

Argatroban, like the other intravenous univalent direct thrombin antagonists inogatran and efegatran, has not undergone phase III testing in ACS. Its use in the management of heparin-induced thrombocytopenia during PCI will be discussed in Chapter 29.

Comparative Benefits of Direct Thrombin Inhibitors

A meta-analysis of clinical trials was performed to obtain additional information and precise estimates of direct thrombin inhibitors in the management of ACS (Direct Thrombin Inhibitor Trialists' Collaborative Group, 2002). A total of 11 randomized trials including 35,970 patients were identified. Compared with UFH, direct thrombin inhibitors were associated with a lower risk of death or MI at the end of treatment (up to 7 days) (4.3% vs. 5.1%, odds ratio 0.85; 95% CI 0.77, 0.94; p = .001) and at 30 days (7.4% vs. 8.2%; odds ratio 0.91; 95% CI 0.84, 0.99; p = .02). There were seven trials, including 30,154 patients with either ACS (unstable angina or non–ST-segment elevation MI) or who were undergoing PCI. In those with ACS, treatment with a direct thrombin inhibitor was associated with a reduction in death or MI compared with UFH (3.7% vs. 4.6%; odds ratio 0.80;

95% CI 0.70, 0.92). Similar reductions were observed in PCI trials (3.0% vs. 3.8%; odds ratio 0.79; 95% CI 0.59, 1.06). There was a statistically insignificant increased rate of major bleeding with direct thrombin inhibitors in trials of ACS (1.6% vs. 1.4%; odds ratio 1.11; 95% CI 0.93, 1.34), but there was a significant difference in PCI trials (3.7% vs. 7.6%; odds ratio 0.46; 95% CI 0.36, 0.59). There were no differences in the rates of intracranial hemorrhage.

The risk reduction in death or MI at the end of treatment was similar in trials comparing hirudin or bivalirudin with UFH, but there was a slight excess with univalent inhibitors (4.7% vs. 3.5%; odds ratio 1.35; 95% CI 0.89, 2.05). When major bleeding outcomes were analyzed by agent, hirudin was associated with an excess of major bleeding compared with UFH (1.7% vs. 1.3%; odds ratio 1.28; 95% CI 1.06, 1.55); whereas both bivalirudin (4.2% vs. 9.0%; odds ratio 0.55; CI 0.34, 0.56) and univalent inhibitors (0.7% vs. 1.3%; odds ratio 0.55; 95% CI 0.25, 1.20) were associated with lower rates of major bleeding.

Oral Direct Thrombin Inhibitors

The Efficacy and Safety of the oral direct thrombin inhibitor ximelagatran in patients with recent myocardial damage (ESTEEM) trial was a placebo-controlled, randomized investigation of 1,900 patients with MI (ST-segment elevation or non–ST-segment elevation, 44% of patients) who received 6 months of treatment with either ximelagatran (24, 36, 48, or 60 mg bid) or placebo (Wallentin et al., 2003). All patients received aspirin (160 mg daily). Oral ximelagatran significantly reduced the composite primary outcome of death (all-cause), nonfatal reinfarction, and severe recurrent ischemia (16.3% vs. 12.7%; hazard ratio 0.76%; 95% CI 0.59–0.98; $p = .03$). A dose response for efficacy was not observed; however, major bleeding, which overall was rare (1.8% in combined ximelagatran group), increased with increasing dose. Elevated hepatic transaminases occurred in approximately 6% of patients receiving ximelagatran with an increased occurrence observed with doses of 36 mg and above (up to 13.0% incidence). There were no cases of irreversible hepatic toxicity. Ximelagatran is not FDA approved for use in patients with ACS.

Fibrinolytic Therapy

Fibrinolytic therapy, although a standard of care for patients with acute coronary occlusion and ST-segment elevation, is contraindicated in the setting of non–ST-segment elevation. ACS is associated with recurrent MI and cardiovascular death (TIMI IIIB Investigators, 1994).

Clinical Constructs

Chest pain is a common complaint among individuals seeking medical care, numbering similar visits yearly in the United States. Although many upon subsequent evaluation do not have heart-related illnesses, nearly 2 million hospital admissions per year are attributed to ACS.

Patient Characteristics

The signs and symptoms of ACS vary considerably; however, a diagnostic approach should include several specific components: (1) the likelihood of underlying coronary artery disease, (2) the presenting history, (3) the 12-lead ECG, and (4) cardiac biomarker determination.

Determining the Probability of Coronary Artery Disease

Risk Factors

Individuals who have one or more traditional risk factors for atherosclerotic CAD or who have previously documented disease (prior MI; coronary angiography with one or more vessels containing a stenosis of ≥70%; revascularization procedure—prior bypass surgery or PCI) are four to five times more likely to be experiencing myocardial ischemia when they present to the hospital with chest pain than those without existing risk factors or previously documented disease.

Electrocardiogram

The surface 12-lead ECG represents an important "first-line" diagnostic test in evaluating patients with suspected myocardial ischemia. It is designed to complement the history and physical examination, providing information that carries considerable predictive value when employed serially in the context of high pretest likelihood of myocardial ischemia (Table 18.19) (Braunwald et al., 2002). Although a normal ECG does not fully exclude a diagnosis of unstable angina or non–ST-elevation MI, the diagnosis should be questioned when serial tracings performed during symptoms remain normal or unchanged. Nevertheless, if the suspicion for myocardial ischemia remains high, observation, biochemical testing, and additional diagnostic testing should be undertaken.

Table 18.19 Patient Characteristics and Electrocardiographic Features Useful in Determining the Probability of Myocardial Ischemia

High probability if:
Known history of myocardial infarction or angina
Male ≥60 or female ≥70 yr of age
Variant angina (coronary vasospasm)
Symmetric T-wave inversion in multiple leads
ST-segment elevation or depression ≥0.5 mm (in two or more leads)
Hypertension, hypercholesterolemia, smoking, family history of coronary artery disease (any combination of these with diabetes mellitus)
Hemodynamic change or electrocardiographic changes during chest pain
Intermediate probability if:
Male <60 or female <70 yr of age
History of peripheral vascular disease
ST-segment depression <0.5 mm (in two or more leads)
T-wave inversion ≥1 mm in leads with dominant R waves
At least two positive risk factors (excluding diabetes mellitus)
Low probability if:
Atypical chest pain
One risk factor (but *not* diabetes mellitus)
Normal electrocardiogram (during symptoms)
Normal physical examination
T-wave flattening or inversion <1 mm in leads with dominant R wave
Age <35 yr for males or <45 yr for females

Risk Stratification

The TIMI Risk Score has emerged as a simple, useful tool for identifying patients at risk for adverse outcomes as well as determining those deriving greatest benefit from GPIIb/IIIa receptor antagonists and an early interventional approach to management (Table 18.20). In general, the higher the TIMI Risk Score is, the greater is the incidence of death, MI, or urgent revascularization, ranging from 4.7% in patients with a score of 0 to 49% in those with a score exceeding 5.

Cardiac Biomarkers

Troponins

Maximum serum levels of troponin T or troponin I are associated with MI and cardiovascular death among patients with non–ST-segment elevation ACS (Antman et al., 1996; Ohman et al., 1996). Because of the lag period for elevation, determinations at 6 and 12 hours from symptom onset are recommended. High sensitivity assays offer diagnostic prognostic, and specific management insights into patients with ele-

Table 18.20 TIMI Risk Score

Age >65 yr of age
Documented coronary stenosis >50% (or prior coronary angiogram)
Three or more cardiac risk factors (age, sex, family history, hyperlipidemia, smoking, hypertension, diabetes mellitus, obesity)
Use of aspirin in the preceding 24 h
ST-segment deviation (transient elevation or persistent depression)
Elevated cardiac biomarkers (CK-MB, troponin)

vated troponin levels who derive particular benefit from GPIIb/IIIa receptor antagonists and early coronary intervention.

C- Reactive Protein

Elevations in C-reactive protein among patients with unstable angina are associated with an increased risk of short- and long-term cardiovascular events including death (Mueller et al., 2002).

CD40L

CD40 signaling in endothelial and smooth muscle cells, monocytes, and platelets promotes a wide variety of proatherogenic and prothrombotic functions in vitro and in vivo. Among patients with non–ST-segment elevation ACS, higher levels of soluble CD40L (a plasma form) identify patients at increased risk for death/MI and the composite outcome of death, MI, or congestive heart failure over the subsequent 10 months (Varo et al., 2003).

Approach to Patients with Non–ST-Segment Elevation ACS

The overall clinical approach to patients with non–ST-segment elevation ACS is summarized to Tables 18.21 and 18.22.

The ACC/AHA recommendations for anticoagulant therapy and antiplatelet therapy are provided in Tables 18.23 and 18.24, respectively.

Conclusions

ACS represents a major clinical manifestation of atherosclerotic coronary artery disease. The development of management guidelines has provided a readily available means to both standardize and achieve optimal care.

Table 18.21 Non ST-Segment Elevation Myocardial Infarction Acute Coronary Syndrome (NSTE-ACS) Site-, Specialty-, and Spectrum-of-Care Strategies for Outcome-Effective Management *CATH Clinical Consensus Panel Guidelines and Recommendations*

ACS CARE LEVEL: A SITE
Interventional cardiology services are available at ACS Care Level A site; revascularization percutaneous coronary intervention [PCI] or coronary artery bypass grafting [CABG] is dominant strategy for appropriately selected ACS patients. ACS care Level A institutions maintain cardiac catheterization facilities and skilled interventional operators capable of performing cardiac catheterization and PCI as well as facilities for performing CABG. As a result, interventional strategies will dominate management of NSTE-ACS patients, and pharmacologic antithrombotic therapy should be considered with this approach.

Level A Site:
Emergency Department
Initiate risk stratification and pharmacologic antithrombotic management
High-risk features present: NSTE-ACS patient with high-risk features and/or treatment-triggered criteria will benefit from an interventional strategy, which is the evidence-based management option of choice for this subgroup of ACS patients. The antithrombotic regimen for NSTE-ACS patients for whom coronary angiographic is planned should include:
- **Aspirin 162–325 mg PO** (immediately)
- **Clopidogrel 300-mg loading dose** (only if it is confirmed that the patient is not a CABG candidate; if CABG is possible, clopidogrel should be withheld until coronary anatomy is defined at time to catheterization)
- **Enoxaparin 30-mg IV bolus** (optional) **followed by 1 mg/kg q12h** (alternative: UFH)

As dictated by clinical presentation and need to implement appropriate measures for acute medical management of ischemic chest pain, pulmonary edema, hypertension, and other hemodynamic abnormalities in the emergency department, the following agents may be initiated according to clinical protocols:
- Nitroglycerin IV/SC/TC/SL
- Morphine sulfate IV   **PLUS** *(GPIIb/IIIa inhibitor)*

If patient is admitted from the emergency department to the hospital and it is anticipated that cardiac catheterization will be performed during the hospitalization, the emergency physician, in consultation with the interventional cardiologist, may initiate antiplatelet therapy with the GPIIb/IIIa receptor antagonist eptifibatide which should be added to the core regimen above:
- **Eptifibatide 180 μg/kg IV bolus, followed by 2.0 μg/kg/min infusion for 18–72 h** (alternative: tirofiban 0.4 μg/kg loading dose, followed by 0.1 μg/kg/min infusion for 48 h

OR

If patient is transferred directly from the emergency department to the cardiac catheterization laboratory to undergo cardiac catheterization for evaluation of coronary architecture and possible PCI, abciximab may be administered in the cardiac catheterization laboratory.
- **Abciximab (0.25 mg/kg bolus IV, followed by 0.125 μg/kg/min [max 10 μg/min] infusion for 12 h)** (alternative GPIIb/IIIa inhibitor for primary PCI: eptifibatide 180 μg/kg IV bolus × 2, 10 min apart, followed by 2.0 μg/kg/min infusion for 18–72 h)

No high-risk features present: For the NSTE-ACS patient who does not have high-risk features or treatment-triggered criteria supporting inclusion of small molecule GPIIb/IIIa receptor antagonist, and in whom cardiac catheterization is not planned, initial management would include:
- **Aspirin 162–325 mg PO QD**
- **Clopidogrel 300 loading dose**
- **Enoxaparin 30 mg IV bolus (optional[1]) followed by 1 mg/kg SC q12h** (alternative: UFH)

As dictated by clinical presentation and need to implement appropriate measures for acute medical management of ischemic chest pain, pulmonary edema, hypertension, and other hemodynamic abnormalities in the emergency department, the following agents may be initiated according to clinical protocols:
- Nitroglycerin IV/SC/TC/SL
- Morphine sulfate IV

(continued)

Table 18.21 (*continued*)

In-Patient Care (Step-Down, Coronary Care/Medical Intensive Care Unit
  Postcardiac catheterization
  In a patient who has undergone cardiac catheterization, has had stent insertion, and is not undergoing CABG:
  • **Aspirin 162 mg PO QD**
  • **Clopidogrel 75 mg PO QD for 1 year** (assumes that 300-mg loading dose already given)
  • **GP IIb/IIIa inhibitor:** (continue 12 h for abciximab; 18 h for eptifibatide or tirofiban)
  As dictated by the presence of ischemic symptoms, abnormal hemodynamic parameters, cardiac risk
  factors, hypertension, diabetes, and/or left ventricular dysfunction, the following agents, if not con-
  traindicated, should be considered for administration during the acute hospitalization, and when indi-
  cated, should be continued for cardioprotection and/or management of symptoms following discharge:
  • Statin therapy (within 96 h of acute ischemic event)   • ACE inhibitors
  • Beta-blockers   • Nitrate therapy

  ***In a patient with anatomy appropriate for surgical revascularization, who is scheduled for and
  awaiting CABG:***
  • **Aspirin 325 mg PO QD**
  • **Clopidogrel** (should be discontinued with a plan to restart at 75 mg PO QD the day following sur-
    gery, provided there is no bleeding)
  • **GPIIb/IIIa inhibitor** (eptifibatide or tirofiban continued up to 4–6 h before induction)
  • **Enoxaparin** (discontinue 24 h before surgery) OR
  • **UFH** (continue up to the time of surgery)
  As dictated by the presence of ischemic symptoms, abnormal hemodynamic parameters, cardiac risk
  factors, hypertension, diabetes, and/or left ventricular dysfunction, the following agents, if not con-
  traindicated, should be considered for administration during the acute hospitalization, and when indi-
  cated, should be continued for cardioprotection and/or management of symptoms following discharge:
  • Statin therapy (within 96 h of acute ischemic event)   • ACE inhibitors
  • Beta-blockers   • Nitrate therapy
  No initial cardiac catheterization
  *Low-risk feature patients with NSTE-ACS who are not undergoing cardiac catheterization and who are
  being managed medically in the hospital:*
  • **Aspirin 162 mg PO QD**
  • **Enoxaparin 1 mg/kg SC q12h (or UFH) × 3–8 d**
  • **Clopidogrel 75 mg PO QD**
  As dictated by the presence of ischemic symptoms, abnormal hemodynamic parameters, cardiac risk
  factors, hypertension, diabetes, and/or left ventricular dysfunction, the following agents, if not con-
  traindicated, should be considered for administration during the acute hospitalization, and when indi-
  cated, should be continued for cardioprotection and/or management of symptoms following discharge:
  • Statin therapy (within 96 h of acute ischemic event)   • ACE inhibitors
  • Beta-blockers   • Nitrate therapy

  *High-risk feature patients with NSTE-ACS who did not undergo cardiac catheterization initially, who are
  being managed medically in the hospital, but in whom cardiac catheterization prior to discharge is planned:*
  • **Aspirin 162 mg PO QD**
  • **Enoxaparin 30 mg IV (optional) followed by 1 mg/kg SC q12h (or UFH) × 3–8 d**
  • **Eptifibatide 180 μg/kg IV bolus followed by 2.0 μg/kg/min infusion for 18–72 h**
    (alternative: tirofiban)
  As dictated by the presence of ischemic symptoms, abnormal hemodynamic parameters, cardiac risk
  factors, hypertension, diabetes, and/or left ventricular dysfunction, the following agents, if not con-
  traindicated, should be considered for administration during the acute hospitalization, and when indi-
  cated, should be continued for cardioprotection and/or management of symptoms following discharge:
  • Statin therapy (within 96 h of acute ischemic event)   • ACE inhibitors
  • Beta-blockers   • Nitrate therapy

ACE, angiotensin-converting enzyme; GP, glycoprotein; UFH, unfractionated heparin.

Interventional Cardiology Consensus Reports 2003.

Table 18.22 Non ST-Segment Elevation Myocardial Infarction Acute Coronary Syndrome (NSTE-ACS) Site-, Specialty-, and Spectrum-of-Care Strategies for Outcome-Effective Management *CATH Clinical Consensus Panel Guidelines and Recommendations*

ACS CARE LEVEL: B SITE

Level B Site:
Medical management is the dominant strategy at ACS Care Level B site, although patient transfer is possible and routinely can be facilitated for individuals with high-risk features requiring invasive care. Level B institution or site-of-care has no facilities for performing percutaneous cardiac catheterization, percutaneous coronary intervention (PCI), or coronary artery bypass grafting (GABG), but interinstitutional communication, physician-to-physician referrals, and transfer networks permit transfer of NSTE-ACS patient to a Level A institution.

Emergency Department
Medical management
Initiate risk stratification
No high-risk features present: For the NSTE-ACS patient who does not have high-risk features or treatment-triggered criteria, initial medical management would include:

- **Aspirin 162–325 mg PO** (immediately)
- **Enoxaparin 30-mg IV bolus** (optional) **followed by 1 mg/kg q12h** (alternative: UFH)
- **Clopidogrel 300-mg loading dose[4]** (assuming low likelihood of surgical revascularization)

As dictated by clinical presentation and need to implement appropriate measures for acute medical management of ischemic chest pain, pulmonary edema, hypertension, and other hemodynamic abnormalities in the emergency department, the following agents may be initiated according to clinical protocols:

- Nitroglycerin IV/SC/TC/SL
- Morphine sulfate IV

High-risk features present: For the NSTE-ACS patient who has high-risk features or treatment-triggered criteria[3], supporting maximal medical therapy, addition of a small molecule GPIIb/IIIa receptor antagonist is recommended.
To above regimen, add small molecule GPIIb/IIIa receptor antagonist **eptifibatide,** 180 μg/kg IV bolus, followed by 2.0 μg/kg/min infusion for 18–72 h (alternative GPIIb/IIIa antagonist tirofiban)
In-Patient Care (Step-Down, Coronary Care/Medical Intensive Care Unit)
Continue medical management and ongoing risk feature evaluation and stratification:
No high-risk features present: During ongoing risk level stratification, in the NSTE-ACS patient who does not manifest high-risk features or treatment-triggered criteria[1] that would support addition of small molecule GPIIb/IIIa receptor antagonist, continuing antithrombotic management should include:

- **Aspirin 162 mg PO QD**
- **Enoxaparin 1 mg/kg SC q12h × 3–8 d** (alternative: UFH)
- **Clopidogrel 75 mg PO QD**

As dictated by clinical presentation and need to implement appropriate measures for acute medical management of ischemic chest pain, pulmonary edema, hypertension, and other hemodynamic abnormalities in the emergency department, the following agents may be initiated according to clinical protocols:

- Nitroglycerin IV/SC/TC/SL
- Beta-blockers
- Statin therapy (within 96 h of acute ischemic event)
- Morphine sulfate IV
- ACE inhibitors

High-risk features present: For the NSTE-ACS patient who has—or during ongoing risk stratification and evaluation develops—high-risk features or treatment-triggered criteria[3] indicating need for maximal medical therapy, addition of a small molecule GPIIb/IIIa receptor antagonist is recommended. It also should be stressed that transfer to ACS Care Level A site is strongly recommended for NSTE-ACS patient with high-risk features.

- **Aspirin 162 mg PO QD**
- **Clopidogrel 75 mg PO QD[4]** (only if not CABG candidate)
- **Enoxaparin 1 mg/kg SC q12h × 3–8 d**

(continued)

Table 18.22 (*continued*)

- **Eptifibatide 180 μg/kg IV bolus,** followed by required 2.0 μg/kg/min infusion for 18–72 h (alternative: tirofiban 0.4 μg/kg loading dose, followed by 0.1 μg/kg/min infusion for 48 h)

As dictated by clinical presentation and need to implement appropriate measures for acute medical management of ischemic chest pain, pulmonary edema, hypertension, and other hemodynamic abnormalities in the emergency department, the following agents may be initiated according to clinical protocols:

- Nitroglycerin IV/SC/TC/SL
- Beta-blockers
- Statin therapy (within 96 h of acute ischemic event)
- Morphine sulfate IV
- ACE inhibitors

Transfer to Cardiac Catheterization Laboratory/PCI (Level A site)

Because ACS Care Level B sites of care do not maintain interventional cardiology capabilities, transfer to an ACS Care Level A site (interventional cardiology, PCI, and CABG services available) is strongly recommended for NSTE-ACS patients who present with or, during ongoing risk feature evaluation manifest, high-risk features and/or aggressive treatment-triggered criteria. Patient outcomes in these high-risk patient subgroups are optimized using an invasive strategy.

ACE, angiotensin-converting enzyme; GP, glycoprotein; UFH, unfractionated heparin.

Interventional Cardiology Consensus Reports 2003.

Table 18.23 ACC/AHA Recommendations for Anticoagulant Therapy in ACS

Class I

Antiplatelet therapy should be initiated promptly. ASA should be administered as soon as possible after presentation and continued indefinitely *(level of evidence: A)*.

Clopidogrel should be administered to hospitalized patients who are unable to take ASA because of hypersensitivity or major gastrointestinal intolerance *(level of evidence: A)*.

In hospitalized patients in whom an early noninterventional approach is planned, clopidogrel should be added to ASA as soon as possible on admission and administered for at least 1 month *(level of evidence: B).**

A platelet GPIIb/IIIa antagonist should be administered, in addition to ASA and heparin, to patients in whom catheterization and PCI are planned. The GPIIb/IIIa antagonist may be also be administered just prior to PCI *(level of evidence: A).**

Class IIa

Enoxaparin is preferable to UFH as an anticoagulant in patients with UA/NSTEMI, in the absence of renal failure and unless CABG is planned within 24 h (level of evidence: A).*†

---

*New indications; not included in the September 2000 guidelines.
†Minor clarification different from full-text version on website.
ACC/AHA, American College of Cardiology/American Heart Association; ACS, acute coronary syndrome; ASA, acetylsalicylic acid; CABG, coronary artery bypass grafting; NSTEMI, non–ST-segment elevation myocardial infarction; UA, unstable angina; UFH, unfractionated heparin.

Braunwald E, Antman EM, Beasley JW, et al. ACC/AHA Guiedlines update for the management of patients with unstable angina and non–ST-segment elevation myocardial infarction: report of the American College of Cardiology/American Heart Association Task Force on Practice Guidelines. J Am Coll Cardiol 2002;40:1366–1374.

Table 18.24 ACC/AHA Recommendations for Anticoagulant Therapy in ACS

Class I
   Anticoagulation with subcutaneous LMWH or intravenous UFH should be added to antiplatelet therapy with ASA and/or clopidogrel (*Level of evidence: A*).
Class IIa
   Enoxaparin is preferable to UFH as an anticoagulant in patients with UA/NSTEMI in the absence of renal failure and unless CABG is planned within 24 hours (*Level of evidence: A*).*†

*New indications; not included in the September 2000 guidelines.
†Minor clarification different from full-text version on website.
ACC/AHA, American College of Cardiology/American Heart Association; ACS, acute coronary syndrome; ASA, acetylsalicylic acid; CABG, coronary artery bypass grafting; LMWH, low-molecular-weight heparin; NSTEMI, non–ST-segment elevation myocardial infarction; UA, unstable angina; UFH, unfractionated heparin.

Braunwald E, Antman EM, Beasley JW, et al. ACC/AHA 2002 Guidelines update for the management of patients with unstable angina and non–ST-segment elevation myocardial infarction: report of the American College of Cardiology/American Heart Association Task Force on Practice Guidelines. J Am Coll Cardiol 2002;40:1366–1374.

References

Abes A, Yamashita T, Miyata M, et al. Early assessment of reperfusion therapy using cardiac troponin T. *J Am Coll Cardiol* 1994;23:1382–1389.

ACC/AHA. Guidelines for the early management of patients with acute myocardial infarction. *J Am Coll Cardiol* 1999;34:890–911.

The Acute Infarction Ramipril Efficacy (AIRE) Study Investigators. Effect of ramipril on mortality and morbidity of survivors of acute myocardial infarction with clinical evidence of heart failure. *Lancet* 1993;342:821–828.

Adams JE III, Sigard GA, Allan BT. Diagnosis of perioperative myocardial infarction with measurement of cardiac troponin I. *N Engl J Med* 1994;330:670–674.

Aguirre FV, Topol EJ, Ferguson JJ, et al. Bleeding complications with the chimeric antibody to platelet glycoprotein IIb/IIIa Integrin in patients undergoing percutaneous intervention. *Circulation* 1995;91:2882.

Allison O, Whooley MA, Oler J, Grady D. Adding heparin to aspirin reduces the incidence of myocardial infarction and death in patients with unstable angina. A meta-analysis. *JAMA* 1996;276:811–815.

Ambrosimi E, Claudio B, Magnaui B, for the Survival of Myocardial Infarction Long-term Evaluation (SMILE) Study Investigators. The effect of the angiotensin-converting-enzyme inhibitor zofenopril on mortality and morbidity after anterior myocardial infarction. *N Engl J Med* 1995;332:80–85.

Andersen HR, Nielsen TT, Rasmussen K, et al. A comparison of coronary angioplasty with fibrinolytic therapy in acute myocardial infarction. *N Engl J Med* 2003;349: 733–742.

Anderson J, Marshall HW, Askins JC, et al. A randomized trial of intravenous and intracoronary streptokinase in patients with acute myocardial infarction. *Circulation* 1984;70:606–618.

Anderson JL, Sorensen SG, Moreno FL, et al. Multicenter patency trial of intravenous anistreplase compared with streptokinase in acute myocardial infarction. The TEAM-2 Study Investigators. *Circulation* 1991;83:126–140.

Anderson JL, Karagounis LA, Becker LC, et al. TIMI perfusion grade 3 but not grade 2 results in improved outcome after thrombolysis for myocardial infarction. Ventriculographic, enzymatic, and electrocardiographic evidence from TEAM-3 Study. *Circulation* 1993;87:1829–1839.

Anderson JL, Karagounis LA, Califf RM. Meta-analysis of five reported studies on the relation of early coronary patency grades with mortality and outcomes after acute myocardial infarction. *Am J Cardiol* 1996;78:1–8.

Antiplatelet Trialists' Collaboration. Collaborative meta-analysis of randomised trials of antiplatelet therapy for prevention of death, myocardial infarction, and stroke in high risk patients. *BMJ* 2002;324:71–86.

Antman E, for the TIMI 9A Investigators. Hirudin in acute myocardial infarction: safety report from the Thrombolysis and Thrombin Inhibition in Myocardial Infarction (TIMI) 9A trial. *Circulation* 1994;90:1624–1630.

Antman EM, Tanasijevic MJ, Thompson B, et al. Cardiac specific troponin I levels predict the risk of mortality in patients with acute coronary syndrome. *N Engl J Med* 1996;335:1343–1349.

Antman E, for the TIMI 11B Investigators. Enoxaparin prevents death and cardiac ischemic events in unstable angina, non-Q wave MI: results of the TIMI 11B trial. *Circulation* 1999;100:1593–1601.

Antman EM, Cohen M, Bradley D, et al. Assessment of the treatment effect of enoxaparin for unstable angina/non-Q-wave myocardial infarction: TIMI 11B-ESSENCE meta-analysis. *Circulation* 1999;100:1602–1608.

Antman EM, Cohen M, McCabe C, et al. Enoxaparin is superior to unfractionated heparin for preventing clinical events at 1-year follow-up of TIMI 11B and ESSENCE. *Eur Heart J* 2002;23:308–314.

Antman EM, Anbe DT, Armstrong PW, et al. ACC/AHA Guidelines for the Management of Patients with ST Segment Elevation MI. *J Am Coll Cardiol* 2004;44:671–719.

Armstrong PW, Baigrie RS, Daly PA, et al. Tissue plasminogen activator: Toronto (TPAT) placebo-controlled randomized trial in acute myocardial infarction. *J Am Coll Cardiol* 1989;13:1469–1476.

ASSENT-2 Investigators. Single bolus tenecteplase compared with front-loaded alteplase in acute myocardial infarction. *Lancet* 1999;354:716–722.

ASSENT-3 Investigators. Efficacy and safety of tenecteplase in combination with enoxaparin, abciximab, or unfractionated heparin: the ASSENT-3 randomized trial in acute myocardial infarction. *Lancet* 2001;358:605–613.

Baird SH, Menown BA, McBride SJ, Trouton TG, Wilson C. Randomized comparison of enoxaparin with unfractionated heparin following fibrinolytic therapy for acute myocardial infarction. *Eur Heart J* 2002;23:627–632.

Barbash GI, Reiner J, White HD, et al., for the GUSTO-1 Investigators. Evaluation of paradoxic beneficial effects of smoking in patients receiving thrombolytic therapy for acute myocardial infarction: mechanism of the "smoker's paradox" from the GUSTO-1 trial, with angiographic insights. *J Am Coll Cardiol* 1995;26:1222–1229.

Bayer AJ, Chadha J, Farag RR, et al. Changing presentation of myocardial infarction with increasing old age. *J Am Geriatr Soc* 1986;34:263–266.

Becker RC, Terrin M, Ross R, et al., and the Thrombolysis in Myocardial Infarction Investigators. Comparison of clinical outcomes for women and men after acute myocardial infarction. *Ann Intern Med* 1994a;120:638–645.

Becker RC, Cyr J, Corraro JM, et al. Bedside coagulation monitoring in heparin-treated patients with acute thromboembolic disease: a coronary care unit experience. *Am Heart J* 1994b;128:719–723.

Becker RC, Charlesworth A, Wilcox RG, for the LATE Investigators. Cardiac rupture associated with thrombolytic therapy: impact of time to treatment in the LATE study. *J Am Coll Cardiol* 1995a;25:1063–1068.

Becker RC, Gore JM, Rubison M, et al., for the National Registry of Myocardial Infarction Investigators. Association between body weight and in-hospital clinical outcome following thrombolytic therapy: a report from the National Registry of Myocardial Infarction. *J Thromb Thrombol* 1995b;2:231–237.

Becker RC, Ball SP, Eisenberg P, for the Antithrombotic Therapy Consortium Investigators. Randomized, multicenter trial of weight-adjusted intravenous heparin dose titration and point-of-care coagulation monitoring in hospitalized patients with active thromboembolic disease. *Am Heart J* 1999;137.59–71.

Becker RC, Spencer FA, Gibson M, Rust JE. Influence of patient characteristics and renal function on factor Xa inhibition pharmacokinetics and pharmacodynamics after enoxaparin administration in non-ST-segment elevation acute coronary syndromes. *Am Heart J* 2002;143:753–759.

Bengston JR, Kaplan AJ, Pieper KS, et al. Prognosis in cardiogenic shock after acute myocardial infarction in the interventional era. *J Am Coll Cardiol* 1992;20:1482–1489.

Bittl JA, Strony J, Brinker JA, et al., for the Hirulog Angioplasty Study Investigators. Treatment with bivalirudin (Hirulog) as compared with heparin during coronary angioplasty for unstable or postinfarction angina. *N Engl J Med* 1995;333: 764–769.

Blazing MA, de Lemons JA, White HD, et al., for the A to Z Investigators. Safety and efficacy of enoxaparin vs unfractionated heparin in patients with non–ST-segment elevation acute coronary syndromes who receive tirofiban and aspirin. A randomized controlled trial. *JAMA* 2004;292:55–64.

Blinc A, Planinsic G, Keber D, et al. Dependence of blood clot lysis on the mode of transport of urokinase into the clot. A magnetic resonance imaging study *in vitro*. *Thromb Haemost* 1990;65:549–552.

Bovill EG, Terrin ML, Stump DC, et al., for the TIMI Investigators. Hemorrhagic events during therapy with recombinant tissue-type plasminogen activator, heparin, and aspirin for acute myocardial infarction. Results of the Thrombolysis in Myocardial Infarction (TIMI) Phase II Trial. *Ann Intern Med* 1991;115:256–265.

Braunwald E, Antman EM, Beasley JW, et al. ACC/AHA 2002 Guidelines update for the management of patients with unstable angina and non–ST-segment elevation myocardial infarction: report of the American College of Cardiology/American Heart Association Task Force on Practice Guidelines. *J Am Coll Cardiol* 2002;40: 1366–1374.

Brouwer MA, van den Bergh PJ, Aengevaeren WRM, et al. Aspirin plus coumarin versus aspirin alone in the prevention of reocclusion after fibrinolysis for acute myocardial infarction: results of the antithrombotics in the Prevention of ReOcclusion in Coronary Thromboysis (APRICOT)-2 trial. *Circulation* 2002;106:659–665.

Burken MI, Whyte JJ. Home international normalized ratio monitoring: where evidence-based medicine is exemplified in the medicate coverage processes. *J Thromb Thrombolysis* 2002;13:5–7.

Burns M, Becker RC, Gore JM, for the NRMI-2 Investigators. Early and predischarge aspirin administration among patients with suspected acute myocardial infarction: current clinical practice in the United States. *J Thromb Thrombolysis* 1999; in press.

Cairns JA, Theroux P, Lewis HD Jr, Ezekowitz M, Meade TW. Antithrombotic agents in coronary artery disease. *Chest* 2001;119(Suppl):228S–252S.

Califf RM, Topol EJ, Stack RS, et al. Evaluation of combination thrombolytic therapy and timing of cardiac catheterization in acute myocardial infarction. Results of Thrombolysis and Angioplasty in Myocardial Infarction—Phase 5 randomized trial. *Circulation* 1991;83:1543–1556.

Cannon CP, Braunwald E. GUSTO, TIMI and the case for rapid reperfusion. *Acta Cardiol* 1994;49:1–8.

Cannon CP, McCabe CH, Gibson CM, et al., for the TIMI 10A Investigators. TNK-tissue plasminogen activator in acute myocardial infarction: results of the TIMI 10A dose ranging trial. *Circulation* 1997;95:351–356.

Cannon CP, Gibson CM, McCabe C, et al., for the TIMI 10B Investigators. TNK-tissue plasminogen activator compared with front-loaded alteplase in acute myocardial infarction: results of the TIMI 10B Trial. *Circulation* 1998;98:2805–2814.

Canto JG, Shlipak MG, Rogers WJ, et al. Prevalence, clinical characteristics, and mortality among patients with myocardial infarction presenting without chest pain. *JAMA* 2000;283:3223–3231.

CAPRIE Steering Committee. A randomised, blinded trial of clopidogrel versus aspirin in patients at risk for ischaemic events (CAPRIE). *Lancet* 1996;348:1329–1339.

Carney RJ, Murphy GA, Brandt TR, et al. Randomized angiographic trial of recomsinant TPA (Alteplasc) in myocardial infarction. RAAMI study investigations. *J Am Coll Cardiol* 1992;20:17–23.

Charbonnier B, Cribier A, Monassier JP, et al. Étude eurpeenne multicentrique et randomisee de l' ASPSAV versus streptokinase dans l'infarctus du myocarde. *Arch Mal Coeur Vaiss* 1989;82:1565–1571.

Chesebro JH, Knatterud G, Roberts R, et al. Thrombolysis in Myocardial Infarction (TIMI) Trial, phase I: a comparison between intravenous tissue plasminogen activator and intravenous streptokinase. *Circulation* 1987;76:142–154.

Chinese Cardiac Study Collaborative Group. Oral captopril versus placebo among 13,634 patients with suspected acute myocardial infarction: interim report from CCS-1. *Lancet* 1995;345:686–687.

Chockalingam A. Impending global pandemic of cardiovascular disease: challenges and opportunities for the prevention and control of cardiovascular disease in developing countries and economies in transition. *Heartbeat* 1999;4:1–5.

Cohen M, Adams PC, Hawkins L, et al. Usefulness of antithrombotic therapy in resting angina pectoris or non-Q-wave myocardial infarction in preventing death and myocardial infarction (a pilot study from the Antithrombotic Therapy in Acute Coronary Syndromes Study Group). *Am J Cardiol* 1990;66:1287–1292.

Cohen M, Adams PC, Parry G, et al. Combination antithrombotic therapy in unstable rest angina and non-Q-wave infarction in non prior aspirin users: primary end points analysis from the ATACS trial: Antithrombotic Therapy in Acute Coronary Syndromes Research Group. *Circulation* 1994;89:81–88.

Cohen M, Demers C, Gurfinkel EP, for the ESSENCE Investigators. A comparison of low-molecular weight heparin with unfractionated heparin for unstable coronary artery disease. *N Engl J Med* 1997;337:447–452.

Cohen M, Théroux P, Borzak S, et al., on behalf of the ACUTE II Investigators. Randomized double-blind safety study of enoxaparin versus unfractionated heparin in patients with non-ST-segment elevation acute coronary syndromes treated with tirofiban and aspirin: the ACUTE II Study. *Am Heart J* 2002;144:470–477.

Collen D, Topol EJ, Tiefenbrunn AJ, et al. Coronary thrombolysis with recombinant human tissue-type plasminogen activator: a prospective, randomized controlled trial. *Circulation* 1984;70:1012–1017.

Collet JP, Montalescot G, Lison L, et al. Percutaneous coronary intervention after subcutaneous enoxaparin pretreatment in patients with unstable angina pectoris. *Circulation* 2001;103:658–663.

CONSENSUS Trial Study Group. Effects of enalapril on mortality in severe congestive heart failure. Results of the Cooperative North Scandinavian Enalapril Survival Study (CONSENSUS). *N Engl J Med* 1987;316:1429–1435.

CONSENSUS Trial Study Group. Effects of the early administration of enalapril on mortality in patients with acute MI. Results of the Cooperative New Scandinavian Enalapril Survival Study II (CONSINSUS II). *N Engl J Med* 1992;327:678–684.

Conti R. Noninvasive assessment of ventricular function at 90 minutes following thrombolytic therapy in patients with infarcting myocardium may predict coronary artery patency and prognosis. *Clin Cardiol* 1994;17:461–462.

Cooper R, Cutler J, Desvigne-Nickens P, et al. Trends and disparities in coronary heart disease, stroke, and other cardiovascular disease in the United States. Findings of the national conference on cardiovascular disease prevention. *Circulation* 2000; 102:3137–3147.

Cribier A, Berland J, Saoudi N, et al. Heparin and intravenous streptokinase in acute infarction: preliminary results of a prospective randomized trial with angiographic evaluation in 44 patients. *Haemostasis* 1986;16:122–129.

Dalby M, Bouzamondo A, Lechat P, Montalescot G. Transfer of primary angioplasty versus immediate thrombolysis in acute myocardial infarction. *Circulation* 2003;108:1809.

Dalen JE, Gore JM, Braunwald E, et al., and the TIMI Investigators. Six- and twelve-month follow-up of the Phase I Thrombolysis in Myocardial Infarction (TIMI) trial. *Am J Cardiol* 1988;62:179–185.

Danchin N, Blanchard D, Steg PG, et al., for the USIC 2000 Investigators. Impact of prehospital thrombolysis for acute myocardial infarction on 1-year outcome: results from the French Nationwide USIC 2000 Registry. *Circulation* 2004;110:1909–1915.

The Danish Study Group on Verapamil in Myocardial Infarction. Effect of verapamil on mortality and major events after acute myocardial infarction (The Danish Verapamil Infarction Trial DAVITT II). *Am J Cardiol* 1990;66:779.

de Chillou C, Riff P, Sadoul N, et al. Influence of cigarette smoking on rate of reopening of the infarct-related coronary artery after myocardial infarction: a multivariate analysis. *J Am Coll Cardiol* 1996;27:1662–1668.

den Heijer P, Vermeer F, Ambrosioni E, et al., on behalf of the In-TIME Investigators. Evaluation of a single-bolus plasminogen activator in patients with myocardial infarction: a double-blind, randomized angiographic trial of lanoteplase versus alteplase. *Circulation* 1998;98:2117–2125.

De Wood MA, Spores J, Notske R, et al. Prevalence of total coronary occlusion during the early hours of transmural myocardial infarction. *N Engl J Med* 1980;303: 897–902.

Direct Thrombin Inhibitor Trialists' Collaborative Group. Direct thrombin inhibitors in acute coronary syndromes: principal results of a meta-analysis based on individual patients' data. *Lancet* 2002;359:294–302.

Dorey A, Patel S, Reese C, et al. Dangers of delay of initiation of either thrombolysis or primary angioplasty in acute myocardial infarction with increasing use of primary angioplasty. *Am J Cardiol* 1998;81:1173–1177.

Ellerbeck EF, Jencks SF, Radford MJ, et al., Quality of care for Medicare patients with acute myocardial infarction. A four-state pilot study from the Cooperative Cardiovascular Project. *JAMA* 1995;273:1509–1514.

Ellis SG, da Silva RB, Heyndrick XGR, et al., for the RESCUE Investigators. The randomized evaluation of salvage angioplasty with combined utilization of endpoints [Abstract]. *Circulation* 1993;88:1–106.

EMERAS Collaborative Group. Randomized trial of late thrombolysis in patients with suspected acute myocardial infarction. *Lancet* 1993;342:767–772.

ESPRIM Trial. Short-term treatment of acute myocardial infarction with molsidomine. European study of prevention of infarct with molsidomine (ESPRIM) group. *Lancet* 1994;344:91–97.

Ferguson JJ, Antman EM, Bates ER, et al., for the NICE-3 Investigators. Combining enoxaparin and glycoprotein IIb/IIIa antagonists for the treatment of acute coronary syndromes: final results of the NICE-3 Study. *Am Heart J* 2003;146:628–634.

Ferguson JJ, Califf RM, Antman EM, et al., for the SYNERGY Trial Investigators. Enoxaparin vs unfractionated heparin in high-risk patients with non-ST-segment elevation acute coronary syndromes managed with an intended early invasive strategy: primary results of the SYNERGY randomized trial. *JAMA* 2004;292:45–54.

FIT Collaborative Group. Indications for fibrinolytic therapy in suspected acute myocardial infarction: collaborative overview of early mortality and major morbidity results from all randomized trials of more than 1,000 patients. *Lancet* 1994;343; 311–322.

Fiore L, Ezekowitz M, Brophy MT, et al. Department of veterans affairs cooperative studies program clinical trial comparing combined warfarin and aspirin with aspirin alone in survivors of acute myocardial infarction. *Circulation* 2002;105: 557–563.

Fox KAA, Poole-Wilson PA, Henderson RA, et al. Interventional versus conservative treatment for patients with unstable angina or non-ST- elevation myocardial infarction: the British heart foundation RITA 3 randomised trial. *Lancet* 2002;360: 743–751.

Freedman B, Richmond DR, Kelly DT. Pathophysiology of coronary spasm. *Circulation* 1982;66:705–709.

FRISC Study Group. Low molecular weight heparin during instability in coronary artery disease. *Lancet* 1996;347:561–568.

FRISC II Investigators. Prolonged low molecular mass heparin (dalteparin) in unstable coronary artery disease: a prospective randomized multicenter trial. *Lancet* 1999; 354:701–707.

Fuster V. Randomized double-blind trial of fixed low-dose warfarin with aspirin after myocardial infarction. Coumadin Aspirin Reinfarction Study (CARS) Investigators. *Lancet* 1997;350;389–396.

Gacioch GM, Ellis SG, Lee L, et al. Cardiogenic shock complicating acute myocardial infarction: the use of coronary angioplasty and the integration of the new support devices into patients' management. *J Am Coll Cardiol* 1992;19:647–653.

Gau GT. Electrocardiology and vectorcardiography. In: Brandenburg F, Fuster V, Guuliani ER, et al., eds: Cardiology: Fundamentals and Practice, Vol 1. Chicago, Year Book Medical Publishers, 1987:268.

Gemmell JD, Hogg KJ, MacIntyre PD, et al. A pilot study of the efficacy and safety of bolus administration of alteplase in acute myocardial infarction. *Br Heart J* 1991; 66:134–138.

GISSI. Effectiveness of intravenous thrombolytic treatment in acute myocardial infarction. *Lancet* 1987;397–402.

GISSI-2. A factoria randomized trial of alteplase versus streptokinase and heparin versus no heparin among 12,490 patients with acute myocardial infarction. *Lancet* 1990;336:65–71.

GISSI-3. Effects of lisinopril and transdermal glyceryl trinitrate singly and together on 6 week mortality and ventricular function after acute MI. *Lancet* 1994;343:1115–1122.

Goodman SG, Langer A, Ross AM for the GUSTO 1 Angiographic Investigators. Non-Q-wave versus Q-wave MI after thrombolytic therapy. *Circulation* 1998;97:449–450.

Goodman SG, Fitchett D, Armstrong PW, et al. Randomized evaluation of the safety and efficacy of enoxaparin versus unfractionated heparin in high-risk patients with non–ST-segment elevation acute coronary syndromes receiving the glycoprotein IIb/IIIa inhibitor eptifibatide. *Circulation* 2003;107:238–244.

Granger CB, Hirsh J, Califf RM, et al. for the GUSTO-1 Investigators. Activated partial thromboplastin time and outcome after thrombolytic therapy for acute myocardial infarction. Results from the GUSTO-1 trial. *Circulation* 1996;93:870–878.

Grines CL, DeMaria AN. Optimal utilization of thrombolytic therapy for acute myocardial infarction. *J Am Coll Cardiol* 1990;16:223–231.

Grines CL, Browne K, Marco J, et al. A comparison of immediate angioplasty with thrombolytic therapy for acute MI. *N Engl J Med* 1993;328:673–678.

Grines CL, Topol EJ, O'Neill WW, et al. Effect of cigarette smoking on outcome after thrombolytic therapy for myocardial infarction. *Circulation* 1995;91:298–303.

Guerci AD, Gerstenblith G, Brinker JA, et al. A randomized trial of intravenous tissue plasminogen activator for acute myocardial infarction with subsequent randomization to elective coronary angioplasty. *N Engl J Med* 1987;317:1613–1618.

Guido B, Topol EJ. Coronary angiography in acute myocardial infarction. *Adv Cardiovasc Med* 1994;1(2).

Gurfinkel EP, Manos EJ, Mejail RI, et al. Low molecular weight heparin versus heparin or aspirin in the treatment of unstable angina and silent ischemia. *J Am Coll Cardiol* 1995;26:313–318.

Gurwitz JH, Goldberg RJ, Gore JM. Coronary thrombolysis for the elderly? *JAMA* 1991;265:1720–1723.

Gurwitz JH, Gore JM, Goldberg RJ, et al. Recent age-related trends in the use of thrombolytic therapy in patients who have had acute myocardial infarction. *Ann Intern Med* 1996;124:283–291.

Gurwitz JH, Gore JM, Goldberg RJ, et al., for the Participants in the National Registry of Myocardial Infarction 2. Risk for intracranial hemorrhage after tPA treatment for the acute myocardial infarction. *Ann Intern Med* 1998;129:597–604.

GUSTO Angiographic Investigators. The comparative effects of tissue plasminogen activator, streptokinase, or both on coronary artery patency, ventricular function and survival after acute myocardial infarction. *N Engl J Med* 1993;329:1615–1622.

GUSTO IIA Investigators. Randomized trial of intravenous heparin versus recombinant hirudin for acute coronary syndromes. *Circulation* 1994;90:1631–1637.

GUSTO IIB Investigators. A comparison of recombinant hirudin with heparin for the treatment of acute coronary syndromes. *N Engl J Med* 1996;335:775–782.

GUSTO III Investigators. A comparison of reteplase with alteplase for acute myocardial infarction. *N Engl J Med* 1997;337:1118–1123.

GUSTO IV Investigators. Effect of the GP IIb/IIIa receptor blocker abciximab on the outcome in patients with acute coronary syndromes without early revascularization. *Lancet* 2001;357:1915–1924.

Hands ME, Rutherford JD, Muller JE, et al. The in-hospital development of cardiogenic shock after myocardial infarction: incidence, predictors of occurrence, outcome and prognostic factors. *J Am Coll Cardiol* 1989;14:40–46.

Hassan WM, Flaker GC, Feutz G, et al. Improved anticoagulation with a weight adjusted heparin nomogram in patients with acute coronary syndromes: a randomized trial. *J Thromb Thrombolysis* 1995;45–49.

Hibbard MD, Holms DR Jr, Bailey KR, et al. Percutaneous transluminal coronary angioplasty in patients with cardiogenic shock. *J Am Coll Cardiol* 1992;19:639–646.

Hilton TC, Thompson RC, William HJ, et al. Technetium 99m sestamibi myocardial perfusion imaging in the emergency room evaluation of chest pain. *J Am Coll Cardiol* 1994;23:1016–1022.

Hochman J. The SHOCK Trial. *Circulation* 1999;100:574.

Hogg KJ, Gemmill JD, Burns J, et al. Angiographic patency study of anistreplase versus streptokinase in acute myocardial infarction. *Lancet* 1990;335:254–258.

Holdright D, Patel D, Cunningham D, et al. Comparison of the effect of heparin and aspirin versus aspirin alone on transient myocardial ischemia and in-hospital prognosis in patients with unstable angina. *J Am Coll Cardiol* 1994;24:39–45.

Hurlen M, Abdelnoor M, Smith P, Erickson J, Arnesen H. Warfarin, aspirin, or both after myocardial infarction. Warfarin Aspirin Reinfarction Study. *N Engl J Med* 2002;347; 969–974.

ISIS-1 Collaborative Group. Mechanism for the early mortality reduction produced by β-blockade started early in acute myocardial infarction: ISIS-1. *Lancet* 1988;1: 921–923.

ISIS-2 Collaborative Group. Randomized trial of intravenous streptokinase, oral aspirin, both, or neither among 17,187 cases of suspected acute myocardial infarction: ISIS-2. *Lancet* 1988;2:349–360.

ISIS-3 Collaborative Group. A randomized comparison of streptokinase vs tissue plasminogen activator vs anistreplase and of aspirin plus heparin vs aspirin alone among 41,299 cases of suspected acute myocardial infarction: ISIS-3. *Lancet* 1992;339:753–770.

ISIS-4 Collaborative Group. A randomized, factorial trial assessing early oral captopril, oral mononitrate, and intravenous magnesium supplementation in 58,050 patients with suspected myocardial infarction. *Eur Heart J* 1994;15:608–619.

Jeremy RW, Hackworthy RA, Bautovicg G, et al. Infarct artery perfusion and changes in left ventricular volume in the month after acute myocardial infarction. *J Am Coll Cardiol* 1987;9:989–995.

Johns JA, Gold HK, Leinbach RC, et al. Prevention of coronary artery reocclusion and reduction in late coronary artery stenosis after thrombolytic therapy in patients with acute myocardial infarction. *Circulation* 1988;78:546–556.

Jugdutt BI. Myocardial salvage by intravenous nitroglycerin in conscious dogs: loss of beneficial effect with marked nitroglycerin-induced hypotension. *Circulation* 1983; 68:673–684.

Jugdutt BI, Warnica JW. Intravenous nitroglycerin therapy to limit myocardial infarct size, expansion and complications. effect of timing, dosage, and infarct location. *Circulation* 1988;78:906–919.

Kahn JK, Ruterford BD, McConahay DR, et al. Usefulness of angioplasty during acute myocardial infarction in patients with prior coronary artery bypass grafting. *Am J Cardiol* 1990;65:698–702.

Karnash SL, Granger CB, White HD, et al., for the GUSTO-1 Investigators. Treating menstruating women with thrombolytic therapy: insights from the global utilization of streptokinase and tissue plasminogen activator for occluded coronary arteries (GUSTO-1) trial. *J Am Coll Cardiol* 1995;26:1651–1656.

Kasper W, Meinertz T, Wollschläger H, et al. Coronary thrombolysis during acute myocardial infarction by intravenous BRL 26921, a new anisoylated plasminogen-streptokinase activator complex. *Am J Cardiol* 1986;58:418–421.

Keeley EC, Boura JA, Grines CL. Primary angioplasty intravenous thrombolytic therapy for acute myocardial infarction: a quantitative review of 23 randomised trials. *Lancet* 2003;361:13–20.

Kennedy JW, Ritchie JL, Davis KB, et al. The Western Washington randomized trial of intracoronary streptokinase in acute myocardial infarction. *N Engl J Med* 1983; 309:1477–1482.

Kennedy JW, Gensini GG, Timmis GC, et al. Acute myocardial infarction treated with intracoronary streptokinase: a report of the Society for Cardiac Angiography. *Am J Cardiol* 1985;55:871–877.

Kersschot IE, Brugda P, Ramentol M, et al. Effects of early reperfusion in acute myocardial infarction on arrhythmias induced by programmed stimulation: a prospective randomized study. *J Am Coll Cardiol* 1986;7:1234–1242.

Killip T, Kimball JT. Treatment of myocardial infarction in a coronary care unit: a two-year experience with 250 patients. *Am J Cardiol* 1967;20:457–464.

Kleiman N, Ohman E, Califf R, et al. Profound inhibition of platelet aggregation with monoclonal antibody 7E3 Fab following thrombolytic therapy: results of the TAMI 8 pilot study. *J Am Coll Cardiol* 1993;22:381–389.

Klein W, Buchwald A, Hillis SE, et al. Comparison of low molecular weight heparin with unfractionated heparin acutely and with placebo for 6 weeks in the management of unstable coronary artery disease. Fragmin in Unstable Coronary Artery Disease Study (FRIC). *Circulation* 1997;96:61–68.

Krumholz HM, Murillo JE, Chen J, et al. Thrombolytic therapy for eligible elderly patients with acute myocardial infarction. *JAMA* 1997;227:1683–1688.

Lagreqvist, B, Husted S, Kintny F, et al. A long-term perspective on the protective effects of an early invasive strategy in unstable coronary artery disease. Two-year follow-up of the FRISC-II invasive study. *J Am Coll Cardiol* 2002;40:1902–1914.

Lamfers EJP, Schut A, Hooghoudt TEH, et al. Prehospital thrombolysis with reteplase: the Nijmegen/Rotterdam study. *Am Heart J* 2003;146:479–483.

LATE Study Group. Late Assessment of Thrombolytic Efficacy (LATE) study with alteplase 6–24h after onset of acute myocardial infarction. *Lancet* 1993;342:759–765.

Latting CA, Silverman ME. Acute myocardial infarction in hospitalized patients over 70. *Am Heart J* 1980;100:311–318.

Lee L, Bates ER, Pitt B, et al. Percutaneous transluminal coronary angioplasty improves survival in acute myocardial infarction complicated by cardiogenic shock. *Circulation* 1988;78:1345–1351.

Lee L, Erbel R, Brown TM, et al. Multicenter registry of angioplasty therapy of cardiogenic shock: initial and long-term survival. *J Am Coll Cardiol* 1991;17:599–603.

Lesnefsky EJ, Lundergren CF, Hodgson J, et al. Increased left ventricular dysfunction in elderly patients despite successful thrombolysis: the GUSTO-1 angiographic experience. *J Am Coll Cardiol* 1996;28:331–337.

Li KS, Santamore WP, Morley DL, et al. Stenotic amplification of vasoconstriction responses. *Am J Physiol* 1989;256:H1044—H1051.

Lincoff AM, Bittl JA, Kleiman NS, et al. The REPLACE 1 trial: a pilot study of bivalirudin versus heparin during percutaneous coronary intervention with stenting and GP IIb/IIIa blockade. *J Am Coll Cardiol* 2002,39(Suppl A):16A.

Lincoff AM, Bittl JA, Harrington RA, et al., for the REPLACE-2 Investigators. Bivalirudin and provisional glycoprotein IIb/IIIa blockade compared with heparin and planned glycoprotein IIb/IIIa blockade during percutaneous coronary intervention: REPLACE-2 randomized trial. *JAMA* 2003;289:853–863.

Lopez-Sendon J, Seabra-Gomes R, Macaya C, et al. Intravenous anisoylated plasminogen streptokinase activator complex versus intravenous streptokinase in myocardial infarction. A randomized multicenter study [Abstract]. *Circulation* 1988;78
(Suppl II).

MacMahan S, Collins R, Peto R. Effects of prophylactic lidocaine in suspected acute myocardial infarction: an overview of results from randomized, controlled trials.
JAMA 1988;260:1910–1916.

Marmur JD, Anand SX, Bagga RS, et al. The activated clotting time can be used to monitor the low molecular weight heparin dalteparin after intravenous administration.
J Am Coll Cardiol 2003;41:394–402.

Mathey DG, Kuck KH, Tilsner V, et al. Nonsurgical coronary artery recanalization in
acute transmural myocardial infarction. *Circulation* 1981;63:489–497.

Maynard C, Martin JS, Hallstrom AP, et al., for the MITI Project Investigators. Changes
in the use of thrombolytic therapy in Seattle area hospitals from 1988 to 1992: results from the Myocardial Infarction Triage and Intervention Registry. *J Thromb
Thrombolysis* 1995a;1:195–199.

Maynard C, Weaver WD, Lambrew C, et al., for the Participants in the National Registry
of Myocardial Infarction. Factors influencing the time to administration of thrombolytic therapy with recombinant tissue plasminogen activator (data from the National Registry of Myocardial Infarction). *Am J Cardiol* 1995b;76:854–862.

Mehta RH, Montoye CK, Faul J, et al. Enhancing quality of care for acute myocardial infarction: shifting the focus of improvement from key indicators to process of care
and tool use. The American College of Cardiology Acute Myocardial Infarction
Guidelines Applied in Practice Project in Michigan: Flint and Saginaw Expansion.
J Am Coll Cardiol 2004;43:2166–2173.

MIAMI Trial Research Group. Metoprolol in Acute Myocardial Infarction (MIAMI): a
randomized placebo-controlled international trial. *Eur Heart J* 1985;6:199–211.

Monnier P, Sigwart U, Vincent A, et al. Anisoylated plasminogen streptokinase activator
complex vs streptokinase in acute myocardial infarction. *Drugs* 1987;3(Suppl 3):
175–178.

Moosvi AR, Khaja F, Villanueva L, et al. Early revascularization improves survival in cardiogenic shock complicating acute myocardial infarction. *J Am Coll Cardiol* 1992;
19:907–914.

Morrow DA, Antman EM, Charlesworth A, et al. TIMI risk score for ST-elevation myocardial infarction: a convenient, bedside, clinical score for risk assessment at presentation: an intravenous nPA for treatment of infarcting myocardium early II trial
substudy. *Circulation* 2000;102:2031–2037.

Mueller C, Buettner HJ, Hodgson JM, et al. Inflammation and long-term mortality after
non-ST elevation acute coronary syndrome treated with a very early invasive strategy in 1042 consecutive patients. *Circulation* 2002;105:1412–1415.

Mukherjee D, Mahaffey KW, Moliterno DJ, et al. The promise of combined low-molecular-weight heparin and platelet glycoprotein IIb/IIIa inhibition—results from PARAGON B. *Am Heart J* 2002:144:995–1002.

Muller JE, Stone PH, Turi SZ, et al., and the MILIS Study Group. Circadian variation in the frequency of onset of acute myocardial infarction. *N Engl J Med* 1985;313: 1315–1322.

Multicenter Diltiazem Postinfarction Trial Research Group (MDPIT). The effect of diltiazem on mortality and reinfarction after acute myocardial infarction. *N Engl J Med* 1988;319:385–392.

National Heart Attack Alert Program Coordinating Committee—60 Minutes to Treatment Working Group. Emergency department: rapid identification and treatment of patients with acute myocardial infarction. *Ann Emerg Med* 1994;23:311–329.

National Heart, Lung, and Blood Institute. Morbidity and mortality: chartbook on cardiovascular, lung and blood diseases. Bethesda, Md.: U.S. Department of Health and Human Services, Public Health Service. National Institute of Health, 1992; Jan.

Neuhaus KL, Tebbe U, Gottwik M, et al. Intravenous recombinant plasminogen activator (rt-PA) and urokinase in acute myocardial infarction: results of the German Activator Urokinase Study (GAUS). *J Am Coll Cardiol* 1988;12:581–587.

Neuhaus KL, Feuerer W, Jeep-Tebbe S, et al. Improved thrombolysis with a modified dose regimen of recombinant tissue-type plasminogen activator. *J Am Coll Cardiol* 1989;14:1566–1569.

Neuhaus KL, von Essen R, Vogt R, et al. Dose finding with a novel recombinant plasminogen activator (BM 06.022) in patients with acute myocardial infarction: results of the German recombinant plasminogen activator study. *J Am Coll Cardiol* 1994;24:55–60.

Neuhaus K-L, von Essen R, Tebbe U, et al. Improved thrombolysis in acute myocardial infarction with front-loaded administration of anistreplase: results of the rt-PA-APSAC patency study (TAPS). *J Am Coll Cardiol* 1992;19:885–891.

Neuhaus K L, von Essen R, Tebbe U, et al. Safety observations from the pilot phase of the randomized r-Hirudin for improvement of thrombolysis (HIT-III) study. *Circulation* 1994;90:1638–1642.

Newby LK, Rutsch WR, Califf RM, et al. for the GUSTO-I Investigators. Time from symptom onset to treatment and outcomes after thrombolytic therapy. *J Am Coll Cardiol* 1996;27:1646–1655.

The Norwegian Multicenter Study Group. Timolol-induced reduction in mortality and reinfarction in patients surviving acute myocardial infarction. *N Engl J Med* 1981; 304:801–807.

OASIS Investigators. Comparison of effects of two doses of recombinant hirudin compared with heparin in patients with acute myocardial ischemia without ST elevation. A pilot study. *Circulation* 1997;96:769–777.

OASIS-2 Investigators. Effects of recombinant hirudin (lepirudin) compared with heparin on death, myocardial infarction, refractory angina, and revascularization procedures in patients with acute myocardial ischaemia without ST elevation: a randomised trial. *Lancet* 1999;353:429–438.

Ohman EM, Armstrong PW, Christenson NH, et al. Cardiac troponin T levels for risk stratification in acute myocardial ischemia. *N Engl J Med* 1996;335:1333–1341.

Ohman EM, Kleiman NS, Gacioch G for the IMPACT-AMI Investigators. Combined accelerated tissue-plasminogen activator and platelet glycoprotein IIb/IIIa integrin receptor blockade with integrin in acute myocardial infarction. *Circulation* 1997; 95:846–854.

O'Rourke M, Baron D, Keogh A, et al. Limitation of myocardial infarction by early infusion of recombinant tissue-factor plasminogen activator. *Circulation* 1988;77: 1311–1315.

Panju AA, Hemmelgarn BR, Guyatt GH, et al. Is this patient having a myocardial infarction? *JAMA* 1998;280:1256–1263.

Petersen JL, Mahaffey KW, Hasselblad V, et al. Efficacy and bleeding complications among patients randomized to enoxaparin or unfractionated heparin for antithrombin therapy in non-ST-segment elevation acute coronary syndromes. A systematic overview. *JAMA* 2004;292:89–96.

Pfeffer MA, Braunwald E, Moye L, et al. Effect of captopril on mortality and morbidity in patients with left ventricular dysfunction after myocardial infarction. Results with left ventricular dysfunction after myocardial infarction. Results of the Survival and Ventricular Enlargement (SAVE) trial. *N Engl J Med* 1992;327:669–677.

Pilote L, Califf RM, Sapp S, et al. for the GUSTO-1 Investigators. Regional variation across the United States in the management of acute myocardial infarction. *N Engl J Med* 1995;333:565–572.

PRIMI Trial Study Group. Randomized double-blind trial of recombinant prourokinase against streptokinase in acute myocardial infarction. *Lancet* 1989;1:863–868.

Puleo PR, Meyer D, Wathen C, et al. Use of a rapid assay of subforms of creatine kinase MB to diagnosis or rule out myocardial infarction. *N Engl J Med* 1994;331:561–566.

Purvis JA, Trouton TG, Roberts MJD, et al. Effectiveness of double bolus alteplase in the treatment of acute myocardial infarction. *Am J Cardiol* 1991;68:1570–1574.

Purvis JA, McNeill AJ, Siddequi RA, et al. Efficacy of 100 mg double bolus alteplase in achieving complete perfusion in the treatment of acute myocardial infarction. *J Am Coll Cardiol* 1994;23:6–10.

Raitt MH, Maynard C, Wagner GS, et al. Appearance of abnormal Q waves early in the course of acute myocardial infarction: implications for efficacy of thrombolytic therapy. *J Am Coll Cardiol* 1995;25:1084–1088.

Rawles JM. Quantification of the benefit of earlier thrombolytic therapy: five-year results of the Grampian Region Early Anistreplase Trial (GREAT). *J Am Coll Cardiol* 1997;30:1181–1186.

Reiner J. The tale of TIMI 2. Presented at the 11th International Workshop of Thrombolysis and Interventional Therapy in Acute Myocardial Infarction. Anaheim, California, Nov. 12, 1995.

Relik-van Wely L, Visser RF, van der Pol J, et al. Angiographically assessed coronary arterial patency and reocclusion in patients with acute myocardial infarction treated with anistreplase: Results of the Anistreplase Reocclusion Multicenter Study (ARMS). *Am J Cardiol* 1991;68:296–300.

Richardson PD, Davies MJ, Born GVR. Influence of plaque configuration and stress distribution on fissuring of coronary atherosclerotic plaques. *Lancet* 1989;2:941–944.

RISC Group. Risk of myocardial infarction and death during treatment with low dose aspirin and intravenous heparin in men with unstable coronary artery disease: the RISC Group. *Lancet* 1990;336:327–330.

Rogers WJ, Bowlby LJ, Chandra NC, et al., for the participants in the National Registry of Myocardial Infarction. Treatment of myocardial infarction in the United States (1990 to 1993). Observations from the National Registry of Myocardial Infarction. *Circulation* 1994a;90:2103–2114.

Rogers WJ, Dean LS, Moore PB, et al., for the Alabama Registry of Myocardial Ischemia Investigators. Comparison of primary angioplasty versus thrombolytic therapy for acute myocardial infarction. *Am J Cardiol* 1994b;74:111–118.

Ross AM, Coyne KS, Morey A for the GUSTO-1 Angiographic Investigators. Extended mortality benefit of early postinfarction reperfusion. *Circulation* 1998;97:1549–1556.

Ross AM, Molhoek P, Lundergan C, et al. Randomized comparison of enoxaparin, a low-molecular-weight heparin, with unfractionated heparin adjunctive to recombinant tissue plasminogen activator thrombolysis and aspirin: second trial of heparin and aspirin reperfusion therapy (HART II). *Circulation* 2001;104:648–652.

Ryan TJ, Antman EM, Brooks NH, et al. 1990 Update: ACC/AHA Guidelines for the management of patients with acute myocardial infarction. A report of the American College Cardiology/American Heart Association Task Force on Practice Guidelines (Committee on Management of Acute Infarction). *J Am Coll Cardiol* 1999;34:890–911.

Sabol MB, Luippold RS, Becker RC, et al. The association between serial measures of systemic blood pressure and early coronary arterial perfusion status following intravenous thrombolytic therapy. *J Thromb Thrombolysis* 1994;1:79–84.

Schmoltz KM, Tebbe O, Herrman C, et al. Frequency of complications of cardiopulmonary resuscitation after thrombolysis during acute myocardial infarction. *Am J Cardiol* 1992;69:724–728.

Sgarbossa EB, Pinski SL, Barbagelata A, et al., for the GUSTO-1 Investigators. Electrocardiographic diagnosis of evolving acute myocardial infarction in the presence of left bundle branch block. *N Engl J Med* 1996a;334:481–487.

Sgarbossa EB, Pinski SL, Gates KB, et al., for the GUSTO-1 Investigators. Early electrocardiographic diagnosis of acute myocardial infarction in the presence of ventricular paced rhythm. *Am J Cardiol* 1996b;77:423–424.

Simes RJ, Topol EJ, Holmes DR, et al. for the GUSTO-1 Investigators. Link between the angiographic substudy and mortality outcomes in a large randomized trial of myocardial reperfusion. Importance of early and complete infarct artery reperfusion. *Circulation* 1995;91:1923–1928.

Simoons ML, Betriu A, Col J, et al. Thrombolysis with tissue plasminogen activator in acute myocardial infarction: no additional benefit from immediate percutaneous coronary angioplasty. *Lancet* 1988;1:197–203.

Simoons ML, Maggioni AP, Knatterud G, et al. Individual risk assessment for intracranial hemorrhage during thrombolytic therapy. *Lancet* 1993;342:1523.

Simoons ML, for the PENTUA Study Group. Pentasaccharide in patients with unstable angina: PENTUA Study. Presented at Plenary X, late breaking clinical trials, scientific sessions, American Heart Association. Anaheim, California, Nov. 14, 2001.

Simoons ML, Bobbink IWG, Boland J, Gardien M, et al., for the PENTUA Investigators. A dose-finding study of fondaparinux in patients with non-ST-segment elevation acute coronary syndromes. The Pentasacharide in Unstable Angina (PENTUA) study. *J Am Coll Cardiol* 2004;43:2183–2190.

Six AJ, Louwerenburg HW, Braams R, et al. A double-blind randomized multicenter dose-ranging trial of intravenous streptokinase in acute myocardial infarction. *Am J Cardiol* 1990;65:119–123.

Smalling RW, Schumacher R, Morris D, et al. Improved infarct-related arterial patency after high dose, weight-adjusted, rapid infusion of tissue-type plasminogen activator in myocardial infarction: results of a multicenter randomized trial of two dosage regimens. *J Am Coll Cardiol* 1990;15:915–921.

Smith P, Arnesen H, Holme I. The effect of warfarin on mortality and reinfarction after myocardial infarction. *N Engl J Med* 1990;323:147–152.

SOLVD Investigators. Effect of enalapril on mortality and the development of heart failure in asymptomatic patients with reduced left ventricular ejection fraction. *N Engl J Med* 1992;327:685–691.

Stace RS, O'Connor CM, Mark DB, et al. Coronary perfusion during acute myocardial infarction with a combined therapy of coronary angioplasty and high-dose intravenous streptokinase. *Circulation* 1988;77:151–161.

Stack RS, Califf RM, Hinohara T, et al. Survival and cardiac event rates in the first year after emergency coronary angioplasty for acute myocardial infarction. *J Am Coll Cardiol* 1988a;111:1141–1149.

Stack RS, O'Connor CM, Mark DB, et al. Coronary perfusion during acute myocardial infarction with a combined therapy of coronary angioplasty and high-dose intravenous streptokinase. *Circulation* 1988b;77:151–161.

Steering Committee of the Physicians' Health Study Research Group. Final report on the aspirin component of the ongoing Physicians' Health Study. *N Engl J Med* 1989; 321:129.

Steg PG, Bonnefoy E, Chabaud S, et al. Impact of time to treatment on mortality after prehospital fibrinolysis or primary angioplasty: data from the CAPTIM randomized clinical trial. *Circulation* 2003;108:2851–2856.

Stone PH. Triggers of transient myocardial ischemia: circadian variation and relation to plaque rupture and coronary thrombosis in stable coronary artery disease. *Am J Cardiol* 1990;66:32G–36G.

SWIFT Trial Study Group. SWIFT trial of delayed elective intervention versus conservative treatment after thrombolysis with anistreplase in acute myocardial infarction. *Br Med J* 1991;302:555–560.

Tebbe U, Transwell P, Seifried E, Feuerer W, Scholtz KH, Herrmann KS. Single bolus injection of recombinant tissue type plasminogen activator in acute myocardial infarction. *Am J Cardiol* 1989;64:448–453.

Tenaglia AN, Califf RM, Candela RJ, et al. Thrombolytic therapy in patients requiring cardiopulmonary resuscitation. *Am J Cardiol* 1991;68:1015–1019.

Terrin ML, Williams DO, Kleiman NS, et al. for the TIMI 11 Investigators. Two- and three-year results of the Thrombolysis in Myocardial Infarction (TIMI) phase II clinical trial. *J Am Coll Cardiol* 1993;22:1763–1772.

Théroux P, Ouimet H, McCans J, et al. Aspirin, heparin, or both to treat acute unstable angina. *N Engl J Med* 1988;319:1105–1111.

Théroux P, Willerson JT, Armstrong PW. Progress in the treatment of acute coronary syndromes: a 50-year perspective (1950–2000). *Circulation* 2000;102:IV-2–13.

Thompson PL, Aylward PE, Federman J, et al. A randomized comparison of intravenous heparin with oral aspirin and dipyridamole 24 hours after recombinant tissue-type plasminogen activator for acute myocardial infarction. *Circulation* 1991;83:1534–1542.

TIMI 11A Trial Investigators. Dose-ranging trial of enoxaparin for unstable angina: results of TIMI 11A. *J Am Coll Cardiol* 1997;29:1474–1482.

TIMI Study Group. The Thrombolysis in Myocardial Infarction (TIMI) trial; phase 1 findings. *N Engl J Med* 1985;312:932–936.

TIMI Research Group. Immediate versus delayed catheterization and angioplasty following thrombolytic therapy for acute myocardial infarction. TIMI IIA results. *JAMA* 1988;260:2849–2858.

TIMI Study Group. Comparison of invasive and conservative strategies after treatment with intravenous tissue plasminogen activator in acute myocardial infarction. Results of the Thrombolysis in Myocardial Infarction (TIMI) phase II trial. *N Engl J Med* 1989;320:618–627.

TIMI IIIB Investigators. Effects of tPA and a comparison of early invasive and conservative strategies in unstable angina and non-Q wave MI. Results of the TIMI IIIB trial. *Circulation* 1994;89:1545–1556.

Tomai F, Crea F, Gaspardone A, et al. Ischemic preconditioning during coronary angioplasty is prevented by glibenclamide, a selective ATP-sensitive K+ channel blocker. *Circulation* 1994;90:700–705.

Topol EJ, Bates ER, Walton JA, et al. Community hospital administration of intravenous tissue plasminogen activator in acute myocardial infarction: improved timing, thrombolytic efficacy and ventricular function. *J Am Coll Cardiol* 1987;10:1173–1177.

Topol EJ, Califf RM, George BS, et al. Coronary arterial thrombolysis with combined infusion of recombinant tissue-type plasminogen activator and urokinase in patients with acute myocardial infarction (TAMI-2). *Circulation* 1988;77:1100–1107.

Topol EJ, George BS, Kereiakes DJ, et al. Comparison of two dose regimens of intravenous tissue plasminogen activator for acute myocardial infarction. *Am J Cardiol* 1988;61:723–728.

Topol EJ, George BS, Kereiakes DJ, et al. A randomized controlled trial of intravenous tissue plasminogen activator and intravenous heparin in acute myocardial infarction (TAMI-3). *Circulation* 1989;79:281–286.

Topol EJ. Thrombolytic intervention. In: Topol EJ, ed, Textbook of Interventional Cardiology. Philadelphia: WB Saunders Co., 1991:76–120.

Topol EJ, Califf RM. Thrombolytic therapy and mortality in acute myocardial infarction. *J Am Coll Cardiol* 1991;18:675–762.

Topol EJ, Califf RM, Weisman HF, et al. for the EPIC Investigators. Use of monoclonal antibody directed against the platelet glycoprotein IIb/IIIa receptor. *N Engl J Med* 1994;330:956–996.

Transhesi B, Chamone DF, Cobbaert C, et al. Coronary recanalization rate after intravenous bolus of alteplase in acute myocardial infarction. *Am J Cardiol* 1991;68:161–165.

Tresch DD, Brady WJ, Aufderheide TP, et al. Comparison of elderly and younger patients with out-of-hospital chest pain. Clinical characteristics, acute myocardial infarction, therapy an outcomes. *Arch Intern Med* 1996;156:1089–1093.

Van de Werf F, Barron HV, Armstrong PW, et al. Incidence and predictors of bleeding events after fibrinolytic therapy with fibrin-specific agents: a comparison of TNK-tPA and rt-PA. *Eur Heart J* 2001;22:2253–2261.

Van Es RF, Jonker JCC, Verheught FWA, et al. Aspirin and Coumadin after acute coronary syndromes (the ASPECT-2 study): a randomized controlled trial. *Lancet* 2002; 360:109–113.

Varo N, de Lemos JA, Libby P, et al. Soluble CD40L: risk prediction after acute coronary syndromes. *Circulation* 2003;108:1049–1052.

Vaska KJ, Whitlow PL. Selective tissue plasminogen activator infusion for chronic total occlusions of native coronary arteries failing angioplasty. *Circulation* 1991;84:II-250.

Verstraete M, Bernard R, Bory M, et al. Randomized trial of intravenous recombinant tissue-type plasminogen activator versus intravenous streptokinase in acute myocardial infarction. Report from the European Cooperative Study Group for Recombinant Tissue-type Plasminogen Activator. *Lancet* 1985a;I:842–847.

Verstraete M, Brower RW, Collen D, et al. Double-blind randomized trial of intravenous tissue-type plasminogen activator versus placebo in acute myocardial infarction (ECSG-1). *Lancet* 1985b;965–969.

Vogt A, von Essen R, Tebbe U, et al. Impact of early perfusion status of the infarct-related artery on short-term mortality after thrombolysis for acute myocardial infarction: retrospective analysis of four German multicenter studies. *J Am Coll Cardiol* 1993; 21:1391–1395.

Vogt A, Von Essen R, Tebbe U, et al. Frequency of achieving optimal reperfusion in acute myocardial infarction (analysis of four German multicenter studies). *Am J Cardiol* 1994;74:1–4.

Vullemenot A, Schiele F, Meneveau N, et al. Efficacy of a synthetic pentasaccharide, a pure factor Xa inhibitor, as an antithrombotic agent—a pilot study in the setting of coronary angioplasty. *Thromb Haemost* 1999;81:214–220.

Wall TC, Califf RM, George BS et al. Accelerated +PA does regimens for thrombolysis: TAMI-7. *J Am Coll Cardiol* 1992; 19482–489.

Wallentin C, Wilcok RG, Emanuelson H, et al., for the ESTEEM Investigators. Oral ximelagatran for secondary prophylaxis after myocardial infarction: the ESTEEM randomized controlled trial. *Lancet* 2003;362:789–797.

Weaver WD, Cerqueira M, Hallstrom AP, et al., for the Myocardial Infarction Triage and Intervention Project Group. Prehospital-initiated versus hospital-initiated thrombolytic therapy. Myocardial triage and intervention trial. *JAMA* 1993;270:1211–1216.

Wharton TP, Grines LL, Turco MA, et al. Primary angioplasty in acute myocardial infarction at hospitals with no surgery on-site (The PAMI-No SOS Study) versus transfer to surgical centers for primary angioplasty. *J Am Coll Cardiol* 2004;43: 1943–1950.

White HD, Cross DB, Williams BF, et al. Safety and efficacy of repeat thrombolytic treatment after myocardial infarction. *Br Heart J* 1990;64:177–181.

White HD, Barbash GI, Modan M, et al., for the Investigators of the International Tissue Plasminogen Activator/Streptokinase Mortality Study. After correcting for worse baseline characteristics, women treated with thrombolytic therapy for acute myocardial infarction have the same mortality and morbidity as men except for a higher incidence of hemorrhage stroke. *Circulation* 1993;88(part I):2097–2103.

Wilcox RG, Olsson CG, Skene AM, et al. Trial of tissue plasminogen activator for mortality reduction in acute myocardial infarction. Anglo-Scandinavian Study of Early Thrombolysis (ASSET). *Lancet* 1988;2:525–530.

Williams DO, Braunwald E, Knatterud G, et al., and TIMI Investigators. One-year result of the Thrombolysis in Myocardial Infarction Investigation (TIMI) phase 11 trial. *Circulation* 1992;85:533–542.

Woodfield SL, Lundergan CF, Reiner JS, et al. Angiographic findings and outcome in diabetic patients treated with thrombolytic therapy for acute myocardial infarction: the GUSTO-1 experience. *J Am Coll Cardiol* 1996;28:1661–1669.

Woods KL, Fletcher S, Roffe C, et al. Intravenous magnesium sulfate in suspected acute myocardial infarction: results of the second Leicester intravenous magnesium intervention trial (LIMIT-2). *Lancet* 1992;339:1553–1558.

Yusuf S, Collins R, MacMohan S. Effect of intravenous nitrates on mortality in acute myocardial infarction: an overview of the randomized trials. *Lancet* 1988;1:1088–1092.

Zabel KM, Granger CB, Becker RC, et al., for the GUSTO-1 Investigators. Use of bedside activated partial thromboplastin time monitor to adjust heparin dosing after thrombolysis for acute myocardial infarction. Results of GUSTO-1. *Am Heart J* 1998;136: 868–876.

Zahn R, Schiele R, Schneider S, et al. Primary angioplasty versus intravenous thrombolysis in acute myocardial infarction: can we define subgroups of patients benefiting most from primary angioplasty? Results from the pooled data of the maximal individual therapy in Acute Myocardial Infarction Registry and the Myocardial Infarction Registry. *J Am Coll Cardiol* 2001;37:1827–1835.

Peripheral Vascular Disease and Stroke

19

More than 25 million persons in the United States have at least one manifestation of atherosclerosis. Throughout the last 50 years, coronary arterial atherosclerosis has been the focus of basic and clinical investigation; however, the systemic nature of atherosclerosis must be acknowledged (Faxon et al., 2004).

Cerebrovascular Disease

Stroke is the third leading cause of death and the principal cause of long-term disability in the United States. There are upward of 600,000 new or recurrent strokes annually. Black populations have a 40% higher stroke rate than white populations and experience a higher mortality.

Aortic Atherosclerosis

The clinical manifestations of aortic atherosclerosis include abdominal aortic aneurysm, aortic dissection, penetrating aortic ulcer, intramural hematoma, and peripheral atheroembolization. Thoracic aortic aneurysms also occur in patients with atherosclerotic risk factors, but are less common.

Peripheral Arterial (Lower Extremity) Disease

The age-adjusted prevalence of peripheral arterial disease (PAD) is approximately 12% and may exceed 20% in persons greater than 70 years of age. An ankle–brachial index of less than or equal to 0.90 is 90% sensitive and 95% specific for PAD, identifying a patient population at risk for claudication, rest pain, skin ulceration, and critical leg ischemia, prompting amputation. A majority of patients with PAD have concomitant coronary artery disease (85%) and many have carotid artery disease (60%).

Renal Artery Atherosclerosis

Although the true prevalence of renal artery disease proceeding to clinical manifestations such as hypertension or renal insufficiency is unknown, autopsy series of patients with cerebrovascular disease and stroke have identified a high incidence of concomitant disease involving at least one renal artery.

Vascular disease of the peripheral arterial circulation, most often caused by atherosclerosis and less commonly by vasculitis (or other nonatherosclerotic arteriopathies), is a chronic process that is responsible for progressive and, at times, incapacitating symptoms, disability, and limb loss. The arterial beds most frequently involved, in order of occurrence, are:

- Femoropopliteal-tibial
- Aortoiliac
- Carotid and vertebral
- Splanchnic and renal
- Brachiocephalic

The causes of acute occlusion include:

- Cardioembolism
- Artery-to-artery
- In situ thrombosis
- Trauma
- Vasospasm

The frequent coexistence of peripheral vascular and coronary artery disease (multibed vascular disease) has been recognized for decades and is clinically important for several reasons. First, it provides a unifying basis for atherosclerosis and its prevention. Second, it offers a biologically plausible explanation for the high cardiovascular mortality (two- to threefold increase) in patients with peripheral vascular disease. Last, the pharmacologic approach to management takes on a more global theme with the objective of preventing atherosclerosis progression and attenuating thrombotic processes, which underlie acute myocardial infarction (MI), stroke, and peripheral arterial occlusion (Adams et al., 2003).

Vascular Disease

The available data, derived from individual clinical trials and a frequently cited meta-analysis conducted by the Antiplatelet Trialists' Collaboration, provide strong support for the benefit of therapies targeting platelet inhibition among patients with vascular disease. In high-risk patients, aspirin therapy (80 mg to 325 mg qd) reduces nonfatal MI by one-third, nonfatal stroke by one-third, and death from all vascular causes by one-sixth (Antiplatelet Trialists' Collaboration, 2002). The benefit applies to a broad range of individuals, including men and women of all ages and those with systemic hypertension or diabetes mellitus.

Cerebrovascular Disease

Ischemic stroke is a major cause of morbidity and mortality worldwide and, in a sizeable proportion of patients, is caused by atherosclerosis involving the carotid (extracranial) and cerebral (intracranial) vasculature. The benefit of platelet antagonists in patients with prior stroke or transient ischemic attack has been documented by several large-scale clinical trials (Table 19.1) and in an overview of all previously conducted trials (CAPRIE Steering Committee, 1996; CAST Collaborative Group, 1997; Gent et al., 1989; International Stroke Trial Collaborative Group, 1997; Multicenter Acute Stroke Trial–Italy Group, 1995). Ticlopidine (or clopidogrel) may offer additional benefit (compared with aspirin) in patients with recent stroke or a fixed neurologic defect, reducing the occurrence of fatal or nonfatal stroke by 15% to 20% (Hass et al., 1989); however, side effects (including neutropenia) are a concern with long-term administration of ticlopidine. Combination aspirin and dipyridamole preparations (Aggrenox) may offer the greatest overall benefit (Diener et al., 1996), but studies investigating the combined administration of clopidogrel and aspirin could potentially identify a preferred strategy.

The primary prevention of stroke with pharmacologic therapy (predominantly platelet antagonists), while efficacious, has limitations. Patients with advanced carotid disease (stenosis >70%) remain at risk for neurologic events and should be considered for carotid endarterectomy; however, antiplatelet therapy should be continued postoperatively. Carotid angioplasty with distal protection is also a potentially important option. Anticoagulant therapy is preferable to antiplatelet therapy following cardioembolic stroke, particularly in the setting of atrial fibrillation.

Peripheral Occlusive Disease

Patients with peripheral vascular (occlusive) disease have specific needs that reflect the widespread nature of atherosclerosis. Intermittent claudication is a manifestation of ischemic muscle that reflects a fixed obstruction to blood flow and periods of heightened intravascular thrombotic activity.

Because of its dynamic pathobiology and clinical expression, the treatment of patients with peripheral vascular disease has included lifestyle changes (risk-factor modification), vasoactive compounds, muscle-metabolism–enhancing drugs, and antithrombotic therapy (aspirin, clopidogrel, or their combination) (Balsano et al., 1989; Belch et al., 1997; Ernst et al., 1990; Lievre et al., 1996).

Critical limb ischemia, as a distinct clinical entity, represents the progression of ischemia to the point of severely compromised nutritive blood flow that threatens tissue viability. The manifestations range from claudication at rest to trophic skin changes, ulceration, overt gangrene, and limb loss (Table 19.2) (Rutherford et

Table 19.1 Randomized Trials in Patients with Either Ischemic Stroke or Transient Ischemic Attacks Receiving Platelet Antagonists

Trial	Patients	Treatment	Comparison(s)	Clinical Outcome(s)	Findings
CAPRIE (1997)	19,185	Clopidogrel 75 mg qd / Peripheral arterial disease, recent stroke, recent MI	ASA 325 mg qd	Ischemic stroke, MI, or vascular death; Stroke; GIH	PAD patients: RRR 23.8% ($p = 0.0028$); RRR 7.3% ($p = 0.26$); 0.52% vs. 0.93% ($p < 0.05$)
CAST (1997)	21,106	ASA 160 mg qd within 48 h	Placebo	Mortality; Death or nonfatal stroke	3.3% vs. 3.9%; or 14% ($p = 0.004$); 5.3% vs. 5.9%; or 12% ($p = 0.03$)
IST (1997)	19,435	ASA 300 mg qd within 48 h	SC heparin; SC heparin + ASA; Neither	Mortality at 14 d; Recurrent stroke; Death or dependence at 6 mo	9.0% vs. 9.4%; not significant; 2.8% vs. 3.9% ($p = 0.01$); Not significant
ESPS-2 (1996)	6,062	ASA 25 mg bid, dipyridamole 200 mg bid, ASA + dipyridamole* / TIA or completed ischemic stroke within 2 mo	Placebo	Mortality; Recurrent stroke	No difference; ASA RRR 18% ($p = 0.013$); Dipyridamole RRR 16% ($p = 0.039$); ASA + dipyridamole RRR 37% ($p = {<}0.001$)
MAST-1 (1995)	622	ASA 300 mg within 6 h	Untreated; Streptokinase; ASA + streptokinase	Mortality	OR 2.7 (1.7–4.3) streptokinase; OR 0.9 (0.6–1.3) ASA + streptokinase
SALT (1991)	1,360	ASA 75 mg qd 1–4 mo after cerebrovascular event	—	Mortality; Stroke; Bleeding event	18% RRR; 18% RRR; 7.2% vs. 3.2% ($p = 0.001$)
UK-TIA (1991)	1,072	ASA 300 mg qd, ASA 600 mg bid	Placebo	Mortality; GI bleeding	15% RRR −3%–29%; 3.3% with 300 mg; 6.4% with 1,200 mg
CATS (1989)	1,072	Ticlopidine 250 mg bid / Recent thromboembolic stroke	Placebo	Stroke, MI, vascular death; As above, but intent-to-treat; Stroke, stoke-related death; Severe side effects	RRR 30.2%; RRR 23.3% ($p = 0.02$); RRR 24.1%; 8.2% vs. 2.8%
TASS (1989)	3,069	Ticlopidine 250 mg bid / TIA, amaurosis fugax, RIND, minor stroke within 3 mo	ASA 650 mg bid	Nonfatal stroke, death; Fatal stroke, nonfatal stroke; Severe neutropenia	17% vs. 19%; RRR 12% (−2%–26%); 10% vs. 13%; RRR 21% (4%–38%); 13/1529 vs. 0/1540

*Extended-release preparations.

ASA, aspirin; GI, gastrointestinal; GIH, gastrointestinal hemorrhage; MI, myocardial infarction; OR, odds ratio; PAD, peripheral arterial disease; RIND, reversible ischemic neurologic deficit; RRR, relative risk reduction; TIA, transient ischemic attack.

Table 19.2 Clinical Classification of Acute Limb Ischemia

		Findings		Doppler Signals	
Category	Description/Prognosis	Sensory Loss	Muscle Weakness	Arterial	Venous
I. Viable	Not immediately threatened	None	None	Audible	Audible
II. Threatened					
a. Marginally	Salvageable if promptly treated	Minimal (toes) or none	None	(Often) inaudible	Audible
b. Imminently	Salvageable with immediate revascularization	More than toes, associated with rest pain	Mild, moderate	(Usually) inaudible	Audible
III. Irreversible[a]	Major tissue loss or permanent nerve damage inevitable	Profound, anesthetic	Profound, paralysis (rigor)	Inaudible	Inaudible

[a]The difference between class IIb and III can be difficult to distinguish at the onset of the leg ischemia.

Rutherford R B, Baker J D, Ernst C, et al. Recommended standards for reports dealing with lower extremity ischemia. J Vasc Surg 1997;26:517–538.

al., 1997). Although revascularization represents the treatment of choice, this is not always technically feasible, raising the question of pharmacologic alternatives. A majority of clinical trials performed to date have focused on vasodilating compounds like cilostazol, many of which also possess antithrombotic properties.

Acute Arterial Insufficiency

The predominant causes of acute arterial insufficiency are trauma, in situ thrombosis, and peripheral embolism. Nontraumatic occlusion can be further classified as thrombotic atherosclerosis and most often involves the lower extremities. In approximately 85% of cases, arterial embolism originates within the heart (atrial fibrillation, valvular heart disease, left ventricular mural thrombus). Noncardiac sources include abdominal aortic or femoral aneurysms, ulcerated atherosclerotic plaques, and paradoxic emboli from lower-extremity venous thrombi that cross into arterial circulation through atrial septal defects, a patent foramen ovale, or ventricular septal defects. The most common sites of involvement, in descending order of frequency, include the iliofemoral, popliteal, and tibial vessels. Diagnostic hallmarks of arterial occlusion are sudden pain with pallor, loss of pulse, and paresthesias. Prolonged ischemia can lead to sensory and motor loss and ultimately tissue necrosis (gangrene).

Acute peripheral emboli are frequently managed with balloon extraction and systemic anticoagulation. The role of anticoagulant therapy (traditionally with unfractionated heparin [UFH]) is to prevent recurrent cardio- and artery-to-artery embolism. It may also reduce in situ thrombosis in areas of endothelial disruption created by the original thrombus and/or balloon extraction–related trauma. Distal (popliteal artery and below) occlusions can be managed with either surgery or selective intraarterial fibrinolytic therapy. Although a consensus has not been reached, fibrinolytic therapy may be most useful in surgically inaccessible small arteries of the forearm, hand, leg, and foot, as well as in patients who are not considered candidates for surgical interventions (STILE Investigators, 1994). The adjunctive role of platelet glycoprotein (GP) IIb/IIIa antagonists is under investigation, but should be considered with recurring thrombosis despite adequate anticoagulation.

A reduction in cardiovascular events, including MI and vascular death, is a primary goal of antithrombotic therapy in patients with peripheral vascular disease. The Antiplatelet Trialists' Collaboration overview documented the benefit of antiplatelet therapy in this particular patient subset defined as having either intermittent claudication, peripheral arterial bypass grafts, or peripheral angioplasty. Cilostazol, which does not offer antithrombotic effects, may reduce claudication. Aspirin or clopidogrel is accepted therapy, with the latter representing a preferable treatment strategy in patients with peripheral vascular disease and known coronary artery disease (dual vascular bed disease). The potential for added benefit with combined strategies of aspirin and clopidogrel has been confirmed in the setting of coronary artery disease.

Peripheral Vascular Reconstructive Surgery

Although the available literature suggests that saphenous veins have patency rates that are superior to polytetrafluorethylene bypass grafts, both are subject to early thrombotic occlusion that stems from in situ thrombogenicity, technical challenges, and, in many patients, poor distal runoff. The importance of flow is highlighted by the comparatively low rates of occlusion involving arteries greater than 6 mm in diameter (aortoiliac, femoral), compared with smaller vessels and flow rates less than 200 mL/minute. Although intermediate and late occlusions may also be thrombotic in origin, neointimal hyperplasia and progressive atherosclerosis dominate the pathobiology.

Because platelets represent the predominant constituent of arterial thrombi, antiplatelet therapy with aspirin or clopidogrel is considered the standard of care for patients undergoing reconstructive procedures (or angioplasty). Systemic anticoagulation with UFH may be protective at the time of intraoperative vessel cross-clamping. The combination of warfarin and aspirin (or an alternative platelet antagonist) should be reserved for high-risk patients (poor vein quality, marginal arterial runoff, and previously failed bypass) (Sarac et al., 1998) (Table 19.3).

Fibrinolytic Therapy in Acute Ischemic Stroke

The "modern reperfusion era" for acute ischemic stroke began in the early 1980s, initially with angiographic studies (and intraarterial fibrinolytic infusions) of the posterior circulation (vertebrobasilar system), followed soon thereafter by studies that focused on the anterior circulation (carotid system). The early experience with streptokinase (SK), urokinase (UK), streptokinase–urokinase combinations, and tissue plasminogen activator (tPA) were characterized by prolonged time to treatment (up to 48 hours from symptom onset), prolonged infusions (up to 48 hours), relatively high recanalization rates (~70%), and high intracerebral hemorrhage rates (10–20%) (Bruckmann et al., 1986; Del Zoppo et al., 1986, 1988; Hacke et al., 1988). It is important to acknowledge that pretreatment computed tomography (CT) scans were not a routine feature of the early clinical experience.

Intravenous fibrinolytic therapy for acute ischemic stroke was embarked upon in the early 1990s with studies designed to determine safety, efficacy, and preferred dosing strategies. In general, the time to treatment was reduced in a majority of

Table 19.3 Antithrombotic Therapy in Peripheral Vascular Disease

Clinical Scenario	Agent	Dosing Range/Comments
Carotid endarterectomy	Aspirin	81–325 mg/d
	Aspirin	50–325 mg/d
	Aspirin/Persantine[++]	25–250 mg bid
	Clopidogrel	75 mg/d
Acute arterial occlusion/ischemia	Unfractionated heparin*	aPTT 2 × control
	Fibrinolytic therapy	tPA
Chronic lower extremity ischemia	Aspirin	81–325 mg/d
	Clopidogrel[†]	75 mg/d
Claudication	Aspirin	81–325 mg/d
	Clopidogrel	75 mg/d
	Cilostazol	50–100 mg bid
Intraoperative anticoagulation during vascular surgery	Unfractionated heparin	aPTT 2–3 × control
Infrainguinal vein bypass	Aspirin	81–325 mg/d
	Clopidogrel	75 mg/d (if aspirin not used)
Infrainguinal prosthetic bypass	Aspirin	81–325 mg/d
Infrainguinal bypass (high thrombotic risk)	Aspirin + warfarin	81–325 mg/d; INR 2.5 (range 2.0–3.0)
Aortoiliac or renal PCI	Aspirin	325 mg/d
	Clopidogrel	75 mg/d (stenting)

*Followed by warfarin to INR (range 2.0–3.0).
†Clopidogrel may be superior to aspirin for reducing vascular complications.
++Extended-release preparation.
aPTT, activated partial thromboplastin time; INR, international normalized ratio; PCI, percutaneous coronary intervention; tPA, tissue plasminogen activator

studies to less than 8 hours and the infusions were abbreviated. Early results raised a note of cautious optimism with consistently high rates of intracerebral hemorrhage (~20%) (Haley et al., 1993; Mori et al., 1992); however, the small number of patients studied precluded a consensus from being reached. As a result, large-scale, placebo-controlled, randomized studies were carried out in the United States and abroad. The findings of three streptokinase trials, Multicenter Acute Stroke Trial–Italy (MAST–I Group, 1995), Multicenter Acute Stroke Trial–Europe (MAST–E Group, 1996), and Australian Streptokinase (ASK) trial (Donnan et al., 1995), alarmed the medical community because of their high mortality rates, often hemorrhagic in nature. Similar concerns accompanied the European Cooperative Acute Stroke Study (ECASS) (Hacke et al., 1995), which used tPA (1.1 mg/kg given over 60 minutes; maximum dose 100 mg). Thirty-day mortality rates and clinical outcomes were no different in treated patients compared with control patients, and there was an alarming 6.3% hemorrhage-related mortality with fibrinolytic therapy.

Careful analysis of the ECASS study suggested that prolonged time to treatment (>3 hours) and a total tPA dose in excess of 0.9 mg/kg body weight contributed to the disappointing outcome. Accordingly, the National Institute of Neurologic Disorders and Stroke (NINDS) study was carried out with several important methodologic features (NINDS Study Group, 1995). Patients were required to have experienced an ischemic stroke with a clearly defined time of onset, a deficit measurable on the National Institute of Health Stroke Scale, and a baseline CT scan of the brain showing no evidence of intracranial hemorrhage (Table 19.4). Treatment with tPA (0.9 mg/kg body weight; maximum 90 mg, 10% given as a bolus with the reminder infused over 60 minutes) or placebo was initiated within 3 hours of symptom onset. Despite the fact that mortality rates did not differ between groups, there was evidence of functional improvement (based on several validated stroke scales) by 3 months in a greater proportion of tPA-treated patients. Individuals treated within 90 minutes from symptom onset derived the greatest overall benefit from treatment. Intracerebral hemorrhage, despite careful screening and relatively early treatment, occurred more frequently with fibrinolytic therapy (6.4% vs. 0.6%) (Albers et al., 2000, 2002; Clark et al., 1999).

Intraarterial fibrinolytic therapy may be of benefit up to 6 hours from symptom onset in cases of acute middle cerebral artery or basilar artery occlusion.

Clinical Construct

With several decades of experience and the benefit of more recent data derived from carefully designed and conducted randomized clinical trials, the question can be asked, "What does fibrinolytic therapy offer patients with acute ischemic stroke?" The pessimist reminds us that one in five large clinical trials showed benefit in favor of fibrinolytics and the incidence of intracerebral hemorrhage was worrisome (10- to 20-fold higher than expected for carefully selected patients with MI receiving fibrinolytic therapy). The optimist replies that carefully chosen patients treated within 180 minutes from symptom onset have a 30% chance for an excellent recovery. The realist acknowledges that fibrinolytic therapy is one of the few treatments available in the early stages of stroke, and therefore represents a step forward, but considerable work remains.

Given that fibrinolytic therapy benefits patients with acute ischemic stroke, and that administration is within 3 hours of symptom onset, there must be a sense of urgency among the general public to seek evaluation promptly and among the staff of medical centers providing treatment. There is little question that stroke, as with acute MI, represents a medical emergency, and the primary goal of therapy is to provide the optimal treatment in a timely manner (Table 19.5).

Many institutions have developed "stroke teams" to facilitate the diagnosis and treatment of patients with acute ischemic stroke (Table 19.6). In essence, the question becomes one of care processes, or, "How is stroke care rendered?" The

Table 19.4 Randomized Placebo-Controlled Trials of Intravenous tPA in Acute Ischemic Stroke

	n	Dose/mg/kg (max)	Treatment Window	Symptomatic ICH (%)		Death		Favorable Clinical Outcome	
				tPA	Placebo	tPA	Placebo	t-PA	Placebo
NINDS	624	0.9 (90)	<3 h	6.4	0.6*	17.4	20.6	39*	26*
ECASS I	620	1.1 (100)	≤6 h	19.8*	6.5*	22	15.6	41	29
ECASS II	800	0.9 (90)	≤6 h	8.8*	3.4*	10.5	10.7	40.3	36.3
ATLANTIS A (0–6 h)	142	0.9 (90)	≤6 h	11.3*	0*	22.5*	7*	47	49
ATLANTIS B (3–5 h)	547	0.9 (90)	3–5 h	7.0*	1.1*	11	6.9	34	32

Statistically significant.
ICH, intracerebral hemorrhage; tPA, tissue plasminogen activator.

Table 19.5 Fibrinolytic Therapy for Acute Ischemic Stroke

Inclusion Criteria
　Age >18 ys
　Clinical diagnosis of stroke with neurologic deficit within prior 180 min
　CT scan without signs of intracranial hemorrhage
Exclusion Criteria
　Minor or rapidly improving symptoms (or signs)
　CT scan evidence of intracranial hemorrhage, cerebral edema, or mass effect
　History of prior intracranial hemorrhage
　History of stroke or serious head trauma within prior 3 mo
　Seizure at stroke onset
　GI or urinary tract bleeding within 3 weeks
　Systolic BP > 180 mmHg, diastolic BP >110 mmHg, or aggressive treatment to lower blood
　　pressure
　Blood sugar <50 mg/dL or >400 mg/dL
　Lumbar puncture within 1 wk
　Arterial puncture (of noncompressible vessel) within 1 wk
　Platelet count <100,000/mm³
　Heparin therapy (with prolonged aPTT) within 48 h
　Pregnancy or lactation
　Oral anticoagulant use with INR >1.7

aPTT, activated partial thromboplastin time; BP, blood pressure; CT, computed tomography; GI, gastrointestinal.

stroke team often includes specialists from neurology, neuroradiology, neurosurgery, and critical care services. The comprehensive approach to management should also include a stroke unit: critical pathways of care; a specialized stroke rehabilitation team with representation from speech, physical, and occupational therapy; neurology; nursing and social services; and specific stroke education programs.

The early experience suggests that stroke teams can have an important impact on overall patient care that translates to (1) reduced time to treatment; (2) reduced complication rates; (3) reduced hospital length of stay, unnecessary diagnostic testing, and cost; (4) improved functional outcome; and (5) improved patient/family understanding (Bowan and Yaste, 1994; Indredavik et al., 1991).

The National Stroke Project (Medicare Quality Improvement Project; unpublished data) identified 14,295 individuals with acute ischemic stroke. Overall, only 1.6% received fibrinolytic therapy (tPA) and, of added concern, nearly 50% of patients in whom criteria for fibrinolytics were documented had one or more deviations from recommended management guidelines. Deep vein thrombosis prophylaxis following the event rarely followed current guidelines (<5%). Clearly, this represents an area where considerable improvement in patient management must be achieved.

Table 19.6 A Clinical Approach to Patients with Acute Ischemic Stroke

Pretreatment Evaluation
   Notify members of the stroke team.
   History
   Physical examination
   CT scan
   Review CT scan with neuroradiology.
   Question exclusion criteria for fibrinolytic therapy.
   Administer tPA under close supervision in stroke unit or ICU.
Posttreatment Evaluation
   Observe in stoke unit or ICU for at least 24 hours.
   Perform daily neurologic examinations (or more frequently as needed).
   Avoid anticoagulants and platelet antagonists for initial 24 after fibrinolytic infusion.
   Provide pneumatic compression boots for DVT prophylaxis.
   Avoid invasive procedures (when possible) for initial 24 h.
   Notify stoke rehabilitation team.

CT, computed tomography; DVT, deep vein thrombosis; ICU, intensive care unit; tPA, tissue plasminogen activator.

Neuroprotection

The brain's response to injury includes a reduction of oxygen and glucose consumption at the ischemic center and surrounding region that remains viable for several hours after stroke onset (ischemic penumbra). Depletion of energy stores serves as a trigger for cytotoxic events that can cause irreversible cellular injury. The available evidence suggests that a build-up of extracellular glutamate causes intracellular calcium overload, leading to free radical formation and, ultimately, cell death.

A wide variety of neuroprotective agents have been investigated with the goal of reducing ischemic injury and cellular death in the penumbral tissue. In theory, one or more of these agents could be administered adjunctively with a fibrinolytic agent (tPA) to maximize the therapeutic response to treatment through prevention of ischemia in viable areas of the brain and by preventing reperfusion injury when flow is restored (Buchan et al., 1993; Diener et al., 1996; RANTTASS Investigators, 1996; SASS Investigators 1994). The potential role of novel anticoagulants and platelet antagonists is worthy of investigation, particularly the latter, which may reduce microvascular occlusion.

Summary

The available evidence provided by phase III and IV clinical trials supports the use of tPA (intravenous) at a dose of 0.9 mg/kg (maximum 90 mg), with 10% of the total dose given as a bolus and the remainder infused over 60 minutes for the treatment of acute ischemic stroke if therapy can be initiated within 3 hours of clearly defined symptom onset.

Patients with angiographically documented occlusion of the middle cerebral artery or basilar artery (and no signs of extensive infarction on the presenting CT scan) who can be treated within 6 hours of symptom onset should be considered for intraarterial fibrinolytic therapy.

Full-dose anticoagulation with heparin preparations (IV or SC) is not recommended in patients with acute ischemic stroke (even if fibrinolytic therapy is not administered).

References

Adams RJ, Chimowitz MI, Alpert JS, et al. Coronary risk evaluation in patients with transient ischemic attack and ischemic stroke. A scientific statement for healthcare professional from the Stroke Council and the Council on Clinical Cardiology of the American Heart Association/American Stroke Association. *Circulation* 2003;108: 1278–1290.

Albers GW, Bates VE, Clark WM, Bell R, Verro P, Hamilton SA. Intravenous tissue-type plasminogen activator for treatment of acute stroke: the Standard Treatment with Alteplase to Reverse Stroke (STARS) study. *JAMA* 2000;283:1145–1150.

Albers GW, Clark WM, Madden KP, Hamilton SA. ATLANTIS Trial: results for patients treated within 3 hours of stroke onset. Alteplase Thrombolysis for Acute Noninterventional Therapy in Ischemic Stroke. *Stroke* 2002;33:493–496.

Antiplatelet Trialists' Collaboration. Secondary prevention of vascular disease by prolonged antiplatelet treatment. *Br Med J (Clin Res Ed)* 2002;296:320–331.

Barsan WG, Brott TG, Olinger CP, et al. Identification and entry of the patient with acute cerebral infarction. *Ann Emerg Med* 1988;17:1192–1195.

Balsano F, Coccheri, Libretti A, et al. Ticlopidine in the treatment of intermittent claudication: a 21-month double-blind trial. *J Lab Clin Med* 1989;114:84–91.

Belch JJ, Bell PR, Creissen D, et al. Randomized, double-blind, placebo-controlled study evaluating the efficacy and safety of AS-013, a prostaglandin E prodrug, in patients with intermittent claudication. *Circulation* 1997;95:2298–2302.

Bowan J, Yaste C. Effect of stroke protocol on hospital costs of stroke patients. *Neurology* 1994;44:1961–1964.

Bruckmann H, Ferbert A, Del Zoppo GJ, et al. Acute vertebral basilar thrombosis: angiologic-clinical comparison and therapeutic implications. *Acta Radiol* 1986; 369:38–42.

Buchan AM, Lesiuk H, Barnes KA, et al. AMPA antagonists: do they hold more promise for clinical stroke trials than NMDA antagonists? *Stroke* 1993;24:1148–1152.

CAPRIE Steering Committee. A randomised, blinded trial of clopidogrel versus aspirin in patients at risk of ischaemic events (CAPRIE). *Lancet* 1996;348:1329–1339.

CAST (Chinese Acute Stoke Trial) Collaborative Group. CAST: randomised placebo-controlled trial of early aspirin use in 20,000 patients with acute ischaemic stroke. *Lancet* 1997;349:1641–1649.

Clark WM, Wissman S, Albers GW, Jhamandas JH, Madden KP, Hamilton S. Recombinant tissue-type plasminogen activator (Alteplase) for ischemic stroke 3 to 5 hours after symptom onset. The ATLANTIS study: a randomized controlled trial. Alteplase Thrombolysis for Acute Noninterventional Therapy in Ischemic Stroke. *JAMA* 1999;282:2019–2026.

Davis PH, Dambrosia JM, Schoenberg BS, et al. Risk factors for ischemic stroke: a prospective stud in Rochester, Minnesota. *Ann Neurol* 1987;22:319–327.

Del Zoppo GJ, Zeumer H, Harker LA. Thrombolytic therapy and stroke: possibilities and hazards. *Stroke* 1986;17:595–607.

Del Zoppo GJ. Thrombolytic therapy in cerebrovascular disease and stroke. *Stroke* 1988;19:1174–1179.

Del Zoppo GJ, Ferbert A, Otis S, et al. Local intra-arterial fibrinolytic therapy in acute carotid territory stroke. A pilot study. *Stroke* 1988;19:307–313.

Del Zoppo GJ, Poeck K, Pessin MS, et al. Recombinant tissue plasminogen activator in acute thrombotic and embolic stroke. *Ann Neurol* 1992;32:78–86.

Diener H, Hacke W, Hennerici M, et al., for the Lubeluzole Study Group. Lubeluzole in acute ischemic stroke: a double-blind, placebo-controlled trial. *Stroke* 1996a;27:76–81.

Diener HC, Cunha L, Forbes C, Sivenius J, Smets P, Lowenthal A. European Stroke Prevention Study. 2. Dipyridamole and acetylsalicylic acid in the secondary prevention of stroke. *J Neurol Sci* 1996b;143:1–13.

Donnan GA, Hommel M, Davis SM, et al. Streptokinase in acute ischemic stroke. Steering committees of the ASK and MAST-E trials. Australian Streptokinase Trial [Letter]. *Lancet* 1995;346:56.

Eickhoiff JH, Buchardt Hansen HJ, Bromme A, et al. A randomized clinical trial of PTFE versus human umbilical vein for femoropopliteal bypass surgery. Preliminary results. *Br J. Surg* 1983;70:85–88.

Ernst E, Kollar L, Matrai A. A double-blind trial of Dextranhaemodilution vs placebo in claudicants. *J Intern Med* 1990;227:19–24.

Faxon DP, Creager MA, Smith SC Jr, et al. Atherosclerotic Vascular Disease Conference Executive Summary: Atherosclerotic Vascular Disease Conference proceeding for healthcare professionals from a special writing group of the American Heart Association. *Circulation* 2004;109:2595–2604.

Fieschi C, Argentino C, Lenzi GL, et al. Clinical and instrumental evaluation of patients with ischemic stroke within the first six hours. *J Neurol Sci* 1989;91:311–322.

Gent M, Blakely JA, Easton JD, et al. The Canadian American Ticlopidine Study (CATS) in thromboembolic stroke. *Lancet* 1989;1:1215–1220.

Hacke W, Zeumer H, Ferbert A, et al. Intra-arterial thrombolytic therapy improves outcome in patients with acute vertebrobasilar occlusive disease. *Stroke* 1988;21: 1216–1222.

Hacke W, Kaste M, Fieschi C, et al., for the ECASS study Group. Intravenous thrombolysis with recombinant tissue plasminogen activator for acute hemispheric stroke. The European Cooperative Acute Stroke Study (ECASS). *JAMA* 1995;274:1017–1025.

Haley EC Jr, Brott TG, Sheppard GL, et al., for the TPA Bridging Study Group. Pilot randomized trial of tissue plasminogen activator in acute ischemic stroke. *Stroke* 1993; 24:1000–1004.

Hass WK, Easton JD, Adams HP, et al. A randomized trial comparing ticlopidine hydrochloride with aspirin for the prevention of stroke in high-risk patients. Ticlopidine Aspirin Stroke Study Group. *N Engl J Med* 1989;321:501–507.

Harvard Stroke Registry. *Neurology* 1978;28:754–762.

Health United States 1992 and Healthy People 2000 Review. Publication 93–12321993. Hyattsville, Md: U.S. Department of Health and Human Services.

Indredavik B, Bakke F, Solberg R, et al. Benefit of a stroke unit: a randomized controlled trial. *Stroke* 1991;22:1026–1031.

International Stroke Trial Collaborative Group. The International Stroke Trial (IST): a randomized trial of aspirin, subcutaneous heparin, both or neither among 19,435 patients with acute ischemic stroke. *Lancet* 1997; 349;1569–1581.

Lievre M, Azoulay S, Lion L, Morand S, Girre JP, Buissel JP. A dose-effect study of beraprost sodium in intermittent claudication. *J Cardiovasc Pharmacol* 1996;27:788–793.

MAST–E Study Group. Thrombolytic therapy with streptokinase in acute ischemic stroke. *N Engl J Med* 1996;335:145–150.

MAST–I Group. Randomized controlled trial of streptokinase aspirin, and combination of both in treatment of acute ischemic stroke. *Lancet* 1995;346:1509–1514.

Matchar DB, Duncan PW. The cost of stroke. *Stroke Clin Updates* 1994;5:9–12.

McCollum C, Kenchington G, Alexander C, Franks PJ, Greenhalgh RM. PTFE or HUV for femoropopliteal bypass: a multicentre trial. *Eur J Vasc Surg* 1991,5.435–443.

Mori E, Yoneda Y, Tabuchi M, et al. Intravenous recombinant tissue plasminogen activator in acute carotid artery territory stroke. *Neurology* 1992;42:976–982.

The National Institute of Neurological Disorders and Stroke Study Group. Tissue plasminogen activator for acute ischemic stroke. *N Engl J Med* 1995;333:1581–1587.

Publications Committee for the Trial of Org 10172 in Acute Stroke Treatment (TOAST) Investigators. Low molecular weight heparinoid Org 10172 (danaparoid) and outcome after acute ischemic stroke: a randomized controlled trial. *JAMA* 1998;279: 1265–1272.

RANTTASS Investigators. A randomized trial of tirilazad mesylate in patients with acute stroke (RANTTASS). *Stroke* 1996;27:1453–1458.

Rutherford RB, Baker JD, Ernst C, et al. Recommended standards for reports dealing with lower extremity ischemia. Revisited version. *J Vasc Surg* 1997;26:517–538.

Sakaguchi S. Prostaglandin E1, intra-arterial infusion therapy in patients with ischemic ulcer of the extremities. *Int Angiol* 1984;3:39–42.

Sarac TP, Huber TS, Back MR, et al. Warfarin improves the outcome of infrainguinal vein bypass grafts at high risk for failure. *J Vasc Surg* 1998;28:446–457.

SASS Investigators. Ganglioside GM1 in acute ischemic stroke. *Stroke* 1994;25:1141–1148.

Schunemann HJ, Cook D, Grimshaw J, et al. Antithrombotic and thrombolytic therapy: from evidence to application: the Seventh ACCP Conference on Antithrombotic and Thrombolytic Therapy. *Chest* 2004;126:688S–696S.

STILE Investigators. Results of a prospective randomized trial evaluating surgery versus thrombolysis for ischemia of the lower extremity. *Ann Surg* 1994;220:251–268

Smith D. Stroke preventions: the importance of risk factors. *Stroke Clin Updates* 1991; 1:17–20.

Wolf PA, Doubler TR, Thomas HE, et al. Epidemiologic assessment of chronic atrial fibrillation and risk of stroke: the Framingham Study. *Neurology* 1987;28:973–977.

Valvular Heart Disease and Atrial Fibrillation

20

Native and Prosthetic Valvular Heart Disease

There are an estimated 250,000 heart valve replacement surgeries performed yearly on a worldwide basis. Mechanical prostheses have an excellent track record of durability (25 years or more), but current models require lifelong anticoagulation. Improved hemodynamics and reduced thrombogenicity characterize bioprosthetic valves; however, there is the disadvantage of degeneration, particularly in younger individuals. The ideal replacement—a tissue engineered "copy" of a native valve—is under development.

The most feared and devastating complications of native or prosthetic valvular heart disease for patients, clinicians, and surgeons are valve thrombosis and systemic embolism. Although the incidence of thromboembolic events has decreased in North America in parallel with the reduced occurrence of rheumatic heart disease, this has not been the case in other parts of the world. Moreover, despite the improvements in design and surgical techniques, thromboembolism remains a serious complication of prosthetic heart valve replacement.

Assessing Thromboembolic Risk

The risk of thromboembolism in patients with native valvular heart disease is influenced strongly by the site of involvement, chamber dimension, ventricular performance, and presence of concomitant risk factors such as atrial fibrillation. Prior thromboembolism is considered a strong risk factor for recurrent events regardless of the valvular pathology.

The risk of thromboembolism in patients with prosthetic valvular heart disease is recognized. Despite methodologic limitations, the available information derived from relatively large studies and an ever-expanding clinical experience allows several conclusions to be drawn:

- Thromboprophylaxis for mechanical prostheses is achieved most effectively with oral anticoagulants.
- Antiplatelet therapy *alone* does not offer adequate protection for patients with mechanical prostheses.
- The thrombogenicity of mechanical heart valves, from greatest to least, is as follows: caged ball > tilting disk > bileaflet.

- High-risk patients (increased risk for thromboembolism) benefit from combination (anticoagulant and platelet antagonist) antithrombotic therapy.
- A "threshold" level of anticoagulation is required for benefit.
- High-intensity anticoagulation (international normalized ratio [INR] >3.5) increases the risk for hemorrhagic complications.
- The risk of thromboembolism following bioprosthetic heart valve replacement is greatest during the first 3 postoperative months (Acar et al., 1996; Horstkotte et al., 1994; Sethia et al., 1986; Vogt et al., 1990).

Risk Stratification

The management of patients with native and prosthetic valvular heart disease must be approached comprehensively, taking into consideration not only the valve itself but the "company that it keeps" as well. Risk stratification, although focused predominantly on the potential risk of thromboembolic events, must consider the likelihood of hemorrhage with systemic anticoagulant therapy as well, particularly in patients with valvular heart disease in whom surgical procedures are being considered (Horstkotte et al., 1998) (Tables 20.1 and 20.2).

Anticoagulant Therapy: Recommendations and Management Guidelines

The recommended approach to patients with native and prosthetic valvular heart disease is based on a composite of clinical trial results and clinical experience (Schunemann et al., 2004); the latter is particularly true of native valvular disease for which few randomized trials have been conducted (Tables 20.3, 20.4, and 20.5).

Bridging Therapy

Decisions regarding periprocedural or "bridging" anticoagulant therapy among patients with mechanical heart valves (and other forms of valvular heart disease or thrombolic disorders requiring long-term anticoagulation) have been complicated by the virtual absence of randomized trials. Cohort studies and institutional data support the safety of low-molecular-weight heparin (LMWH) (when anticoagulant therapy is required) for relatively brief periods of time (up to 7 days) (Montalescot et al., 2000). There are insufficient data to confirm the safety and efficacy of LMWH (or other anticoagulants) in pregnant patients with mechanical heart valves (APPCR Panel, 2002).

Table 20.1 Thromboembolic Risk Scale[†]

Low Risk
  Atrial fibrillation
  Bioprosthetic heart valve (>3 mo postop)
  St. Jude mechanical heart valve (aortic position) (>6 mo postop)
  Dilated cardiomyopathy (ejection fraction <35%)
Intermediate Risk
  Atrial fibrillation and prior thromboembolism (>3 mo)
  St. Jude mechanical heart valve (aortic position) plus atrial fibrillation or ejection fraction <35%
  Dilated cardiomyopathy and prior thromboembolism (>3 mo)
  Two low-risk factors
  Anterior myocardial infarction <3 mo (no other risk factors)
  St. Jude mechanical heart valve ≤6 mo postop or in mitral position
  Bjork-Shiley (tilting disc) mechanical heart valve (aortic position)
High Risk
  Atrial fibrillation and prior thromboembolism (<3 mo)
  Dilated cardiomyopathy and prior thromboembolism (< 3 mo)
  Bjork-Shiley mechanical heart valve (mitral position) and any other risk factor
  St. Jude mechanical heart valve (aortic position) and ≥1 intermediate-risk factor
  Caged-ball mechanical heart valve (mitral position)
Very High Risk
  Antiphospholipid syndrome plus prior event or additional risk factors
  Cardioversion ≤2 wk
  Arterial thromboembolic event ≤1 mo
  Caged-ball mechanical heart valve (any position) plus additional risk factors
  Any combination ≥2 risk factors

[†] *Becker/Spencer Risk Scale.*

Pregnant Women with Mechanical Prosthetic Heart Valves

The use of LMWH preparations in pregnant women with mechanical heart valves has not been studied sufficiently to determine their overall safety and efficacy. If used, frequent evaluation and monitoring of peak (1.0–1.5 AXa units) and trough (0.5–1.0 AXa units) levels are recommended.

Strategies for bridging therapy are being developed; however, the safety of thromboprophylaxis during pregnancy requires further study to establish "best practice."

Rheumatic Mitral Valve Disease

Focused Summary of Recommendations

1. It is strongly recommended that long-term warfarin therapy sufficient to prolong the INR in the range of 2.0 to 3.0 be used in patients with rheumatic mitral valve disease who have either a history of systemic embolism or who have paroxysmal or chronic atrial fibrillation (AF).

Table 20.2 Hemorrhagic Risk Scale[†]

Low Risk
    Dental procedures*
    Cataract surgery
    Angiography (diagnostic)
    Cystoscopy
    Breast biopsy
    Arthroscopic surgery
Intermediate Risk
    Total hip replacement
    Total knee replacement
    Laparoscopic surgery
    Maxillofacial surgery
    Transurethral prostate removal
    Hysterectomy
    Colonoscopy with biopsy
    Prostate biopsy
    Skin graft
High Risk
    Major abdominal surgery
    Major thoracic surgery
    Brain/central nervous system surgery
    Radical prostatectomy
    Skin graft
    Liver biopsy
    Kidney biopsy

[†] *Becker/Spencer Risk Scale.*
Exception: multiple extractions.

Table 20.3 Antithrombotic Therapy for Patients with Native Valvular Heart Disease

Native Valvular Heart Disease	Recommendations
Rheumatic Mitral Valvular Disease	
Prior thromboembolism	Oral anticoagulant, INR 2.5
Paroxysmal or chronic AF	Oral anticoagulant, INR 2.5
LA diameter >5.5 cm	Oral anticoagulant, INR 2.5
MVA <1.0 cm^2, LA enlargement	Oral anticoagulant, INR 2.5
Recurrent embolism (despite oral anticoagulant)	Add aspirin (80–100 mg qd) or clopidogrel (75 mg qd)
Mitral Annular Calcification	
Uncomplicated	No antithrombotic therapy
AF or systemic embolism	Oral anticoagulant, INR 2.5
Mitral Valve Prolapse	
Uncomplicated	No antithrombotic therapy
TIA	Aspirin (325 mg qd)
Recurrent TIAs	Oral anticoagulant, INR 2.5, or clopidogrel (75 mg qd)
Systemic embolism	Oral anticoagulant, INR 2.5
Aortic Valvular Disease	
Sinus rhythm	No antithrombotic therapy
Chronic AF or systemic embolism	Oral anticoagulant, INR 2.5

AF, atrial fibrillation; INR, international normalized ratio; LA, left atrium; MVA, mitral valve area; TIA, transient ischemic attack.

Table 20.4 Antithrombotic Therapy for Patients with Bioprosthetic Heart Valves or Valve Repair

Valve Type/Position	INR	Duration of Treatment
Mitral position	2.5	3 mo
Aortic position	2.5	3 mo
Atrial fibrillation	2.5	Long-term
LA thrombosis	2.5	3–6 mo
Systemic embolism	2.5	3–12 mo
Systemic embolism despite anticoagulant therapy	2.5	Minimum 12 mo
Valve repair†	2.5	3 mo

*Add aspirin (80–100 mg qd) or clopidogrel (75 mg qd).
† With or without annuloplasty ring.
INR, international normalized ratio; LA, left atrium (includes left atrial appendage).

2. It is recommended that long-term warfarin therapy (INR 2.0–3.0) be considered in patients with rheumatic mitral valve disease and normal sinus rhythm if the left atrial diameter exceeds 55 mm.

3. It is recommended that patients who experience systemic embolism despite adequate warfarin therapy should also receive aspirin (80–100 mg/day). For patients unable to take aspirin, alternative strategies include (a) increasing the target INR to between 2.5 and 3.5; (b) adding dipyridamole 400 mg/day; or (c) adding ticlopidine 250 mg twice daily.

Aortic Valve Disease

It is strongly recommended that long-term antithrombotic therapy not be given to patients with aortic valve disease unless they also have concomitant mitral valve disease, AF, or a history of systemic embolism.

Mitral Valve Prolapse

Focused Summary of Recommendations

1. It is strongly recommended that long-term antithrombotic therapy not be given to patients with mitral valve prolapse (MVP) who have not experienced systemic embolism, unexplained transient ischemic attacks (TIAs), or AF.

2. It is recommended that patients with MVP who have documented but unexplained TIAs receive long-term low-dose aspirin therapy (160–325 mg/day).

Table 20.5 Summary of Recommendations for Patients with Mechanical Heart Valves

Valve Type/Position	INR Target
Bileaflet, aortic	2.5 (3.0 if AF, LA >5.5 cm, or LVEF <35%)
Tilting disc, aortic	3.0
Bileaflet, mitral	3.0 or 2.5 + aspirin 80–100 mg qd
Tilting disc, mitral	3.0 or 3.0* + aspirin 80–100 mg qd
Caged-ball/disc	3.0 + aspirin 80–100 mg qd
Systemic embolism despite anticoagulant therapy	3.0 + aspirin 80–100 mg qd

*With additional risk factors.
AF, atrial fibrillation; INR, international normalized ratio; LA, left atrium; LVEF, left ventricular ejection fraction.

3. It is recommended that patients with MVP who have (a) documented systemic embolism, (b) chronic or paroxysmal AF, or (c) recurrent TIAs despite aspirin therapy received long-term warfarin therapy (INR 2.0–3.0).

Mitral Annular Calcification

1. It is recommended that long-term antithrombotic therapy not be given to patients with mitral annular calcification (MAC) who lack a history of thromboembolism or AF.
2. It is recommended that patients with MAC complicated by (a) systemic embolism or (b) AF be treated with long-term warfarin therapy (INR 2.0–3.0).

Patent Foramen Ovale and Atrial Septal Aneurysm

1. It is strongly recommended that anticoagulant therapy not be given to patients with either asymptomatic patent foramen ovale (PFO) or atrial septal aneurysm.
2. It is strongly recommended that patients with unexplained systemic embolism or TIAs and demonstrable venous thrombosis or pulmonary embolism (PE) and either a PFO or atrial septal aneurysm be treated with long-term warfarin therapy (unless venous interruption or closure of the PFO is considered preferable). In the case of an atrial septal aneurysm, the possibility of both paradoxical embolism and systemic embolism from the arterial side of the aneurysm should be considered in choosing therapy.

Infective Endocarditis

1. It is strongly recommended that anticoagulant therapy not be given to patients in normal sinus rhythm with uncomplicated infective endocarditis involving either a native or a bioprosthetic valve.
2. It is recommended that long-term warfarin therapy be continued for endocarditis in patients with a mechanical prosthetic valve unless there are specific contraindications (high risk for bleeding).
3. The indications for anticoagulant therapy when systemic embolism occurs during the course of infective endocarditis involving either a native or bioprosthetic heart valve are uncertain. The decision should consider comorbid conditions, including AF, evidence of left atrial thrombus, evidence and size of valvular vegetations, and particularly the success of antibiotic therapy in controlling the infective process.

Nonbacterial Thrombotic Endocarditis

1. It is recommended that patients with nonbacterial thrombotic endocarditis and systemic or pulmonary embolism be treated with heparin (followed by warfarin).
2. It is recommended that heparin therapy be considered for patients with disseminated cancer or debilitating disease who are found to have aseptic vegetations (on echocardiography).

Atrial Fibrillation

Atrial fibrillation affects upward of 5% of the U.S. population (Rosenthal, 2004), increasing steadily with age (Stewart et al., 2002). Although there is limited information on the prevalence of AF according to race, the available data suggest that black Americans may be at slightly lower risk than Caucasians (Go et al., 2001). According to current estimates, by the year 2015 more than half of all individuals with AF will be 80 years of age or older, representing a total of nearly 4 million cases (Braunwald, 1997; Go et al., 2001).

The estimated lifetime risks for developing AF (including atrial flutter) were determined in 3,999 men and 4,726 women participating in the Framingham Heart Study. Excluding individuals with either congestive heart failure or myocardial infarction (MI), lifetime risks for AF were approximately 16% (one in six) (Lloyd-Jones et al., 2004).

There are a variety of contributing factors and comorbid illnesses related to AF. One in particular, hypertensive heart disease, accounts for approximately

15% of all cases. Similarly, patients with hypertensive heart disease have a fourfold increased risk for developing the arrhythmia. Coronary artery disease accounts for another 8% of cases among men. Independent risk factors for AF include increased age, male sex, valvular disease (particularly mitral stenosis), congestive heart failure, systemic hypertension (which doubles the risk of AF in both men and women), and diabetes mellitus. Additional risk factors and associated conditions are hyperthyroidism, alcohol abuse (acute/chronic), cardiomyopathies (dilated, hypertrophic), atrial septal defects, acute pulmonary embolism, pericarditis, sick sinus syndrome, and Wolff-Parkinson-White (WPW) syndrome. Common contributors among hospitalized patients are pneumonia, hypoxia, hypoglycemia, bacteremia, hypokalemia, hypothermia, MI, and cardiac surgery (Benjamin et al., 1994).

Thromboembolism and Atrial Fibrillation

The available data suggest that as many as 15% of all strokes in the United States may be attributable to AF. Nonvalvular AF, currently the most common form of this arrhythmia, increases the risk of stroke nearly fivefold (Go et al., 2001; Wolf et al., 1978, 1987) (Figure 20.1), particularly among the elderly. In contrast, valvular AF, particularly when associated with mitral stenosis, increases the risk even further to approximately 20-fold.

Figure 20.1 Stroke incidence increases with age for the general population; however, the overall incidence is particularly high in aging adults with atrial fibrillation. (From Wolf PA, Dawber TR, Thomas HE Jr, Kannel WB. Epidemiologic assessment of chronic atrial fibrillation and risk of stroke: the Framingham study. *Neurology* 1978;28:973–977.)

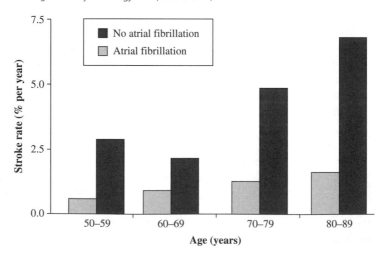

Genetic Polymorphisms and Thromboembolic Risk

The association between genetic polymorphisms and thromboembolic risk has been a subject of increased interest. In the majority of studies, no relationship between the most common inherited thrombophilic conditions (factor V Leiden mutation, prothrombin G20210A mutation) and thromboembolic stroke has been identified among patients with AF (Feinberg et al., 1999; Poli et al., 2003). In contrast, the α-fibrinogen Thr312Ala polymorphism has been linked to increased poststroke mortality (Carter et al., 1999). The potential interface between AF, inflammation, and thrombosis attributable to factor XIII polymorphisms is under investigation.

Antithrombotic Therapy for the Prevention of Thromboembolism

Anticoagulants

Vitamin K Antagonists

There is incontrovertible evidence that AF, by several integrated mechanisms including stasis of blood flow, coagulation factor activation, heightened state of inflammation, reduced local fibrinolytic activity, and concomitant hemodynamic abnormalities associated with systemic disorders and/or organic heart disease, fosters thrombus development and subsequent thromboembolism.

Large-scale randomized trials performed over the past decade and a half have shown convincingly that anticoagulant therapy with vitamin K antagonists (predominantly warfarin) and, more recently, the direct thrombin inhibitor ximelagatran prevents cardioembolic stroke with a very low risk for major hemorrhage (Figure 20.2). A meta-analysis of randomized trials (Atrial Fibrillation Investigators, 1994) demonstrated that anticoagulant therapy reduced the risk of stroke by 68%, with a relatively small increase in the frequency of intracranial hemorrhage or major bleeding.

Current National Rates of Warfarin Use

The National Stroke Medicare Quality Improvement Project evaluated vitamin K antagonist use among over 12,000 patients with AF. Treatment at the time of hospital discharge barely reached 50% and decreased with increased patient age, particularly among black American and Asian populations. These observations underscore the tremendous opportunity for improvement in stroke prevention for patients with AF.

253

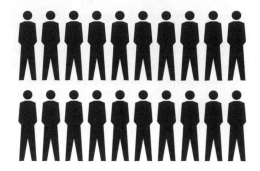

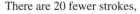

There are 20 fewer strokes,

Figure 20.2 The benefit of anticoagulation therapy translates to 20 fewer strokes at the risk of one additional major hemorrhage. (From Hylek EM, Skates SJ, Sheehan MA, Singer DE. An analysis of the lowest effective intensity of prophylactic anticoagulation for patients with nonrheumatic atrial fibrillation. *N Eng J Med* 1996;335:540–545; and Hylek EM, Singer DE. Risk factors for intracranial hemorrhage in outpatients taking warfarin. *Ann Intern Med* 1994;120:897–902.)

but only 1 more major bleeding event.

Low-Molecular-Weight Heparin

Low-molecular-weight heparin preparations vary in molecular weight from 2,000 to 10,000 daltons. Accordingly, they contain both short and long polysaccharide chains with antifactor Xa and antifactor IIa inhibiting potential, respectively.

The absorption of LMWH is near complete at a wide range of subcutaneous doses, its bioavailability exceeds 90% (minimal plasma protein and vascular endothelial cell binding), and the plasma half-life varies from 5 to 8 hours (compounds with a greater proportion of short polysaccharide chains [molecular weight] are cleared more slowly via renal mechanisms). Following subcutaneous administration, peak antifactor Xa activity is achieved within 5 to 8 hours, with persistently measurable anticoagulant activity for 12 to 16 hours (longer in patients with renal insufficiency).

It is important to acknowledge that each LMWH preparation has a distinct pharmacokinetic and pharmacodynamic profile, which may impact dosing, dosing strategies, and efficiency in thrombotic disorders. Their use in the setting of AF is discussed in the section on cardioversion.

Ximelagatran

The challenges of vitamin K antagonist titration and the clear relationship between intensity of anticoagulation and both thromboembolic and hemorrhagic risk has generated enthusiasm for the development of alternative anticoagulants with predictable pharmacokinetics and pharmacodynamics, permitting administration at fixed doses (no requirement for titration). Ximelagatran is an oral direct thrombin inhibitor that is rapidly absorbed and metabolized to the active compound melagatran. It is the first oral anticoagulant to have been developed in the past 50 years. Following oral administration, peak plasma activity is reached in 40 minutes with a plasma half-life of approximately 4 to 5 hours. There is minimal plasma protein binding and elimination occurs through renal mechanisms (Eriksson et al., 2003). The pharmacokinetics of ximelagatran are predictable, stable over time, and unaffected by body weight, age, sex, or ethnic origin (Johansson et al., 2003; Sarich et al., 2003). Unlike vitamin K antagonists, it has a low potential for drug interactions and no known food interactions. As a result, coagulation monitoring and dose adjustment will not be required during routine clinical use.

A comprehensive program of clinical investigation was undertaken to evaluate ximelagatran (Exanta) in the setting of AF. Stroke Prevention by Oral Thrombin Inhibitor in Atrial Fibrillation (SPORTIF) II, a modestly sized phase II study, randomized 254 high-risk patients with nonvalvular atrial fibrillation to receive 20, 40, or 60 mg of ximelagatran twice daily. Overall, the drug was well tolerated at all doses with one nonfatal ischemic stroke and one transient ischemic attack reported during the 12-week study period (Petersen et al., 2003).

SPORTIF III was a randomized, open label, phase III study that included 3,407 high-risk patients treated with either fixed-dose ximelagatran (36 mg twice daily) or warfarin (target INR 2.5; range 2.0–3.0). After a mean follow-up of 17 months, 1.6% (per year treated) of patients randomized to ximelagatran had experienced either ischemic/hemorrhagic stroke or systemic thromboembolism, compared to 2.3% (per year treated) among those receiving warfarin (relative risk reduction 29%). The combined incidence of major and minor hemorrhage was lower with ximelagatran than with warfarin (relative risk reduction 14%). The concentrations of alanine aminotransferase (ALT) rose above three times the upper limit of normal in 6.0% of ximelagatran-treated patients, typically beginning between 2 and 6 months from treatment initiation (Olson and the Executive Steering Committee on behalf of the SPORTIF III Investigators, 2003).

The SPORTIF V trial randomized 3,922 individuals to receive either ximelagatran (36 mg twice daily) or warfarin (target INR 2.0–3.0). Treatment allocation was double blind. During 6,405 patient years of exposure (mean 20 months), the primary endpoint (composite of all strokes [ischemic and hemorrhagic] and systemic embolic events) occurred at rates of 1.6% per year and 1.2% per year, respectively (The Executive Steering Committee on behalf of the SPORTIF V Investigators, 2003). Rates of disabling fatal stroke, hemorrhagic stroke, and major hemorrhage did not differ between groups. Hepatic enzymes (ALT) increased to three times the upper limit of normal in 6.0% of patients on ximelagatran within the first 6 months of treatment. At least one case of drug-related filament hepatic failure was reported. Ximelagatran is not currently FDA approved for thrombo-prophylaxis among patients with atrial fibrillation.

Antiplatelet Therapy

The pathobiology of cardioembolism associated with AF may intuitively support a treatment approach favoring anticoagulants; however, platelet activation occurs in this setting as well, and platelet aggregates represent a crucial template for thrombin generation and thrombus propagation.

Several clinical trials have evaluated antiplatelet therapy in AF. In two randomized trials, Atrial Fibrillation Aspirin Coagulation (AFASAK) (Peterson et al., 1989) and the European Atrial Fibrillation Trial (EAFT) (European Atrial Fibrillation Trial Study Group, 1995), aspirin treatment reduced the risk of cardioembolic stroke by 16% and 17%, respectively (not statistically significant). In contrast, the American Stroke Prevention in Atrial Fibrillation (SPAF)-1 trial (Stroke Prevention in Atrial Fibrillation Investigators, 1991) identified a significant reduction (42%) with aspirin treatment. A pooled analysis of the previously mentioned aspirin trials demonstrated a 21% reduction in the rate of ischemic stroke.

In studies comparing antiplatelet and anticoagulant therapy, the latter has consistently shown greater benefit in high-risk patients. For example, stroke rates were reduced by 40% to 50% among patients receiving warfarin (compared to aspirin) in the AFASAK and EAFT trials. The SPAF-3 trial investigated to efficacy of fixed-dose, low-intensity warfarin therapy (INR 1.2–1.5; maximum daily dose 3 mg) plus aspirin, compared to standard adjusted-dose warfarin (target INR 2.5; range 2.0–3.0). The trial was terminated because of a clear difference in event rates between the two groups (7.9% per year and 1.9% per year, respectively) (Stroke Prevention in Atrial Fibrillation Investigators, 1996).

The available data led to the following conclusions: (1) aspirin therapy is beneficial in low-risk patients; and (2) the combination of low-intensity anticoagulant and aspirin therapy is inferior to moderate-intensity warfarin among high-risk patients.

The potential role of dual antiplatelet therapy with aspirin and clopidogrel (Plavix), an adenosine diphosphate antagonist used widely in the setting of arterial thrombotic disorders, is undergoing investigation among patients with AF.

Antithrombotic Therapy during Cardioversion

The risk of thromboembolic events following cardioversion for AF in the absence of adequate anticoagulant therapy approaches 7% (Arnold et al., 1992). For AF of more than 48 hours in duration, current guidelines advocate the use of anticoagulation for at least 3 weeks before and 4 weeks after the procedure (Fuster et al., 2001). Transesophageal echocardiography (TEE) can reduce the overall duration of anticoagulation by approximately 3 weeks with the exclusion of left atrial/left atrial appendage thrombus (Klein et al., 2001). Low-molecular-weight heparin has been used in the setting of cardioversion; however, clinicians, particularly those practicing in the United States, have voiced concern because of limited randomized data.

The Anticoagulation in Cardioversion Using Enoxaparin (ACE) trial (Stellbrink et al., 2004) was a randomized, prospective, multicenter study of 496 patients undergoing elective cardioversion for AF who received either enoxaparin (1 mg/kg SC twice daily for 3–8 days, followed by 40 mg twice daily in patients <65 kg and 60 mg twice daily for those ≥65 kg) or intravenous unfractionated heparin for a minimum of 72 hours, followed by phenprocoumon [target INR 2.0–3.0]). The study's primary endpoint, a composite of embolic events, all-cause mortality, and major hemorrhage, occurred in 3.2% of enoxaparin-treated patients and 5.7% of unfractionated heparin/phenprocoumon-treated patients. The overall event rates were lower in both groups when a TEE-based strategy was employed.

The available data suggest that enoxaparin, and possibly other LMWH preparations, can be used in the setting of cardioversion for AF. Given its ease of administration and rapid achievement of predictable states of systemic anticoagulation, hospitalization costs and adverse events may be reduced, particularly when used along with a strategy that includes TEE (Klein et al., 2004) (Figure 20.3).

Safe and Effective Use of Oral Vitamin K Antagonists

Vitamin K antagonists, despite their wide-scale availability and established track record in the management of AF, are best classified as narrow therapeutic index drugs. The available information suggests strongly that a minimum threshold of anticoagulation, as determined by the prothrombin time–INR, must be surpassed to protect against thromboembolism; however, high-intensity states of inhibition place patients at risk for major hemorrhagic events including intracranial hemorrhage (Hylek and Singer, 1994; Hylek et al., 1996) (Figure 20.4).

The effect of anticoagulation intensity may also influence outcome following thromboembolic stroke. Based on a cohort of 13,559 patients with AF, an INR less than 2.0 at the time of hospital admission for stroke independently increased the odds of a severe event and death within 30 days (compared to those with an INR ≥2.0) (Hylek et al., 2003).

The initiation of anticoagulant therapy with vitamin K antagonists is particularly challenging for clinicians, and the first 6 weeks of treatment represent the time during which complications are most likely to occur. The reason relates to starting dose, frequency of INR monitoring, titration strategies, and a wide variety of potential interactions that influence anticoagulant response ranging from comorbid disease states to diet, activity, and concomitant medications (Table 20.6).

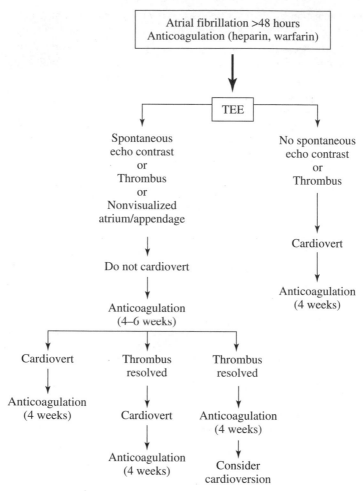

Figure 20.3 Transesophageal echocardiography (TEE) can be used in the elective management of patients with atrial fibrillation (AF).

Management Guidelines

An ability to utilize the knowledge gained through scientific investigation and carefully conducted, large-scale clinical trials is required to impact the standard of patient care. Management guidelines, based on the available evidence and expert consensus, currently represents the best available means to achieve optimal patient outcomes on a wide scale (Table 20.7).

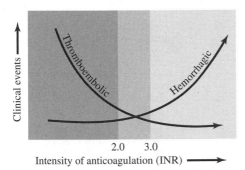

2.0   3.0
Intensity of anticoagulation (INR) ⟶

Figure 20.4 Thromboembolic events may occur at an international normalized ratio (INR) value of less than 2.0. Conversely, hemorrhagic risk increases with a greater intensity of systemic anticoagulation. (From Hylek EM, Skates SJ, Sheehan MA, Singer DE. An analysis of the lowest effective intensity of prophylactic anticoagulation for patients with nonrheumatic atrial fibrillation. *N Eng J Med* 1996;335:540–545; and Hylek EM, Singer DE. Risk factors for intracranial hemorrhage in outpatients taking warfarin. *Ann Intern Med* 1994;120:897–902.)

The American College of Chest Physicians' (ACCP) Antithrombotic Therapy Guidelines for Nonvalvular AF (Schunemann et al., 2004) include a practical classification scheme and treatment recommendations based on risk category (risk for stroke and systemic thromboembolism). Joint recommendations developed by the American Heart Association/American College of Cardiology/European Society of Cardiology are similar to those of the ACCP; however, they include additional patient subsets in a "highest risk" category (rheumatic heart disease, prosthetic heart valves, and persistent atrial thrombus on TEE) where target INRs ranging from 2.5 to 3.5 (or higher) may be appropriate (but not commonly sought in routine clinical practice), and a "lowest risk" category (lone atrial fibrillation) that may not require antithrombotic therapy (aspirin is optional).

Table 20.6 Stroke Predictors with Atrial Fibrillation: Risk-Stratification Scheme

Stratification	Clinical Features	Stroke Rate (%/yr)
High risk	Prior stroke or TIA or systemic embolism; age >75, hypertension, poor LV systolic function; rheumatic mitral valve disease or prosthetic heart valve	4–12
Moderate risk	Age 65–75; CAD with preserved LV function, thyrotoxicosis	2–4
Low risk	No high- or moderate-risk features, age <65, no cardiovascular disease	1

CAD, coronary artery disease; LV, left ventricular; TIA, transient ischemic attack.

Fintel D, Hofmann C. The American Physicians Guide to Preventing Strokes and Lowering Health Risks in Patients with Atrial Fibrillation. Lisle, Ill.: Illinois Academy of Family Physicians 2000; and Singer DE, Albers GW, Dalen JE, et al. Antithrombotic therapy in atrial fibrillation. Chest 2004; 126:429S–456S.

Table 20.7 Antithrombotic Therapy in Nonvalvular Atrial Fibrillation

Age (yr)	Risk Factors*	Recommendations
<65	Absent	Aspirin
	Present	Warfarin (target INR 2.5, range 2.0–3.0)
65–75	Absent	Aspirin or warfarin
	Present	Warfarin (target INR 2.5, range 2.0–3.0)
>75	All patients	Warfarin (target INR 2.5, range 2.0–3.0)

*Prior transient ischemic attack, systemic embolus or stroke, hypertension, poor left ventricular function, rheumatic mitral valve disease, or prosthetic heart valve.
INR, international normalized ratio

Singer DE, Albers GW, Dalen JE, et al. Antithrombotic therapy in atrial fibrillation. Chest 2004; 126: 429S–456S.

Rate vs. Rhythm Control

Many primary care physicians and cardiologists managing patients with AF practice with the belief that achieving sinus rhythm definitively addresses the risk of cardioembolic events including stroke. Published results from two clinic trials, Atrial Fibrillation Follow-up Investigation of Rhythm Management (AFFIRM) (Wyse et al., 2002) and Rate Control Versus Electrical Cardioversion for Persistent Atrial Fibrillation (RACE) (Van Gelder et al., 2002), challenge this widely taught dogma. Beyond the overall study results, which did not favor one management strategy over the other, two-thirds of patients in the RACE trial who experienced thromboembolic events had an INR less than 2.0, and three-quarters had atrial AF at the time of their event. In AFFIRM, 72% of patients with an ischemic stroke had either an INR less than 2.0 or had discontinued therapy. Most striking, a majority of patients in the rhythm control group (by definition, no anticoagulant therapy) were believed to be in sinus rhythm. An on-treatment analysis of the AFFIRM data revealed that warfarin use improved survival (AFFIRM Investigators, 2004).

Thus, the available information suggests that anticoagulant therapy should be considered strongly in high-risk patients with AF, even with rhythm control.

Summary

Atrial fibrillation is an increasingly common arrhythmia that causes several million strokes each year in the United States. The benefits of antithrombotic therapy are recognized, particularly among high-risk patients in whom vitamin K antagonists reduce event rates by nearly 70%. Moderate-risk patients benefit from either anticoagulant or platelet-directed therapy; however, careful risk assessment must be undertaken serially to avoid underestimating overall risk (and optimal treatment). Electrical cardioversion, preferably combined with a strategy of TEE in patients at risk for hemorrhagic complications, is associated with thromboembolic events, necessitating anticoagulation with either enoxaparin or unfractionated heparin (followed by a vitamin K antagonist). Data with the oral direct thrombin inhibitor, ximelagatran, were encouraging and, in all likelihood, represent the beginning of a new era in the treatment of thrombotic disorders. It is possible that a fixed-dose alternative (to warfarin) will increase the overall number of patients with AF who are offered therapy. In addition, the management of individuals with INR variability, a requirement for frequent testing, and a medication profile that includes multiple interacting drugs, could be optimized. Last, a drug (or drug strategy) with a favorable safety and efficacy profile may provide an option for patients unable to take warfarin

References

Acar J, Iung B, Boissel JP, et al. AREVA: multicenter randomized comparison of low-dose versus standard dose anticoagulation in patients with mechanical prosthetic heart valves. *Circulation* 1996;94:2107–2112.

AFFIRM Investigators. Relationships between sinus rhythm, treatment, and survival in the Atrial Fibrillation Follow-Up Investigation of Rhythm Management (AFFIRM) study. *Circulation* 2004;109:1509–1513.

Anticoagulation in Prosthetic Valves and Pregnancy Consensus Report (APPCR) Panel. Anticoagulation and enoxaparin use in patients with prosthetic heart valves and/or pregnancy. An evidence-based review and focused analysis of current controversies and clinical strategies. Consensus Panel Statements for Outcome-Effective and Evidence-Based Patient Management. *Am Health Consultants* 2002;3:1–20.

Arnold AZ, Mick MJ, Mazurek RP, Loop FD, Trohman RG. Role of prophylactic anticoagulation for direct current cardioversion in patients with atrial fibrillation or atrial flutter. *J Am Coll Cardiol* 1992;19:851–855.

Atrial Fibrillation Investigators. Risk factors for stroke and efficacy of antithrombotic therapy in atrial fibrillation. Analysis of pooled data from five randomized controlled trials. *Arch Intern Med* 1994;154:1449–1457.

Benjamin EJ, Levy D, Vaziri SM, D'Agostino RB, Belanger AJ, Wolf PA. Independent risk factors for atrial fibrillation in a population-based cohort. The Framingham Heart Study. *JAMA* 1994;271:840–844.

Braunwald E. Shattuck lecture—cardiovascular medicine at the turn of the millennium: triumphs, concerns, and opportunities. *N Eng J Med* 1997;337:1360–1369.

Carter AM, Catto AJ, Grant PF. Association of the α-fibrinogen Thr312Ala polymorphism with poststroke mortality in subjects with atrial fibrillation. *Circulation* 1999; 99:2423–2426.

Eriksson UG, Bredberg U, Hoffmann KJ, et al. Absorption, distribution, metabolism, and excretion of ximelagatran, an oral direct thrombin inhibitor, in rats, dogs, and humans. *Drug Metab Dispos* 2003;31:294–305.

European Atrial Fibrillation Trial Study Group. Optimal oral anticoagulation therapy in patients with nonrheumatic atrial fibrillation and recent cerebral ischemia. *N Engl J Med* 1995;333:5–10.

The Executive Steering Committee on behalf of the SPORTIF V Investigators. Stroke prevention using the oral direct thrombin inhibitor ximelagatran in patients with nonvalvular atrial fibrillation (SPORTIF V) [Abstract]. *Circulation* 2003;108:2723.

Feinberg WM, Pearce LA, Hart RG, et al. Markers of thrombin and platelet activity in patients with atrial fibrillation. Correlation with stroke among 1531 participants in the Stroke Prevention in Atrial Fibrillation III Study. *Stroke* 1999;30:2547–2553.

Fintel D, Hofmann C. *The American Physicians Guide to Preventing Strokes and Lowering Health Risks in Patients with Atrial Fibrillation.* Lisle, Ill.: Illinois Academy of Family Physicians 2000.

Fuster V, Ryden LE, Asinger RW, et al. ACC/AHA/ESC guidelines for the management of patients with atrial fibrillation: executive summary. A report of the American College of Cardiology/American Heart Association Task Force on Practice Guidelines and the European Society of Cardiology Committee for Practice Guidelines and Policy Conferences (committee to develop guidelines for the management of patients with atrial fibrillation) developed in collaboration with the North American Society of Pacing and Electrophysiology. *Circulation* 2001;104:2118–2150.

Go AS, Hylek EM, Phillips KA, et al. Prevalence of diagnosed atrial fibrillation in adults: national implications for rhythm management and stroke prevention: the AnTicoagulation and Risk Factors in Atrial Fibrillation (ATRIA) Study. *JAMA* 2001;285: 2370–2375.

Horstkotte D, Schulte HD, Bircks W, Strauer BE. Lower intensity anticoagulation therapy results in lower complication rates with the St. Jude medical prosthesis. *J Thorac Cardiovasc Surg* 1994;107:1136–1145.

Horstkotte D, Piper C, Weimer M. Optimal frequency of patient monitoring and intensity of oral anticoagulation therapy in valvular heart disease. *J Thromb Thrombolysis* 1998;5:S19–S24.

Hylek EM, Singer DE. Risk factors for intracranial hemorrhage in outpatients taking warfarin. *Ann Intern Med* 1994;120:897–902.

Hylek EM, Skates SJ, Sheehan MA, Singer DE. An analysis of the lowest effective intensity of prophylactic anticoagulation for patients with nonrheumatic atrial fibrillation. *N Engl J Med* 1996;335:540–545.

Hylek EM, Go AS, Chang Y, et al. Effect of intensity of oral anticoagulation on stroke severity and mortality in atrial fibrillation. *N Engl J Med* 2003;349:1019–1026.

Johansson LC, Frison L, Logren U, Fager G, Gustafsson D, Eriksson UG. Influence of age on the pharmacokinetics and pharmacodynamics of ximelagatran, an oral direct thrombin inhibitor. *Clin Pharm* 2003;42:381–392.

Klein AL, Grimm RA, Murray RD, et al. Assessment of Cardioversion Using Transesophageal Echocardiography Investigators. Use of transesophageal echocardiography to guide cardioversion in patients with atrial fibrillation. *N Engl J Med* 2001; 344:1411–1420.

Klein AL, Murray RD, Becker ER, et al. for the ACUTE Investigators. Economic analysis of a transesophageal echocardiography-guided approach to cardioversion of patients with atrial fibrillation. *J Am Coll Cardiol* 2004;43:1217–1224.

Lloyd-Jones DM, Wang TJ, Leip EP, et al. Lifetime risk for development of atrial fibrillation. The Framingham Heart Study. *Circulation* 2004;110:1042–1046.

Montalescot G, Polle V, Collet JP, et al. Low molecular weight heparin after mechanical heart valve replacement. *Circulation* 2000;101:1083–1086.

Olsson SB, Executive Steering Committee on behalf of the SPORTIF III Investigators. Stroke prevention with the oral direct thrombin inhibitor ximelagatran compared with warfarin in patients with non-valvular atrial fibrillation (SPORTIF III): randomised controlled trial. *Lancet* 2003;362:1691–1698.

Petersen P, Grind M, Adler J, SPORTIF II Investigators. Ximelagatran versus warfarin for stroke prevention in patients with nonvalvular atrial fibrillation. SPORTIF II: a dose-guiding, tolerability, and safety study. *J Am Coll Cardiol* 2003;41:1445–1451.

Peterson P, Boysen G, Godtfredsen J, Anderson ED, Anderson B. Placebo controlled randomized trial of warfarin and aspirin for prevention of thromboembolic complications in chronic atrial fibrillation. The Copenhagen AFASAK study. *Lancet* 1989; 1:175–179.

Poli D, Antonucci E, Cecchi E, et al. Thrombophilic mutations in high-risk atrial fibrillation patients: high prevalence of prothrombin gene G20210A polymorphism and lack of correlation with thromboembolism. *Thromb Haemost* 2003;90:1158–1162.

Rosenthal L. Atrial fibrillation [Online]. Accessed April 8, 2004. Available at: www .emedicine.com/med/topic184

Sarich TC, Teng R, Peters GR, et al. No influence of obesity on the pharmacokinetics and pharmacodynamics of melagatran, the active form of the oral direct thrombin inhibitor ximelagatran. *Clin Pharm* 2003;42:485–492.

Schunemann HJ, Cook D, Grimshaw J, et al. Antithrombotic and thrombolytic therapy: from evidence to application: the Seventh ACCP Conference on Antithrombotic and Thrombolytic Therapy. *Chest* 2004;126:688S–696S.

Sethia B, Turner MA, Lewis S, Rodger RA, Bain WH. Fourteen years' experience with the Björk-Shiley tilting disc prosthesis. *J Thorac Cardiovasc Surg* 1986;91:350–361.

Singer DE, Albers GW, Dalen JE, et al. Antithrombotic therapy in atrial fibrillation. *Chest* 2004; 126:429S–456S.

Stellbrink C, Nixdorff U, Hofmann T, et al. on behalf of the ACE (Anticoagulation in Cardioversion using Enoxaparin) Study Group. Safety and efficacy of enoxaparin compared with unfractionated heparin and oral anticoagulants for prevention of thromboembolic complications in cardioversion of nonvalvular atrial fibrillation. *Circulation* 2004;109:997–1003.

Stewart S, MacIntyre K, Chalmers JW, et al. Trends in case-fatality in 22968 patients admitted for the first time with atrial fibrillation in Scotland, 1986–1995. *Int J of Cardiol* 2002;82:229–236.

Stroke Prevention in Atrial Fibrillation Investigators. Stroke Prevention in Atrial Fibrillation study. Final results. *Circulation* 1991;84:527–539.

Stroke Prevention in Atrial Fibrillation Investigators. Adjusted-dose warfarin versus low-intensity, fixed-dose warfarin plus aspirin for high-risk patients with atrial fibrillation: stroke prevention in atrial fibrillation III randomized clinical trial. *Lancet* 1996;348:633–638.

Van Gelder IC, Hagens VE, Bosker HA, et al. Rate Control versus Electrical Cardioversion for Persistent Atrial Fibrillation Study Group. A comparison of rate control and rhythm control in patients with recurrent persistent atrial fibrillation. *N Engl J Med* 2002;347:1834–1840.

Vogt S, Hoffmann A, Roth J, et al. Heart valve replacement with the Björk-Shiley and St. Jude medical prosthesis: a randomized comparison in 178 patients. *Eur Heart J* 1990;11:583–591.

Wolf PA, Dawber TR, Thomas HE Jr, Kannel WB. Epidemiologic assessment of chronic atrial fibrillation and risk of stroke: the Framingham study. *Neurology* 1978;28: 973–977.

Wolf PA, Abbott RD, Kannel WB. Atrial fibrillation: a major contributor to stroke in the elderly: the Framingham Study. *Arch Intern Med* 1987;147:1561–1564.

Wyse DG, Waldo AL, DiMarco JP, et al., Atrial Fibrillation Follow-up Investigation of Rhythm Management (AFFIRM) Investigators. A comparison of rate control and rhythm control in patients with atrial fibrillation. *N Engl J Med* 2002;347: 1825–1833.

Plaque-Stabilizing Therapies

21

The association between elevated low density lipoprotein (LDL) cholesterol and atherothrombotic vascular disease is well established. Lipid-lowering therapies reduce cardiovascular events; however, the mechanism of benefit attributable to HMG CoA reductase inhibitors likely transcends lipids alone by directly or indirectly affecting inflammatory response, endothelial cell resistance, apoptosis, and progenitor cell behavior.

HMG CoA Reductase Inhibitors (Statins)

Although collectively in the same class of drugs, statins have unique pharmacokinetic profiles (Table 21.1). They may also differ in their ability to impact inflammatory responses, endothelial performance including enhanced thromboresistance capability, plaque vulnerability, and vascular thrombosis (Table 21.2, Figure 21.1). Unlike the LDL cholesterol–lowering effect, the "nonlipid"-related properties of statins are less closely tied to dose (Table 21.3) (Undas et al., 2005).

Clinical Trials and Registries

Support for a multifactorial benefit from statin therapy has been derived from a number of clinical trials revealing a nonlinear correlation between LDL cholesterol reduction and protection from clinical events. In the Anglo-Scandinavian Cardiac Outcomes Trial–Lipid Lowering Arm (ASCOT-LLA), 1,934 hypertensive patients (ages 40–75) with at least three other cardiovascular risk factors and either average or below average total cholesterol levels received either atorvastatin (10 mg) or placebo. By 3.3 years of follow-up, there was a marked reduction in cardiovascular death, nonfatal myocardial infarction (MI), and stroke (fatal and nonfatal) in patients receiving low-dose atorvastatin (Sever et al., 2003). Several studies and registries have also shown a benefit attributable to statin use among patients with acute coronary syndromes. Many, with the exception of the Myocardial Ischemia Reduction with Aggressive Cholesterol Lowering (MIRACL), have been post hoc, retrospective analyses or observational studies (Arntz et al., 2000; Aronow et al., 2001; Bybee et

Table 21.1 Pharmacokinetic Profiles of Statins

	Lovastatin	Simvastatin	Pravastatin	Fluvastatin	Atorvastatin
Metabolized CYP 450	yes	yes	no	yes	yes
Lipophilic	yes	yes	no	yes	yes
Protein binding (%)	>95	95–98	50	>98	>98
Elimination half-life (h)	22	23	22	23	22

Table 21.2 Multidimensional Properties of HMG CoA Reductase Inhibitors (Statins)

Inflammatory Response
    Reduce CRP, IL-6, TNF-α
    Attenuate metalloproteinase activity
Endothelial Performance/Thromboresistance
    Prevent endothelial cell apoptosis
    Enhance migration and differentiation of endothelial progenitor cells
    Stimulate nitric oxide release
    Upregulate eNOS
Plaque Vulnerability
    Attenuate matrix metalloproteinase activity
    Reduce monocyte/macrophage burden
Thrombolic Potential
    Reduce monocyte tissue factor expression
    Reduce platelet aggregation
    Augment fibrinolytic potential

CRP, C-reactive protein; IL, interleukin; TNF, tumor necrosis factor; eNOS, endotheilial nitric oxide synthase.

Table 21.3 Major Effects of Statin Use on Blood Coagulation

Process/Reaction	Effect
Tissue factor expression	Decrease
FVII production/FVII activation	Decrease
Thrombin generation	Decrease
FV activation	Decrease
Fibrinogen cleavage	Decrease
FXIII activation	Decrease
Fibrinogen synthesis	No change
Thrombomodulin expression	Increase
Inactivation of FVa	Increase
TFPI production/activity	Decrease

F, factor; TFPI, tissue factor pathway inhibitor.

Adapted from: Undas A, Brummel-Ziedins KE, Mann KG. Statins and Blood coagulation. Arterioscler Thromb Vasc Biol *2005;25: 287–294.*

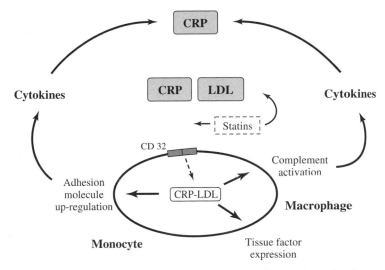

Figure 21.1 C-reactive protein (CRP) and its participation in atherothrombotic vascular disease. In response to cytokine stimulation, it colocalizes with low-density lipoprotein (LDL) cholesterol, facilitating monocyte entry via CD32, a cell surface receptor. Once internalized, the CRP–LDL–cholesterol complex incites complement activation tissue factor expression, and surface adhesion molecule up-regulation. Statins appear to interrupt this initiating step at several sites.

al., 2001; Schwartz et al., 2001). However, in the PROVE-IT (Pravastatin or Atorvastatin Evaluation and Infection Therapy) trial (Cannon et al., 2004), 4,162 patients treated with either pravastatin (40 mg daily—moderate-intensity statin therapy) or atorvastatin (80 mg daily—intensive therapy) within 10 days of an acute coronary syndrome (ACS) had a 16% reduction in the likelihood of death (any cause), MI, ACS requiring hospitalization, revascularization, or stroke with more intensive treatment.

Statin Withdrawal Phenomenon

The cellular effects of statin therapy may underlie a withdrawal or "rebound" phenomenon that has been associated with an increased incidence of death and nonfatal reinfarction following sudden discontinuation (Heeschen et al., 2002). The specific mechanisms and potential for occurrence with dose reduction (after initial therapy with high-dose treatment) are under investigation.

References

Arntz HR, Agrawal R, Wunderlich W, et al. Beneficial effects of pravastatin ($\pm$ cholestyramine/niacin) initiated immediately after a coronary event (the randomized lipid-coronary artery disease [L-CAD] study). *Am J Cardiol* 2000;86:1293–1298.

Aronow HD, Topol EJ, Roe MT, et al. Effect of lipid-lowering therapy on early mortality after acute coronary syndromes: an observational study. *Lancet* 2001;357: 1063–1068.

Bybee KA, Wright RS, Williams BA, et al. Effect on concomitant or very early statin administration on in-hospital mortality and reinfarction in patients with acute myocardial infarction. *Am J Cardiol* 2001;87:771–774.

Cannon CP, Braunwald E, McCabe CH, , et al. for the Pravastatin or Atorvastatin Evaluation and Infection Therapy-Thrombolysis in Myocardial Infarction 22 Investigators. Intensive versus moderate lipid lowering with statins after acute coronary syndromes. *N Eng J Med* 2004;350:1495–1504.

Heeschen C, Hamm CW, Laufs U, et al. Withdrawal of statins increases event rates in patients with acute coronary syndromes. *Circulation* 2002;105:1446–1452.

Schwartz GG, Olsson AG, Ezekowitz MD, et al. for the Myocardial Ischemia Reduction with Aggressive Cholesterol Lowering (MIRACL) Study Investigators. Effects of atorvastatin on early recurrent events in acute coronary syndromes: the MIRACL study: a randomized controlled trial. *JAMA* 2001;285:1711–1718.

Sever PS, Bahlöf B, Poulter NR, et al. Prevention of coronary and stroke events with atorvastatin in hypertensive patients who have average or lower-than-average cholesterol concentrations, in the Anglo-Scandinavian Cardiac Outcomes Trial—Lipid Lowering Arm (ASCOT-LLA): a multicentre randomized controlled trial. *Lancet* 2003; 361:1149–1158.

Undas A, Brummel-Ziedins KE, Mann KG. Statins and blood coagulation. *Arterioscler Thromb Vasc Biol* 2005;25:287–294.

Part V
Management of Venous Thrombotic Disorders

Venous Thromboembolism Prophylaxis

22

Venous thromboembolism represents a true worldwide medical problem that is encountered within all realms of practice.

Epidemiology

Venous thromboembolism (VTE) occurs in approximately 100 patients per 100,000 population yearly in the United States and increases exponentially with each decade of life (White, 2003) (Table 22.1). Approximately one-third of patients with symptomatic deep vein thrombosis (DVT) experience a pulmonary embolism (PE). Death occurs within 1 month in 6% of patients with DVT and 12% of those with PE. Early mortality is associated strongly with presentation as PE, advanced age, malignancy, and underlying cardiovascular disease.

Risk Factors for Venous Thromboembolism

An experience dating back several decades has provided a better understanding of disease states and conditions associated with VTE (Table 22.2) (Anderson and Spencer, 2003).

Venous Thromboembolism Prophylaxis

Given the potential morbidity and mortality associated with VTE, it is apparent that prophylaxis represents an important goal in clinical practice. A variety of anticoagulants including unfractionated heparin, low-molecular-weight heparin (LMWH), and warfarin have been studied. More recently, two new agents have been developed that warrant discussion.

Fondaparinux

Fondaparinux underwent a worldwide development program in orthopedic surgery for the prophylaxis of VTE (Figure 22.1). The program consisted mainly of four large, randomized, double-blind phase II studies comparing fondaparinux

Table 22.1 Epidemiology of Venous Thromboembolism

Variable	Finding
Incidence in total population (assuming >95% Caucasian)	70–113 cases/100,000/yr
Age	Exponential increase in VTE with age, particularly after age 40 yr
25–35 yr	30 cases/100,000 persons
70–79 yr	300–500 cases/100,000 persons
Gender	No convincing differences between men and women
Race/ethnicity	2.5–4-fold lower risk of VTE in Asian-Pacific Islanders and Hispanics
Relative incidence of PE vs. DVT	Absent autopsy diagnosis: 33% PE; 66% DVT
	With autopsy: 55% PE; 45% DVT
Seasonal variation	Possibly more common in winter and less common in summer
Risk factors	25–50% "idiopathic" depending on exact definition
	15–25% associated with cancer; 20% following surgery (3 mo)
Recurrent VTE	6-month incidence: 7%; higher rate in patients with cancer
	Recurrent PE more likely after PE than after DVT
Death after treated VTE	30-day incidence 6% after DVT
	30-day incidence 12% after PE
	Death strongly associated with cancer, age, and cardiovascular disease

DVT, deep vein thrombosis; PE, pulmonary embolism; VTE, venous thromboembolism.

White R. The epidemiology of venous thromboemolism. Circulation *2003;107:14–18.*

(SC), at a dose of 2.5 mg starting 6 hours postoperatively, with the two enoxaparin regimens approved for VTE prophylaxis—40 mg qd or 30 mg twice daily beginning 12 hours postoperatively. The results support a greater protective effect with fondaparinux, yielding a 55.2% relative risk reduction of VTE (Bauer et al., 2001; Eriksson et al., 2001; Lassen et al., 2002; Turpie et al., 2001, 2002;).

Ximelagatran

A European program of three large-scale clinical trials (MElagatran for THRombin inhibition in Orthopedic surgery [METHRO] I, II, and III, and EXpanded PROphylaxis Evaluation Surgery Study [EXPRESS]) (Eriksson et al., 2002a, b, 2003a, b) evaluated the safety and efficacy of subcutaneous melagatran followed by oral ximelagatran compared with LMWH for thromboprophylaxis following total hip replacement (THR) and total knee replacement (TKR) surgery. In METHRO II, patients received either 5,000 IU subcutaneous dalteparin once daily or a combination of one of four doses (from 1 to 3 mg) of subcutaneous melagatran twice daily started immediately before surgery, followed by one of four doses (from 8 to 24 mg) of oral ximelagatran bid started 1 to 3 days after surgery. Of 1,900 patients, 1,495

Table 22.2 Established Risk Factors for VTE

Strong risk factors (odds ratio >10)
Fracture (hip or leg)
Hip or knee replacement
Major general surgery
Major trauma
Spinal cord injury
Moderate risk factors (odds ratio 2–9)
Arthroscopic knee surgery
Central venous lines
Chemotherapy
Congestive heart or respiratory failure
Hormone replacement therapy
Malignancy
Oral contraceptive therapy
Paralytic stroke
Pregnancy/postpartum
Previous VTE
Thrombophilia
Weak risk factors (odds ratio <2)
Bed rest >3 d
Immobility due to sitting (e.g., prolonged car or air travel)
Increased age
Laparoscopic surgery (e.g., cholecystectomy)
Obesity
Pregnancy/antepartum
Varicose veins

VTE, venous thromboembolism.

*Anderson FA, Spender FA. Risk factors for venous thrombo-
embolism. Circulation 2003;107:I9–I16.*

were assigned to four dose categories of subcutaneous melagatran from just before surgery (1 mg, 1.5 mg, 2.25 mg, or 3 mg twice daily) followed from the day after surgery by oral ximelagatran (8 mg, 12 mg, 18 mg, or 24 mg twice daily). Three-hundred-eighty-one patients were assigned subcutaneous dalteparin 5,000 IU once daily, from the evening before surgery. In METHRO II, there was a highly significant dose-response relationship for subcutaneous melagatran plus ximelagatran, with the highest dose combination superior to dalteparin in the prevention of VTE.

In METHRO III (Eriksson et al., 2003a), a randomized, double-blind study, 2,788 patients undergoing THR or TKR were randomly assigned to receive for 8 to 11 days either 3 mg of subcutaneous melagatran started 4 to 12 hours postoperatively, followed by 24 mg of oral ximelagatran twice daily, or 40 mg of subcutaneous enoxaparin once daily, started 12 hours preoperatively. Ximelagatran was to be initiated within the first 2 postoperative days. The primary efficacy endpoint was VTE

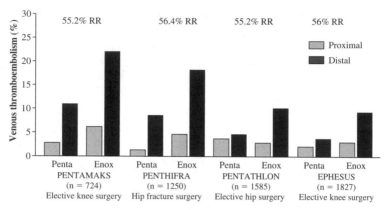

Figure 22.1 Comparative event rates for fondaparinux and enoxaparin in the prevention of venous thromboembolism (VTE) following orthopedic surgery. Enox, enoxaparin; Penta, pentasaccharide; RR, relative risk. (Data compiled from phase III clinical trials PENTAMAKS, PENTHIFRA, PENTATHLON 2000, and EPHESUS.)

or unexplained death. The main safety endpoint was bleeding. Venous thromboembolism occurred in 31% and 27.3% of patients in the ximelagatran and enoxaparin group, respectively, a difference in risk of 3.7% in favor of enoxaparin ($p = .053$). This difference was entirely accounted for by a higher frequency of distal DVT with ximelagatran compared to enoxaparin in THR patients. Bleeding was comparable between the two groups.

EXPRESS (Ericksson et al., 2003b) was a phase III comparator-controlled, double-blind, parallel-group, multicenter study conducted in 2,835 patients undergoing THR or TKR. Patients were randomized to receive either 40 mg of subcutaneous enoxaparin daily beginning the evening prior to THR or TRK surgery, or 2 mg started immediately before surgery, followed by 3 mg of subcutaneous melagatran the evening of surgery, and then oral 24 mg ximelagatran twice daily. Ximelagatran/melagatran was superior to enoxaparin in preventing VTE with a relative risk reduction in proximal DVT plus PE of 63% ($p = .001$). The relative risk reduction for total VTE was 23.6% ($p = .001$). Efficacy was maintained for both TKR and THR. There were no differences in clinically important bleeding events (fatal bleeding, critical organ bleeding, and bleeding requiring reoperation).

A phase III study of an oral-only regimen of ximelagatran after TKR was performed in 680 patients who had undergone TKR; patients received either oral ximelagatran, 24 mg twice daily starting on the morning after surgery, or warfarin (target international normalized ratio [INR], 2.5 [range 1.8–3.0]), starting on the evening of the day of surgery for a total treatment period of 7 to 10 days. The incidence of

VTE was 19.2% in the ximelagatran group and 25.7% in the warfarin group (difference was –6.5 percentage points [95% confidence interval (CI), –13.5 to 0.6 percentage points]; $p = .070$). In the ximelagatran and warfarin groups, respectively, major bleeding occurred in 1.7% and 0.9% of patients and minor bleeding occurred in 7.8% and 6.4% of patients (Francis et al., 2002a).

A double-blind phase III trial of patients undergoing TKR included fixed-dose oral ximelagatran, 24 or 36 mg twice daily, or warfarin (target INR 2.5; range 1.8–3.0) for 7 to 12 days (Francis et al., 2002b). Warfarin was initiated the evening of the day of surgery, and ximelagatran, the morning after surgery. Efficacy was assessed in the 1,851 patients with adequate bilateral venography; symptomatic objectively confirmed VTE or death and bleeding were adjudicated by an independent central committee. Ximelagatran 36 mg PO twice daily was superior to warfarin for the composite endpoint of distal and/or proximal DVT, and/or confirmed symptomatic DVT/PE, and/or all-cause mortality (relative risk reduction 26%; $p = .003$).

Ximelagatran is approved for VTE prophylaxis following knee surgery in several European countries.

Venous Thromboembolism Prophylaxis Guidelines

A modified and abbreviated summary of VTE prophylaxis guidelines for trauma, surgery, and medical conditions according to the American College of Chest Physicians (Schunemann et al., 2004) appears in Table 22.3.

Long-Term Prophylaxis

Recurrent VTE affects 25% to 30% of patients who suffer idiopathic DVT or PE. In the past several years, two large-scale clinical trials specifically addressed the net clinical utility of long-term prophylaxis. The Prevention of Recurrent Thromboembolism (PREVENT) trial (Ridker et al., 2003) investigated a low- to moderate-intensity warfarin strategy (INR 1.5–2.0) against placebo among patients who had completed at least 3 months of therapy. A total of 508 patients were followed for, on average, 2.1 years. The trial was stopped by the Data and Safety Monitoring Board after a highly significant 64% reduction in risk for recurrent VTE emerged (hazard ratio 0.36). Major bleeding was infrequent among warfarin-treated patients.

The Extended Low-Intensity Anticoagulation for Thrombo-Embolism (ELATE) trial (Kearon et al., 2003) included 738 patients who were followed for 2.4 years while receiving warfarin to a target INR of either 1.5 to 2.0 or 2.0 to 3.0. Fewer recurrent events were observed in the moderate-intensity treatment group (0.7 events per 100 person years vs. 1.9 events per 100 patient years) (hazard ratio 2.5 for low-

Table 22.3 Recommendations for Venous Thromboembolism Prophylaxis

General Recommendations
1. We recommend that every hospital develop a formal strategy that addresses the prevention of thromboembolic complications. This should generally be in the form of a written thrombo-prophylaxis policy especially for high-risk groups.
2. For all patient groups, we do not recommend aspirin for prophylaxis, because other measures are more efficacious (grade 1A).
3. In all patients having spinal puncture or epidural catheters placed for regional anesthesia or analgesia, we recommend that antithrombotic therapy or prophylaxis be used with caution (grade 1C+).

General Gynecologic and Urologic Surgery
General Surgery
1. In low-risk general surgery patients (Table 2) who are undergoing minor procedures, are <40 yr of age, and have no additional risk factors, we recommend the use of no specific prophylaxis other than early ambulation (grade 1C).
2. Moderate-risk general surgery patients are those undergoing minor procedures but have additional thrombosis risk factors, those having nonmajor surgery between the ages of 40 and 60 yr with no additional risk factors, or those undergoing major operations who are younger than 40 yr with no additional clinical risk factors. We recommend prophylaxis with LDUH, LMWH, ES, or IPC (all grade 1A in comparison to no prophylaxis).
3. Higher-risk general surgery patients are those having nonmajor surgery over the age of 60 yr or with additional risk factors or patients undergoing major surgery over the age of 40 yr or with additional risk factors. We recommend thrombosis prophylaxis with LDUH, LMWH, or IPC (all grade 1A in comparison to no prophylaxis).
3.1 In higher-risk general surgery patients with a greater than usual risk of bleeding, we recommend the use of mechanical prophylaxis with ES or IPC, at least initially (grade 1C).
4. In very-high-risk general surgery patients with multiple risk factors, we recommend that effective pharmacologic methods (LDUH or LMWH) be combined with ES or IPC (grade 1C based on small studies and on extrapolation of data from other patient groups).
5. In selected very-high-risk general surgery patients, we recommend that clinicians consider postdischarge LMWH or perioperative warfarin (INR 2.0–3.0) (grade 2C).

Gynecologic Surgery
1. For gynecologic surgery patients undergoing brief procedures for benign disease, we recommend early mobilization alone (grade 1C).
2. We recommend that patients having major gynecologic surgery for benign disease, without additional risk factors, receive twice-daily LDUH (grade 1A). Alternatives include once-daily LMWH or IPC, started just before surgery and continued for at least several days postoperatively (grade 1C+).
3. For patients undergoing extensive surgery for malignancy, we recommend routine prophylaxis with three daily doses of LDUH (grade 1A). Alternative considerations include the combination of LDUH plus mechanical prophylaxis with ES or IPC, or higher doses of LMWH, since these options may provide additional protection (grade 1C).

Urologic Surgery
1. In patients undergoing transurethral or other low-risk urologic procedures, we recommend that no specific prophylaxis other than prompt ambulation be used (grade 1C).
2. For patients with major, open urologic procedures, we recommend routine prophylaxis with LDUH, ES, IPC, or LMWH (all grade 1B in comparison to no prophylaxis).
3. For patients at the highest risk, we recommend combining ES plus or minus IPC, with LDUH or LMWH (grade 1C).

Table 22.3 (continued)

Major Orthopedic Surgery
Elective Hip Replacement*
1. For patients undergoing elective THR surgery, we recommend either SC LMWH therapy (started 12 h before surgery, 12–24 h after surgery, or 4–6 h after surgery at half the usual high-risk dose and then continuing with the usual high-risk dose the following day), or adjusted-dose warfarin (INR target 2.5, range 2.0–3.0; started preoperatively or immediately after surgery) (all grade 1A).
2. Adjusted-dose heparin therapy (started preoperatively) is an acceptable but more complex alternative (grade 2A).
3. Adjuvant prophylaxis with ES or IPC may provide additional efficacy (grade 2C).
4. Although other agents such as LDUH, aspirin, dextran, and IPC alone may reduce the overall incidence of VTE, they are less effective, and we do not recommend that these options be used.

Elective Knee Replacement*
1. For patients undergoing elective TKR surgery, we recommend either LMWH or adjusted-dose warfarin (grade 1A).
2. Optimal use of IPC is an alternative option (grade 1B recommendation because of the few trials and small sample sizes).
3. LDUH is not recommended (grade 1C+).

Hip Fracture Surgery*
1. For patients undergoing hip fracture surgery, we recommend either LMWH or adjusted-dose warfarin prophylaxis (grade 1B because the available data are limited).
2. The use of LDUH may be an alternative option, but this is a grade 2B recommendation based on the very limited available data.
3. We do not recommend the use of aspirin alone because it is less efficacious than other approaches (grade 2A).

Other Prophylaxis Issues for Major Orthopedic Surgery
1. The optimal duration of anticoagulant prophylaxis after THR or TKR surgery is uncertain, although at least 7–10 d of prophylaxis is recommended (grade 1A).
2. Extended out-of-hospital LMWH prophylaxis (beyond 7–10 d after surgery) may reduce the incidence of clinically important thromboembolic events, and we recommend this approach at least for high-risk patients (grade 2A because of uncertainty regarding cost-effectiveness).
3. We do not recommend routine duplex ultrasonography screening at the time of hospital discharge or during outpatient follow-up in asymptomatic THR or TKR patients (grade 1A).

Neurosurgery, Trauma, and Acute SCI
Neurosurgery
1. We recommend the use of IPC with or without ES in patients undergoing intracranial neuro-surgery (grade 1A).
2. LDUH or postoperative LMWH are acceptable alternatives (grade 2A because of concerns about clinically important intracranial hemorrhage).
3. The combination of physical (ES or IPC) and pharmacologic (LMWH or LDUH) prophylaxis modalities may be more effective than either modality alone in high-risk patients (grade 1B).

Trauma
1. Trauma patients with an identifiable risk factor for thromboembolism should receive prophylaxis if possible. If there is no contraindication, we recommend that clinicians use LMWH, starting treatment as soon as it is considered safe to do so (grade 1A).
2. We recommend that initial prophylaxis with a mechanical modality (ES and/or IPC) be used if LMWH prophylaxis will be delayed or is contraindicated because of concerns about the patient's risk of bleeding (grade 1C).

(continued)

Table 22.3 (continued)

   3. In patients at high risk for thromboembolism who have received suboptimal prophylaxis, consideration should be given to screening with duplex ultrasound (grade 1C).
   4. We recommend that IVC filter insertion be used if proximal DVT is demonstrated and anti-coagulation is contraindicated (grade 1C+). We do not recommend the use of IVC filter insertion for primary prophylaxis (grade 1C).

Acute SCI
   1. In patients with acute SCI, we recommend prophylaxis with LMWH (grade 1B).
   2. LDUH, ES, and IPC appear to be relatively ineffective when used alone, and we do not recommend these modalities (grade 1C).
   3. ES and IPC might have benefit if used in combination with LMWH or LDUH or if anti-coagulants are contraindicated early after injury (grade 2B).
   4. In the rehabilitation phase of acute SCI, we recommend the continuation of LMWH therapy or conversion to full-dose oral anticoagulation (INR target 2.5, range 2.0–3.0) (grade 1C).

Medical Conditions
Acute MI
   1. We recommend that most patients with acute MI receive prophylactic or therapeutic anti-coagulant therapy with SC LDUH or IV heparin (grade 1A).
Ischemic Stroke
   1. For patients with ischemic stroke and impaired mobility, we recommend the routine use of LDUH, LMWH, or the heparinoid danaparoid (all grade 1A).
   2. If anticoagulant prophylaxis is contraindicated, we recommend mechanical prophylaxis with ES or IPC (grade 1C+).
Other Medical Conditions
   1. In general medical patients with risk factors for VTE (including cancer, bed rest, heart failure, severe lung disease), we recommend LDUH or LWMH (grade 1A).

* *Fondaparinux is also an option.*
DVT, deep vein thrombosis; ES, elastic stockings; INR, international normalized ratio; IPC, intermittent pneummic compression; IVC, inferior vena cava; LDUH, ; LMWH, low-molecular-weight heparin; MI, myocardial infarction; SCI, spinal cord injury; THR, total hip replacement; TKR, total knee replacement; VTE, venous thromboembolism.

intensity treatment). The risk for major hemorrhage was increased modestly for those receiving moderate-intensity anticoagulation (hazard ratio 1.2).

A choice of one anticoagulation strategy over another must be determined on a case-by-case basis after careful assessment of thrombotic and hemorrhagic risk.

References

Anderson FA Jr, Spencer FA. Risk factors associated with venous thromboembolism. *Circulation* 2003;107:I9–I16.

Bauer KA, Eriksson BI, Lassen MR, for the Pentamaks Steering Committee. Fonda-parinux compared with enoxaparin for the prevention of VTE after elective major knee surgery. *N Engl J Med* 2001;345:1305–1310.

Eriksson BI, Bauer KA, Lassen MR, Steering Committee for the Pentasaccharide in Hip Fracture Surgery Study. Fondaparinux compared with enoxaparin for the prevention of VTE after hip fracture surgery. *N Engl J Med* 2001;345:1298–1304.

Eriksson BI, Arfwidsson AC, Frison L, et al. A dose-ranging study of the oral direct thrombin inhibitor ximelagatran and its subcutaneous form melagatran compared with dalteparin in the prophylaxis of thromboembolism after hip or knee replacement: METHRO I. MElagatran for THRombin inhibition in Orthopaedic surgery. *Thromb Haemost* 2002a;87:231–237.

Eriksson BI, Bergqvist D, Kalebo PK, et al. Ximelagatran and melagatran compared with dalteparin for prevention of venous thromboembolism after total hip or knee replacement: the METHRO II randomized trial. *Lancet* 2002b;360:1441–1447.

Eriksson BI, Agnelli G, Cohen AT, et al., for the METHRO III Study Group. Direct thrombin inhibitor melagatran followed by oral ximelagatran in comparison with enoxaparin for prevention of venous thromboembolism after total hip or knee replacement. *Thromb Haemost* 2003a;89:288–296.

Eriksson BI, Agnelli G, Cohen AT, et al., for the EXPRESS Study Group. The direct thrombin inhibitor melagatran followed by oral ximelagatran compared with enoxaparin for the prevention of venous thromboembolism after total hip or knee replacement: the EXPRESS study. *J Thromb Haemost* 2003b;1:2490–2496.

Francis CW, Berkowitz DS, Comp PC, et al. Randomized, double-blind, comparison of ximelagatran, an oral direct thrombin inhibitor and warfarin to prevent venous thromboembolism (VTE) after total knee replacement (TKR). *Blood* 2002a;100:82a.

Francis CW, Davidson BL, Berkowitz DS, et al. Ximelagatran versus warfarin for the prevention of venous thromboembolism after total knee arthroplasty. A randomized, double-blind trial. *Ann Intern Med* 2002b;137:648–655.

Kearon C, Ginsberg JS, Kovacs MJ, et al., for the Extended Low-Intensity Anticoagulation for Thrombo-Embolism Investigators. Comparison of low-intensity warfarin therapy with conventional-intensity warfarin therapy for long-term prevention of recurrent venous thromboembolism. *N Engl J Med* 2003;349:631–639.

Lassen MR, Bauer KA, Eriksson BI, for the EPHESUS Steering Committee. Post-operative fondaparinux versus pre-operative enoxaparin for the prevention of VTE in elective hip replacement surgery. *Lancet* 2002;359:1715–1720.

Ridker PM, Goldhaber SZ, Danielson E, et al., for the PREVENT Investigators. Long-term, low-intensity warfarin therapy for the prevention of recurrent venous thromboembolism. *N Engl J Med* 2003;348:1425–1434.

Schunemann HJ, Cook D, Grimshaw J, et al. Antithrombotic and thrombolytic therapy: from evidence to application: the Seventh ACCP Conference on Antithrombotic and Thrombolytic Therapy. *Chest* 2004;126:688S–696S.

Turpie AG, Gallus AS, Hoek JA, for the Pentasaccharide Investigators. A synthetic pentasaccharide for the prevention of DVT following total hip replacement. *N Engl J Med* 2001;344:619–625.

Turpie AG, Bauer KA, Eriksson BI, Lassen MR, for the PENTATHALON 2000 Study Steering Committee. Postoperative fondaparinux versus postoperative enoxaparin for prevention of VTE after elective hip-replacement surgery: a randomised double-blind trial. *Lancet* 2002;359:1721–1726.

White RH. The epidemiology of venous thromboembolism. *Circulation* 2003;107:I4–I8.

Venous Thromboembolism Treatment

The potential morbidity and mortality associated with venous thromboembolism (VTE) dictates rapid diagnosis and effective treatment.

Anatomic Considerations

An understanding of basic anatomy permits a strategic approach to diagnosis and decisions regarding initial therapy. VTE can include the superficial or deep venous systems of the lower (most common) and upper extremities (Figure 23.1). Because deep vein thrombosis (DVT) of the proximal vessels (iliac, femoral veins) is associated with the greatest risk of pulmonary embolism (PE) (as well as chronic compli-. cations such as postphlebitic [thrombotic] syndrome), a proactive response, which may include anticoagulant therapy pending a definitive diagnosis, is recommended.

Natural History

Many DVTs begin in the calf veins and most, in all likelihood, resolve spontaneously. The probability of extension to the popliteal vein or above (where embolism is more likely) is determined by the prothrombotic environment. Proximal thrombi resolve slowly with anticoagulant therapy, and may be detectable in up to 50% of patients 1 year later. Approximately 10% of patients develop postphlebitic syndrome within 5 years—a complication from progressive valvular damage that increases in prevalence with recurrent events (Anderson et al., 1991). Approximately 10% of all PEs are rapidly fatal, and an additional 5% of patients die even after treatment is initiated. Up to 5% of patients develop pulmonary hypertension because of limited thrombus resolution (Kearon, 2003) (Table 23.1).

Diagnosis

The diagnosis of DVT and PE is difficult and requires a mixture of clinical suspicion and objective testing. A complete history with attention to specific symptoms

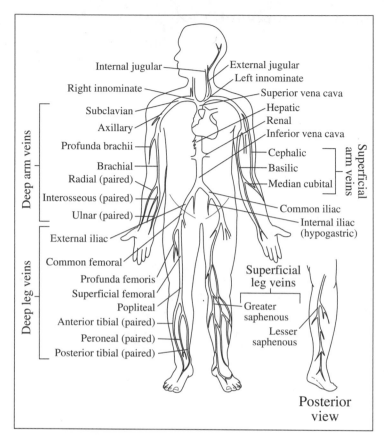

Figure 23.1 Superficial and deep venous systems of the upper and lower extremities. (From Fahey VA, ed. *Vascular nursing,* 3rd ed. Philadelphia: WB Saunders Co, 1999:23.)

and signs should be recorded; a thorough family history is also invaluable. The laboratory evaluation is critical in establishing an unequivocal diagnosis, but most of the tests currently used are not of uniform high sensitivity and specificity. Thus, an accurate diagnosis requires experience and attention to detail (Figure 23.2).

Signs and Symptoms of Deep Vein Thrombosis

The cardinal symptoms of DVT are pain and swelling in the lower extremity. The pain may be sharp and sudden in onset or come on more gradually and be reported

Table 23.1 Natural History of VTE: Implications for Patient Management

Primary Prophylaxis
Because most patients who die from PE do not have preceding symptoms of DVT, primary prophylaxis is a high priority.
Patient-related and surgical risk factors identify candidates for primary prophylaxis.
A minimum duration of prophylaxis may be required after high-risk procedures to facilitate spontaneous lysis of thrombi that form during or shortly after surgery (e.g., 7–10 d after major orthopedic surgery).
Extended prophylaxis (e.g., 3 wk after hospital discharge) may be indicated after surgical procedures associated with a prolonged risk of VTE (e.g., hip replacement).
Diagnosis
Most calf DVT that extend to the proximal veins can be detected by ultrasound 1 wk after an initial normal examination.
Detection of asymptomatic DVT can be used to diagnose PE in patients with a nondiagnostic lung scan or helical CT.
Incomplete resolution of previous DVT or PE may reduce the specificity of diagnostic testing for recurrent VTE.

CT, computed tomography; DVT, deep vein thrombosis; PE, pulmonary embolism; VTE venous thromboembolism.

Kearm C. Natural history of venous thromboembolism. Circulation 2003;107:122–130.

as restricting in character. There may be little or no swelling, or the entire lower extremity may be markedly enlarged. On examination, there is frequently reddish-purple discoloration of the leg in comparison with the noninvolved side. One may also observe a prominent venous pattern on the affected limb. In cases of upper extremity DVT, swelling of the dorsal aspect of the hand is seen frequently; when accompanied by proximal progression, prominence of the veins in the upper chest and arm may be seen. If there is associated superficial phlebitis, there is often tenderness over the vein itself and a cord may be palpable; otherwise, diffuse calf tenderness and warmth of the leg may be present. The Homans' sign (pain in the calf with dorsiflexion of the foot) is present in only about half of the cases and is neither sensitive nor specific for DVT.

Once a diagnosis of DVT has been established, it is important to determine whether the thrombotic event is idiopathic or secondary to a defined risk factor such as surgery, trauma, malignancy, antiphospholipid antibody syndrome, or an inherited thrombophilia. If the latter is suspected, blood samples should be obtained for measurements of proteins C and S, antithrombin III, lupus anticoagulant, anticardiolipin antibodies, homocysteine, and genetic testing for factor V Leiden (FVL) and the prothrombin 20210A mutation (see Chapter 24).

Treatment for acute DVT is usually initiated with low-molecular-weight heparin (LMWH). In the past 10 years, more than a dozen controlled, double-blind, clinical trials have compared various LMWH with unfractionated heparin (UFH) in

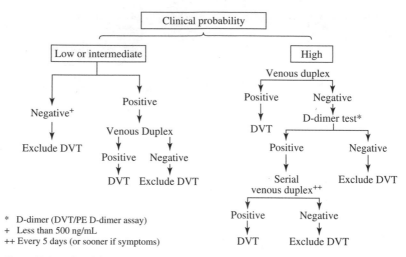

Figure 23.2 A clinical diagnostic algorithm for patients with suspected deep vein thrombosis (DVT). PE, pulmonary embolism.

the management of acute DVT. Lensing and associates (1995) performed a meta-analysis of 10 studies and noted that there was statistically significant risk reduction in symptomatic thromboembolic complications, clinically important bleeding, and mortality with the use of LMWH. Oral vitamin K antagonist therapy can be initiated early (day 1 or 2) in a majority of patients.

Low-molecular-weight heparin should be continued for at least 3 to 5 days and until the international normalized ratio (INR) has been above 2.0 for 48 hours.

Outpatient Therapy

Patients with acute DVT may be treated at home if several criteria are met:

- The thrombus should be distal to the iliac vein. Iliac vein thrombi usually cause considerable leg swelling and discomfort, and are more likely to embolize to the lungs.
- The presence of pulmonary emboli warrants close supervision for at least 72 hours, until the patient is hemodynamically stable and further risk of embolization has lessened.
- Patients with risk factors for bleeding, such as liver disease, peptic ulcer, and thrombocytopenia, should be given anticoagulants with close observation in the hospital setting.

- The patient or caregiver must be instructed on the technique for administering the LMWH, and must be considered reliable.
- There must be provision for obtaining prothrombin times in the outpatient setting.
- The patient should be geographically accessible in the event of thrombus recurrence, bleeding, or other untoward reactions to medications.

Duration of Treatment

Following a transition from LMWH to an oral anticoagulant, a decision must be made concerning the duration of oral anticoagulation (Table 23.2). The British Thoracic Society (Research Committee of the British Thoracic Society, 1992) conducted a study comparing 4 weeks of anticoagulation with 3 months of therapy. Approximately 350 patients were randomized to each treatment. Of those treated for 4 weeks, 7.8% had recurrent thrombosis vs. 4% of those receiving anticoagulants for 3 months ($p = .04$), prompting a recommendation that at least 3 months of treatment be given. Prandoni and colleagues (1996) found that the recurrence rate of DVT in patients treated for 3 months was 10% at 1 year and 20% at 2 years, suggesting that a longer treatment period might be beneficial. Six weeks of anticoagulation were compared with 6 months of therapy by Schulman and colleagues (1995); the 6-month group experienced half the recurrences of the 6-week group. Kearon and colleagues (1999) randomized patients to receive either 3 months or at least 6 months of anticoagulation. The study was stopped when it was observed that 17 of 83 patients whose anticoagulation was discontinued after 3 months had recurrent thromboembolism (as compared with only one of 79 patients continued on anticoagulation) ($p = .001$). A second study by the same investigators (Shulman et al., 1997) compared 6 months of treatment with prolonged (indefinite) therapy among patients with a second episode of venous thromboembolism. There was a 24% and 4% cumulative probability of recurrence at 4 years in the two study groups, respectively.

Patients with idiopathic VTE who had received full-dose anticoagulation therapy with warfarin for at least 6 months were then randomized to either placebo or low-intensity anticoagulation (target INR 1.5–2.0) (Ridker et al., 2003). The trial

Table 23.2 Low-Molecular-Weight Heparins Used for the Treatment of Venous Thromboembolism

Drug (Trade)	Dose
Dalteparin (Fragmin)	100 U/k q12h; 200 U/kg daily
Enoxaparin (Lovenox)	1 mg/kg q12h; 1.5 mg/kg daily
Tinzaparin (Innohep)	175 U/kg daily

was terminated after a total of 508 patients (mean follow-up 2.1 years) were randomized due to a 64% risk reduction in recurrent VTE favoring low-intensity warfarin treatment. A higher intensity of anticoagulation (INR 2.0–3.0) may offer greater protection against recurrent thrombotic events.

Novel Therapies: Ximelagatran

The potential of ximelagatran to be used in the treatment of acute DVT was investigated in the Thrombin Inhibitor in Venous Thromboembolism (THRIVE) studies. THRIVE I was a randomized, controlled trial evaluating the safety and tolerability of ximelagatran (24, 36, 48, or 60 mg twice daily) compared with dalteparin followed by warfarin for 2 weeks. Evaluation of paired venograms from 295 of 350 patients showed regression of thrombus in 69% of patients in both groups. Change in thrombus size according to the Marder Score and safety were also similar (Eriksson et al., 2003a).

Based on the encouraging results of THRIVE I, a large, multicenter, randomized double-blind study (THRIVE Treatment Study) was performed. A total of 2,489 patients with acute DVT (37% had confirmed PE) were assigned to receive either oral ximelagatran 36 mg twice daily for 6 months or enoxaparin 1 mg/kg subcutaneous (minimum 5 days) followed by warfarin (INR 2.0–3.0). Recurrent venous thromboembolism occurred in 2.1% and 2.0% of patients, respectively. Major bleeding (on treatment analysis) was experienced in 1.3% and 2.2% of patients, respectively (Huisman and the THRIVE Treatment Study Investigators, 2003).

The THRIVE III study included 1,233 patients with confirmed VTE who had received standard anticoagulant therapy for 6 months. They were then randomized to either ximelagatran (24 mg twice daily) or placebo for another 18 months. Recurrent events occurred in 12 patients receiving ximelagatran and 71 patients on placebo (hazard ratio 0.16; $p < .0001$). Six patients given the active study drug experienced a major hemorrhagic event (none were fatal or involved the central nervous system) (Eriksson et al., 2003b). Ximelagatran is not currently approved for the treatment of VTE.

Recommended Approach to the Treatment of Venous Thromboembolism during Pregnancy

Based on available safety data, LMWH and UFH are the preferred drugs for treating VTE during pregnancy (Ginsberg and Bates, 2003). As the pregnancy progresses (and most women gain weight), the volume of distribution for LMWH changes. In addition, the glomerular filtration rate increases in pregnancy. Because LMWHs are cleared through the kidney, changes in renal function could also affect the pharmacokinetics of these agents. Therefore, monthly heparin (anti-fXa) levels 4 to 6 hours after the morning dose and with adjustment of the LMWH dose to achieve a level between 0.5 to 1.2 U/mL is recommended. Alternatively, UFH initiated as an IV bolus, followed by a continuous infusion to maintain the activated partial thromboplastin time (aPTT) in the therapeutic range for at least 5 days, followed by adjusted-dose subcutaneous UFH (typically every 8–12 hours) for the remainder of the pregnancy, can be used. Dose adjustment should be based on a mid-dose aPTT determination. The administration of warfarin during the first (and early second) trimester has been associated with fetal abnormalities.

Management of Anticoagulant Therapy at the Time of Delivery

Therapeutic doses of LMWH or UFH should be discontinued 24 hours prior to elective induction of labor (to avoid an unwanted anticoagulant effect during delivery). Women with a prior very high risk of recurrent VTE (e.g., proximal DVT or PE within 4 weeks) can receive therapeutic doses of IV UFH with its discontinuation 4 to 6 hours prior to the expected time of delivery. If spontaneous labor occurs in women receiving adjusted-dose subcutaneous UFH, close monitoring of the aPTT is required, and if prolonged at the time of delivery, protamine sulfate should be considered to reduce the risk of bleeding. Women receiving therapeutic doses of LMWH should have an anti-Xa level. If the assay is not available, a dose (1 mg/kg) has been given within the past 8 hours, or the level is greater than 1.0 U/mL, several precautions should be taken. First, epidural analgesia should be avoided. Second, judicious use of protamine sulfate should be considered. Finally, the obstetrician should be made aware of the potential for bleeding and make efforts to minimize risk.

UFH or LMWH therapy can be reinstituted after delivery as soon as it is safe, usually within 12 hours in the absence of complications. Warfarin can be started at the same time. Heparin is continued until an INR of 2.0 or greater is reached. Anticoagulants should be given for at least 4 weeks following delivery (unless there is an indication for more prolonged treatment).

Anticoagulation before and after Elective Surgery

Patients requiring warfarin therapy for venous or arterial thromboembolism create a challenge in management when elective surgical procedures are planned. The approach to decision making is based on the clinician's ability to determine the risk of thromboembolism on the one hand and hemorrhagic risk on the other (Kearon and Hirsh, 1997).

After warfarin is discontinued it usually takes between 3 and 4 days for the INR to drop below 1.5 (considered safe for most surgical procedures). After warfarin is restarted it takes approximately 3 day to reach an INR of 2.0. Thus, the practice of holding warfarin for 4 days before surgery and restarting either the evening of or day after the surgery is associated with a subtherapeutic INR for approximately 2 days.

The estimated rates of thromboembolism associated with acute DVT/PE, recurrent venous thromboembolism, nonvalvular atrial fibrillation (with or without prior embolism), mechanical heart valves, and acute arterial embolism are summarized in Table 23.3.

The risk of recurrent arterial or venous thromboembolism is greatest during the first month. Accordingly, patients undergoing surgical procedures should be protected with heparin (IV UFH or LMWH), to be started when the INR drops below 2.0. Typically, heparin is discontinued 4 to 6 hours prior to surgery. Heparin is restarted postoperatively (usually without a bolus in the case of UFH) when hemostasis has been achieved and continued until the INR exceeds 2.0 on 2 consecutive days. In the second and third months after venous thromboembolism, preoperative heparin is usually not required; however, it should be used postoperatively given the marked increase risk of venous thrombosis in the postoperative setting. The risk of embolism in most patients with either mechanical heart valves or atrial fibrillation is sufficiently low that routine preoperative heparin administration is not recommended. Venus thromboembolism prophylaxis should be offered and warfarin should be restarted when hemostasis has been achieved.

A recommended approach to anticoagulation prior to and after elective surgery is outlined in Table 23.4. Patients with acute venous or arterial thrombosis in whom surgery must take place within 2 weeks should be considered for inferior vena cava (IVC) filter placement. A retrievable model is recommended whenever

Table 23.3 Estimated Rates of Thromboembolism Associated with Various Indications for Oral Anticoagulation, and the Reduction in Risk Due to Anticoagulant Therapy

Indication	Rate without Therapy (%)	Risk Reduction with Therapy (%)
Acute venous thromboembolism		
Month 1	40	80
Months 2 and 3	10	80
Recurrent venous thromboembolism*	15	80
Nonvalvular atrial fibrillation*	4.5	66
Nonvalvular atrial fibrillation and previous emboli*	12	66
Mechanical heart valve*	8	75
Acute arterial embolism	15	66
Month 1		

* 1-year rates.

Kearon C, Hirsh J. Management of anti coagulation before and after elective surgery. N Engl J Med 1997;336:1506–1511.

Table 23.4 Recommendations for Preoperative and Postoperative Anticoagulation in Patients Who Are Taking Oral Anticoagulants

Indication	Before Surgery	After Surgery
Acute venous thromboembolism		
Month 1	IV heparin	IV heparin
Months 2 and 3	No change	IV heparin
Recurrent venous thromboembolism	No change	SC heparin
Acute arterial embolism		
Month 1	IV heparin	IV heparin
Mechanical heart valve	No change	SC heparin
Nonvalvular atrial fibrillation	No change	SC heparin

Kearon C, Hirsh J. Management of anticoagulation before and after elective surgery. N Engl J Med *1997;336:1506–1511.*

possible. A similar approach should be taken for patients at high risk for both thrombosis and bleeding.

Summary—Venous Thromboembolism

Patients with acute VTE including those with uncomplicated pulmonary embolism can be treated with LMWH or IV UFH. Low-molecular-weight heparin is preferred because of its predictable pharmacokinetics and pharmacodynamics as well as the absence for need for routine monitoring. Patients with severe renal insufficiency should probably receive IV UFH; however, frequent anti-Xa monitoring and modified dosing may permit LMWH use in these patients. Further investigation is needed. Patients should be considered for abbreviated hospitalization or home therapy when the appropriate management system and follow-up services are in place.

Oral vitamin K antagonists (or in the future ximelagatran) should be continued for 3 to 6 months; however, long-term prevention strategies using a lower intensity of anticoagulant is appropriate for high-risk patients. Long-term treatment with LMWH probably has advantages over oral vitamin K antagonists in the setting of malignancy.

Pulmonary Embolism

Pathophysiology

In patients with acute PE, the pulmonary artery circuit is compromised by existing thrombus, lowering its capacitance and causing a sudden rise in pulmonary arterial pressure. The rise in pressure is greater than the actual extent of cross-sectional obstruction, a phenomenon that may be related to neurohumoral factors that provoke arterial constriction (McIntyre and Susahara, 1997). Because alveolar function, at least initially, is normal, the reduction in blood flow causes ventilation (V)/perfusion (Q) mismatching and, as a result, an oxygen gradient between alveolar and arterial blood. Elevated pulmonary artery pressure causes right heart strain, accompanied by progressive dilation of the right ventricle, tricuspid regurgitation, and clinical stigmata of right heart failure. This, in turn, causes a reduction in left ventricular preload and stroke volume. In an attempt to maintain cardiac output, heart rate increases. Needless to say, the sequence of events can be more or less profound depending on the extent of embolization, neurohumoral response, and underlying cardiopulmonary reserve.

Diagnosis Approach

The initial diagnostic approach to PE begins with a clinician's high index of suspicion. An autopsy finding of multiple, small emboli in patients without hemodynamic compromise or a prior history of PE is not uncommon, emphasizing the critical nature of maintaining a high index of suspicion in patients with sudden unexplained cardiopulmonary signs and symptoms (PIOPED Investigators, 1990).

Physical Signs and Symptoms

The signs and symptoms of PE are variable and have prompted clinicians over the years to refer to it as the "Great Masquerader." Most patients with acute thromboembolism are tachycardic, tachypneic, and dyspneic. Fever, syncope, pleuritic chest pain, hemoptysis, and hypotension are less common presenting features; however, they still must be entertained as potential signs of PE.

The physical examination may be entirely normal with small emboli, particularly in patients with normal cardiopulmonary reserve. Although the physical signs of PE are not specific, when present they do have a significant role in narrowing the list of possibilities. They include distended neck veins, loud pulmonic component of the second heart sound (P_2), right-sided (ventricular) S_3 gallop, and right ventricular heave. The predictive value of any of the prior findings is, needless to say, markedly enhanced when they develop suddenly in an individual deemed at risk.

The Prospective Investigation of Pulmonary Embolism diagnosis (PIOPED) study (PIOPED Investigators, 1990) revealed that V/Q scans alone are not sufficient to secure the diagnosis of PE. The PIOPED Investigators grouped physicians' clinical suspicion into three categories: high (80–100%), intermediate (20–79%), and low (0–19%) suspicion (that the patient had experienced a PE). The physicians were correct 91% of the time when they placed suspicions in the low category, but were correct only 68% of the time when their suspicion was high. Table 23.5 outlines the percentage of patients with angiographically confirmed PE by V/Q scan results and physician suspicion. Carefully considered, it is clear that the V/Q "probability" and the physician's "suspicion" are complementary. The importance of "pretest probability" was highlighted among 1,239 patients with suspected PE. A scoring system was developed using well-established risk factors for VTE, clinical signs and symptoms, and determination of whether an alternative diagnosis was likely (Wells et al., 1998). Low, moderate, and high pretest probability was associated with 3.4%, 27.8%, and 78.4% rates of PE, respectively. Figure 23.3 provides a diagnostic algorithm for patients with suspected PE.

Biochemical Testing

Biochemical tests may also aid in the diagnosis. D-dimer is a degradation product of cross-linked fibrin that can be measured in plasma. Measurements of D-dimer using enzyme-linked immunosorbent assay (ELISA) techniques yield high sensitivity and low specificity for the diagnosis of PE (97% vs. 45%, respectively, using a cutoff value of 500 ng/L). A D-dimer level less than 500 ng/L is uncommon in the setting of acute PE. In other words, a low D-dimer concentration has a strong negative predictive value; however, due to its low specificity, the positive predictive value for elevated levels (>500 ng/L) is poor. Accordingly, D-dimer measurement is clinically useful when attempting to *exclude* the diagnosis of PE.

Table 23.5 Importance of Physician Suspicion in the Context of Ventilation/Perfusion Scan Probability of Pulmonary Embolism

Scan Probability	Suspicion		
	High	Intermediate	Low
High	96%[a]	88%	56%
Intermediate	66%	28%	16%
Low	40%	16%	4%
Normal/near normal	0%	6%	2%

[a]The percentages represent pulmonary embolism confirmed by pulmonary angiography.

PIOPED Investigators. Value of the ventilation/perfusion scan in acute pulmonary embolism: results of the Prospective Investigation of Pulmonary Embolism Diagnosis (PIOPED). JAMA 1990;263:2753–2759.

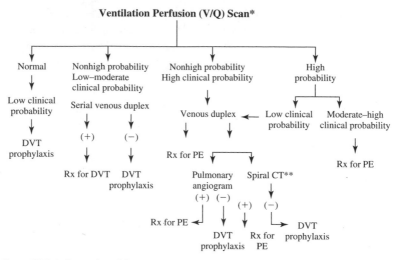

Figure 23.3 A diagnostic and therapeutic approach to acute pulmonary embolism (PE). *In patients with low clinical probability, a negative deep vein thrombosis (DVT)/PE D-dimer assay *may* exclude PE. **Spiral computed tomography (CT) scan of chest with contrast (specify PE protocol). The utilization of contrast CT or magnetic resonance imaging (MRI) as a *first-line* diagnostic strategy is under investigation and may, with time, replace ventilation (V)/perfusion (Q) scanning. Clinical probability (increased with): respiratory: dyspnea, pleuritic chest pain: O_2 saturation <92% (on room air with suboptimal correction with supplemental O_2), hemoptysis, pleural rub. Risk factors: surgery <12 weeks, immobilization (for 3 or more days), prior DVT/PE, malignancy, trauma, postpartum, family history of DVT/PE, stroke, spinal cord injury, obesity.

Pulmonary Angiography

Since Forssman first introduced a catheter into his own heart in 1928, the use of cardiac catheterization as a diagnostic and therapeutic procedure has expanded substantially. Pulmonary angiography represents the gold standard for determining the existence of thrombi within the pulmonary vasculature. The only absolute contraindication to pulmonary angiography is radiographic contrast-induced anaphylaxis, which can usually be prevented with steroids given prior to the procedure. Recent myocardial infarction, arrhythmias, renal failure, and poorly controlled hypertension remain strong relative contraindications. In 1980, Mills and colleagues (1980) reported an experience of 1,350 patients over an 11-year span in which a 5% morbidity and 0.2% mortality was attributed to the procedure. In the three reported deaths, patients exhibited severe pulmonary hypertension and irreversible hypotension after injection of contrast dye. Therefore, caution among patients with markedly elevated right ventricular end-diastolic pressure is recommended.

Pulmonary angiography involves the delivery of contrast (iodinated dye) under pressure into a subsection of lung under fluoroscopic visualization. Manipulation of the catheter tip into a specific pulmonary vascular bed allows a comprehensive evaluation with less contrast (total volume) delivery to the patient. This particular technique, in contrast to a balloon occlusion method, allows both direct and detailed visualization of both the proximal and peripheral vessels. At least two projections are recommended to secure a diagnosis.

Echocardiography

Transthoracic echocardiography has been evaluated for the diagnosis of PE (Table 23.6). It is a widely available and sensitive technique for identifying acute right ventricular pressure overload with massive PE (Cheriex et al., 1994). In addition to right ventricular dilatation and hypokinesis, septal flattening and paradoxical septal motion are often observed (Jardin et al., 1987).

The findings of a nationwide, multicenter registry suggest that clinicians turn to echocardiography often and early in the evaluation of patients with suspected PE (Kasper et al., 1997). From a total of 1,001 consecutive patients enrolled in the German Registry, 74% underwent echocardiography, and the information was used in deciding candidacy for fibrinolytic therapy.

Treatment

The management of patients with PE must be individualized. We recommend an approach based on the presenting stability of hemodynamic status. The hemodynamically stable patient should receive IV UFH with a target aPTT two times that of the control or SC LMWH (e.g., enoxaparin 1 mg/kg SC bid or 1.5 mg/kg qd) while further diagnostic testing is being scheduled and performed. In contrast, unstable patients should be considered for reperfusion therapy (Jerjes-Sanchez et al., 1995). The ultimate goal of fibrinolytic therapy is prompt dissolution of pulmonary arterial thrombus with a subsequent reduction of right ventricular afterload. A decrease in pulmonary artery pressure leads to improved right ventricular function, increased left ventricular preload, and hemodynamic stability. There is evidence that fibrinolytic therapy leads to more rapid radiographically determined clot reso-

Table 23.6 Echocardiographic Features of Right Ventricular Dysfunction[a] in Acute Pulmonary Embolism

Right ventricular hypokinesis
Right ventricular dilation
Septal flattening and paradoxical motion
Tricuspid regurgitation
Lack of or decrease in inspiratory collapse of the inferior vena cava

[a]*Manifestations of right ventricular pressure overload.*

lution and improvement in hemodynamic parameters compared with heparin alone (Levine, 1995). The studies performed to date have included a relatively small sample size, and therefore are underpowered in their ability to reliably detect an improvement in overall survival.

Incomplete thrombus dissolution has been associated with chronic pulmonary hypertension and right ventricular dysfunction. It has also been reported that patients with residual right ventricular dysfunction after PE are at increased risk for recurrent thromboembolism and death compared to patients with preserved right ventricular function (Lualdi and Goldhaber, 1995). Accordingly, successful fibrinolysis should reduce the incidence of chronic pulmonary hypertension and recurrent thromboembolism. This has not yet been confirmed in a randomized study.

A variety of factors influence fibrinolytic response. Thrombi that are proximal in location, more recently formed (fresh), and smaller in size (reduced clot burden) typically undergo rapid and complete dissolution. Not withstanding, there is reported angiographic benefit with treatment initiated up to 14 days after the clinical onset of PE (Goldhaber, 1995). The management algorithm outlined in Figure 23.4 is designed to individualize patient treatment on the basis of presenting clinical features (Table 23.7).

The potential benefit of fibrinolytic therapy among patients with submassive PE as been investigated (Konstantinides et al., 1997, 2002). A total of 256 patients with PE accompanied by pulmonary hypertension or right ventricular dysfunction (but not hypotension) randomly received either alteplase (100 mg over 2 hours) plus UFH or UFH alone. Fibrinolytic therapy was associated with a lower incidence of death and a need for escalation of therapy due to clinical determinants (catecholamine infusion, need for fibrinolysis, endotracheal intubation, cardiopulmonary resuscitation [CPR] or emergency embolectomy [surgical or catheter-based]).

Unstable patients with an absolute contraindication to fibrinolysis or who have failed a course of fibrinolytic therapy should be considered for mechanical (extraction) or surgical thrombectomy. Patients with acute PE complicated by cardiopulmonary arrest should be considered for immediate surgical intervention. Unstable patients who are not considered candidates for either fibrinolytic or surgical treatment should, at the very least, be considered for treatment with a heparin compound (LMWH or UFH) unless it is also contraindicated. In this case, IVC interruption (filter placement) should be considered (Table 23.8). Unless contraindications exist, patients should receive anticoagulant therapy with warfarin for 6 to 12 months (or longer if required) to minimize clot burden in the proximal deep veins and the likelihood of the "postphlebitic" syndrome (chronic venous stasis, pain, edema) in the lower extremities.

While considering the available therapeutic options, including fibrinolytic therapy, anticoagulation, and surgical intervention, the clinician must concomitantly address the patient's hemodynamic status. Hypotension should be managed

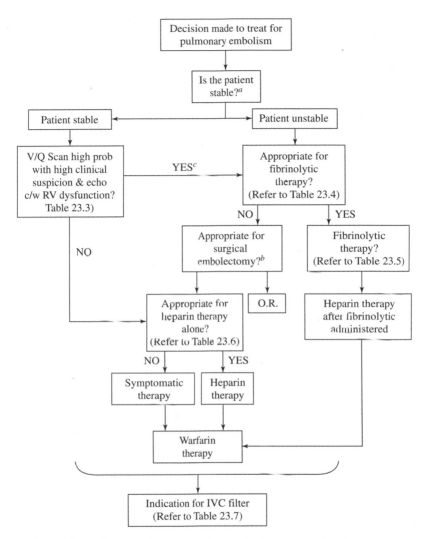

Figure 23.4 A stepwise approach to the management of patients with confirmed pulmonary embolism that incorporates the use of echocardiography in the treatment decision. [a]Hypotension; severe hypoxemia. [b]Surgical thrombectomy should be considered when the patient has absolute contraindications to or has failed fibrinolytics. Patients in cardiac arrest require a surgical approach. [c]Use of fibrinolytics in the stable patient is controversial. Prob, probability; V/Q, ventilation/perfusion scan; IVC, inferior vena cava; c/w, compatible with; RV, right ventricular.

Table 23.7 Contraindications to Fibrinolytic Therapy

Absolute
  Suspected or diagnosed aortic dissection
  Acute pericarditis
  Active internal or uncontrolled external bleeding
  History of prior intracranial hemorrhage
  History of intracerebral disease
    Aneurysm
    A-V malformation
    Cerebral neoplasm
Relative
  GI/GU hemorrhage within the past 2 mo
  Ischemic stroke within the past 12 mo
  Major surgery or trauma, organ biopsy, minor head trauma, or puncture of a noncompressible
    vessel in the past 2 mo
  Prolonged CPR in a patient with evidence of chest trauma or who is unresponsive
  Diabetic proliferative retinopathy
  Severe uncontrolled hypertension (systolic BP >180 mmHg or diastolic BP >100 mmHg)
  History of bleeding diathesis, hepatic dysfunction, or active malignancy
  Pregnancy (including early postpartum period)[a]

[a]*Some authorities consider pregnancy to be an absolute contraindication to fibrinolytic therapy.*
A-V, arteriovenous; BP, blood pressure; CPR, cardiopulmonary resuscitation; GI, gastrointentinal; GU, genitourinary.

with IV fluid as a means to increase ventricular preload and systemic blood pressure. If vasopressors are needed, dobutamine, with its positive inotropic properties and pulmonary vasodilation, should be considered the drug of choice. Profound hypotension (mean arterial blood pressure <65 mmHg) frequently necessitates the use of either dopamine or norepinephrine. Patients with underlying cardiopulmonary disease commonly experience a more substantial reduction in cardiac output without prominent elevations in central venous pressure when compared to normal individuals.

Profound hypoxemia, with a large alveolar–arterial (A-a) oxygen gradient, often accompanies massive PE and also can be seen to a lesser degree of clot burden in the presence of concomitant cardiopulmonary disease. High concentrations of supplemental oxygen, at times necessitating endotracheal intubation and positive end-expiratory pressure, may be a vital component of initial treatment.

Summary

Pulmonary embolism is a potentially fatal thrombotic disorder that requires a prompt diagnosis and immediate treatment. Anticoagulant therapy with heparin (UFH or LMWH) is the mainstay of treatment and designed to prevent recurrent events. Fi-

Table 23.8 Indication for IVC Filter†

Contraindication to fibrinolytic and/or anticoagulant therapy
Resistance to anticoagulant therapy or recurrent pulmonary embolism despite adequate anti-
    coagulation profile
Large proximal thrombus burden or "free-floating" thrombus in vena cava
Chronic recurrent pulmonary embolism with subsequent pulmonary hypertension
During concurrent performance of surgical pulmonary embolectomy or pulmonary endarterectomy

IVC, inferior vena cava.
† Consider retrievable filters when appropriate

brinolytic therapy should be considered in patients with hemodynamic instability
and possibly in those with evidence of right ventricular dysfunction.

References

Anderson FA Jr, Wheeler HB, Goldberg RJ, et al. A population-based perspective of the
    hospital incidence and case-fatality rates of venous thrombosis and pulmonary
    embolism: the Worcester DVT Study. *Arch Intern Med* 1991;151:933–938.
Cheriex FC, Sreeram N, Eussen YFJM, et al. Cross sectional Doppler echocardiography
    as the initial technique for the diagnosis of acute pulmonary embolism. *Br Heart J*
    1994;72:52–57.
Eriksson H, for the THRIVE Investigators. A randomized, controlled, dose-guiding study
    of the oral direct thrombin inhibitor ximelagatran compared with standard ther-
    apy for the treatment of acute deep vein thrombosis. THRIVE I. *J Thromb Haemost*
    2003a;1:41–47.
Eriksson H, Wahlander K, Lundstrom T, et al., for the THRIVE III Investigators. Ex-
    tended secondary prevention with the oral direct thrombin inhibitor ximelagatran for
    18 months after 6 months of oral anticoagulation in patients with venous thrombo-
    embolism: a randomized placebo-controlled trial [Abstract]. *J Thromb Haemost*
    2003b;1(suppl 1).
Fahey VA. *Vascular nursing,* 3rd ed. Philadelphia: WB Saunders Co. 1999;23.
Ginsberg S, Bates SM. Management of venous thromboembolism during pregnancy.
    J Thromb Haemost 2003;1:1435–1442.
Goldhaber SZ. Thrombolytic therapy in venous thromboembolism. Clinical trials and
    current indications. *Clin Chest Med* 1995;16:307–320.
Huisman MV for the THRIVE Treatment Study Investigators. Efficacy and safety of the
    oral direct thrombin inhibitor ximelagatran compared with current standard therapy
    for acute, symptomatic deep vein thrombosis with or without pulmonary embolism:
    a randomized, double-blind, international study [Abstract]. *J Thromb Haemostas*
    2003;1(suppl 1).

Jardin F, Dubourg O, Gueret P, et al. Quantitative two-dimensional echocardiography in massive pulmonary embolism: emphasis on ventricular interdependence and leftward septal displacement. *J Am Coll Cardiol* 1987;10:1201–1206.

Jerjes-Sanchez C, Ramirez-Rivera A, Garcia M de L, et al. Streptokinase and heparin versus heparin alone in massive pulmonary embolism: a randomized controlled trial. *J Thromb Thrombolysis* 1995;2:227–229.

Kasper W, Konstantinides S, Geibel A, et al. Management strategies and determinants of outcome in acute major pulmonary embolism: results of a multicenter registry. *J Am Coll Caridol* 1997;30:1165–1171.

Kearon C. Natural history of venous thromboembolism. *Circulation* 2003;107:I22–I30.

Kearon C, Hirsh J. Management of anticoagulation before and after elective surgery. *N Engl J Med* 1997;336:1506–1511.

Kearon C, Gent M, Hirsh J, et al. A comparison of three months of anticoagulation with extended anticoagulation for a first episode of idiopathic venous thromboembolism [published correction appears in *N Engl J Med* 1999;341:298]. *N Engl J Med* 1999; 340:901–907.

Konstantinides S, Geibel A, Olschewiski M, et al. Impact of thrombolytic treatment on the prognosis of hemodynamically stable patients with major pulmonary embolism: results of a multicenter registry. *Circulation* 1997;96:882–888.

Koinstantinides S, Geibel A, Heusel G, et al. Heparin plus alteplase compared with heparin along in patients with submassive pulmonary embolism. *N Engl J Med* 2002; 347:1143–1150.

Lensing AW, Prins MH, Davidson BL, Hirsh J. Treatment of deep venous thrombosis with low-molecular weight heparins. A meta-analysis. *Arch Intern Med* 1995;155: 601–607.

Levine MN. Thrombolytic therapy for venous thromboembolism, complications and contraindications. *Clin Chest Med* 1995;16:321–328.

Lualdi JC, Goldhaber SZ. Right ventricular dysfunction after acute pulmonary embolism: pathophysiologic factors detection, and therapeutic implications. *Am Heart J* 1995; 130:1276–1282.

McIntyre KM, Susahara AA. The homodynamic response to pulmonary embolism in patients without cardiopulmonary disease. *Am J Cardiol* 1997;28:288–294.

Mills SR, Jackson DC, Older RA, et al. The incidence, etiologies, and avoidance of complications of pulmonary angiography in a large series. *Radiology* 1980;136:295–299.

PIOPED Investigators. Value of the ventilation/perfusion scan in acute pulmonary embolism: results of the Prospective Investigation of Pulmonary Embolism Diagnosis (PIOPED). *JAMA* 1990;263:2753–2759.

Prandoni P, Lensing AW, Cogo A, et al. The long-term clinical course of acute deep venous thrombosis. *Ann Intern Med* 1996;125:1–7.

Research Committee of the British Thoracic Society. Optimum duration of anticoagulation for deep-vein thrombosis and pulmonary embolism. *Lancet* 1992;340:873–876.

Ridker PM, Goldhaber SZ, Danielson E, et al. for the PREVENT Investigators. Long-term, low-intensity warfarin therapy for the prevention of recurrent venous thromboembolism. *N Engl J Med* 2003;348:1425–1434.

Schulman S, Rhedin AS, Lindmarker P, et al. A comparison of six weeks with six months of oral anticoagulant therapy after a first episode of venous thromboembolism. Duration of Anticoagulation Trial Study Group. *N Engl J Med* 1995;332:1661–1665.

Schulman S, Granqvist S, Holmstrom M, et al. The duration of oral anticoagulant therapy after a second episode of venous thromboembolism. Duration of Anticoagulation Trial Study Group. *N Engl J Med* 1997;336:393–398.

Wells PS, Ginsberg JS, Anderson DR, et al. Use of a clinical model for safe management of patients with suspected pulmonary embolism. *Ann Intern Med* 1998;129·997–1005.

Part VI
Genomics, Proteomics, and
Suspected Thrombophilias

Fundamentals and Patient Evaluation

24

Thrombophilia is the term used to describe a tendency toward developing thrombosis. This tendency may be inherited, involving polymorphism in gene coding for platelet or clotting factor proteins, or acquired due to alterations in the constituents of blood and/or blood vessels.

Basis for Further Investigation

An inherited thrombophilia is likely if there is a history of repeated episodes of thrombosis or a family history of thromboembolism. One should also consider an inherited thrombophilia when there are no obvious predisposing factors for thrombosis or when clots occur in a patient under the age of 45. Repeated episodes of thromboembolism occurring in patients over the age of 45 raise suspicion for an occult malignancy.

Inherited Thrombophilia

A summary of inherited thrombophilias are summarized in Table 24.1. This list continues to grow, as new genetic polymorphisms and combined mutations are being detected.

Epidemiology

The prevalence of common thrombophilias is shown in Figure 24.1. Factor V Leiden (FVL) mutation and hyperhomocysteinemia are present in nearly 5% of the general population and are often found in patients with venous thrombosis, while deficiencies of antithrombin (AT), protein C, and protein S are relatively uncommon. Elevated levels of factor VIII (FVIII) are uncovered frequently in the general population and in patients with thrombosis. This is not surprising as FVIII is an acute-phase reactant that increases rapidly after surgery or trauma; however, prospective studies have shown that FVIII elevation in some patients cannot be

Table 24.1 A Summary of Inherited and
Acquired Thrombophilias

Inherited
 Factor V Leiden mutation
 Prothrombin 20210A mutation
 MTHFR 677, CS mutation
 Mutations in protein C gene
 Mutations in protein S gene
 Mutations in antithrombin gene
 Mutations in TM and TFPI gene
 Increased FVIII, IX XI
 Mutations in fibrinogen genes
 Mutations in plasminogen gene
 Platelet GP1A mutation
 Increased PAI-1
 Mutant heparin cofactor II
Acquired
 Hyperhomocysteinemia
 Antiphospholipid antibodies
 Pregnancy, estrogens, oral contraceptives
 Hyperlipidemias
 Nephrotic syndrome
 Malignancy
 Trauma
 Immobilization
 Myeloproliferative disorders
 Thrombotic microangiopathies
 Heparin-induced thrombocytopenia
 Endotoxemia

*F, factor; GP, glycoprotein; MTHFR, methylenetetra-
hydrofolate reductase; PAI, plasminogen activator
inhibitor; TFPI, tissue factor pathway inhibitor; TM,
thrombomodulin.*

attributed to a stress reaction and probably represents mutations in the genes regulating FVIII synthesis or release (Kyrle et al., 2000). The same may be true for factors IX and XI.

The relative risks for thrombosis among patients with inherited thrombophilias have been determined. While AT mutations are the least common, they are associated with a substantial risk of venous thrombosis; similar risk is seen with protein C and S deficiency. In contrast, the lifetime risk of having a thromboembolic
event in an individual heterozygous for FVL is comparatively low (Martinelli et al.,
1998). Incidence rates markedly increase with age, and are highest among those with
AT deficiency, followed by protein C and protein S, and least with FVL. FVL occurs
with the highest frequency in persons of Northern European ancestry (3–8%), followed by Southern European (0.6–2.9%), and is rare in Asians and Africans. In the
United States, the prevalence is 4% to 6% (Price and Ridker, 1997).

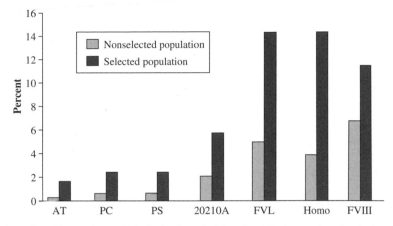

Figure 24.1 The prevalence of inherited and acquired thrombophilias in nonselected and selected patient populations. AT, antithrombin; FVIII, factor VIII; FVL, factor V Leiden; Homo, hyperhomocysteinemia; PC, protein C; PS, protein S; 20210, prothrombin 20210A. (From Lensing AW, et al. *Lancet* 1999;353:479–485.)

Mechanisms of Thrombosis

Mutations in the genes for either clotting factors (gain of function) or their inhibitors (loss of function) may increase the risk of thrombosis. A gene mutation may also result in increased production of a procoagulant protein, such as FVIII or prothrombin, or lead to a mutated factor that is resistant to inactivation by its natural inhibitor (factor V and activated protein C [APC]), causing resistance to inactivation. An alteration in the amino acid sequence of antithrombin prevents heparin from binding to and activating this anticoagulant. Mutant fibrinogens may be resistant to profibrinolytic enzymes. Lastly, patients not infrequently have more than one mutation, greatly increasing their risk of thrombosis.

Inherited Thrombophilias

Antithrombin Deficiency

Antithrombin is a 67,000 kd glycoprotein that accounts for 75% of the total AT activity of plasma. A naturally occurring accelerator of heparin-like species (e.g., heparan sulfate) on the vascular endothelial surface, AT is essential for physiologic thromboresistance. In typical cases, AT deficiency is inherited as an autosomal dominant disorder with proportionately decreased AT antigenic and functional activities of 25% to 60% of normal (type I deficiency). However, qualitative deficiencies may occur as well (type II deficiency). Acquired AT deficiency (quantitative or qualitative) has been described in patients with nephrotic syndrome, advanced liver disease, and disseminated intravascular coagulation (DIC), and following high-dose intravenous nitroglycerin administration (Becker et al., 1990).

The most frequently observed clinical symptoms are recurrent deep vein thrombosis (DVT) and pulmonary embolism, occurring for the first time in the second or third decades of life. Other sites may be involved as well, including the renal, mesenteric, hepatic, retinal, and cerebral veins (Winter et al., 1982). In contrast, arterial thrombosis is much less common, with rare cases of myocardial infarction (MI) appearing in the medical literature (Innerfield et al., 1976; Matsuda et al., 1977; O'Brien, 1974).

Protein C Deficiency

Protein C, a 62,000 kDa glycoprotein precursor of APC, participates in vascular thromboresistance by proteolytically inactivating coagulation factors Va and VIIIa in the presence of thrombomodulin. Activated protein C also has fibrinolytic properties (Clouse and Comp, 1986; Esmon, 1983). An insufficient amount of protein C would, therefore, be expected to increase local thrombus formation. Indeed, protein C deficiency, a codominantly inherited disorder, is associated with thromboembolic events that most often come to clinical attention during the second and third decades of life (Bovill et al., 1989). The clinical spectrum typically includes recurrent DVT and pulmonary embolism; however, involvement of other venous sites, albeit less common, can occur as well. As with AT deficiency, arterial thrombosis, including MI and stroke, occurs rarely (Hacker et al., 1991).

Protein S Deficiency

Protein S, like protein C, is a vitamin K–dependent protein that serves as a cofactor for the anticoagulant and fibrinolytic effects of APC (de Fouw et al., 1986; Walker, 1980). Protein S exists in two forms within plasma, either as a free protein (40%) or complexed with C4b-binding protein (an inhibitor of the complement system). Only free protein S is functionally active. A majority of patients with inherited protein S deficiency have decreased plasma levels; however, some have normal antigen levels, but the molecules are bound to C4b-binding protein, rendering them functionally inactive. Acquired protein S deficiency has been described in pregnancy, oral contraceptive use, DIC, advanced liver disease, nephrotic syndrome, chronic viral illnesses (e.g., HIV), and type I diabetes mellitus (Schwarz et al., 1987; Vigano-D'Angelo et al., 1987).

As with AT and protein C deficiency states, patients with protein S deficiency can experience recurrent thromboembolic events, most commonly DVT and pulmonary embolism. Arterial thrombosis has also been described, but is uncommon.

Dysplasminogenemias

The fibrinolytic system is a proteolytic enzyme system with a diversity of physiologic functions, of which degradation of fibrin deposits in the cardiovascular system is the most well known and widely investigated. Plasminogen variants have been identified in patients with thromboembolic disease, including DVT, pulmonary embolism, mesenteric vein thrombosis, cerebral vein thrombosis, and less commonly, stroke and MI. To date, 12 reported variants have been described. Congenital dysplasminogenemias are characterized by decreased plasminogen functional activity. In contrast, familial hypoplasminogenemia exhibits a proportional decrease in both antigenic and functional activity.

Abnormal Plasminogen Activation

Large epidemiologic studies that have included middle-aged men and other patient populations at risk for atherosclerotic coronary artery disease (CAD), have, thus far, failed to demonstrate a clear relationship between deficient fibrinolytic activity and cardiovascular events. However, in patients with typical angina pectoris, or those with a previous MI, a number of cross-sectional studies have identified an association between impaired fibrinolytic potential and major cardiac events, including recurrent infarction and death. Fibrinolytic impairment secondary to either decreased vascular tissue plasminogen activator (tPA) release or increased circulating plasminogen activator inhibitor (PAI)-1 concentration has been observed commonly, particularly in young survivors of MI. Prospective studies are needed to define more clearly the role of impaired fibrinolysis in predicting cardiac events.

Activated Protein C Resistance

In a majority of patients experiencing venous thromboembolism, an inherited thrombophilic disorder (e.g., AT, protein C or S deficiency) is not uncovered; however, recent advances have increased awareness that the predisposition to thrombosis may have its origin within an individual's genotype. Activated protein C resistance represents greater than 50% of all inherited thrombophilias and is uncovered in 25% of patients with recurrent venous thromboembolism. In at least 90% of cases, APC resistance is caused by a single point mutation in the factor V gene (G $\rightarrow$ A at nucleotide 1691) (FVL). This mutation causes the replacement of Arg506 by Gln in one of the APC-cleavage sites of the heavy chain of factor V by APC and the promotion of its procoagulant activity. Data from the Leiden Thrombophilia Study suggest that APC resistance is associated with a sevenfold increased risk of DVT (Bertina et al., 1995) and a four- to fivefold increased risk of recurrent thrombosis (Ridker et al., 1997).

The diagnosis of APC resistance is suggested by an abnormally low APC sensitivity ratio [aPTT (+APC)/aPTT (–APC)] (typically <0.84) and confirmed by DNA-based genotyping. When an abnormal functional test is not accompanied by the FVL genotype, alternative genetic mutations should be considered.

Factor II (Prothrombin) G20210A

A mutation involving a Gly to Arg substitution within nucleotide 20210 of the factor II (prothrombin) gene has been identified (Poort et al., 1996) and may be responsible for up to 18% of selected patients and 6.2% of unselected patients with venous thromboembolism. The calculated relative risk for thrombosis associated with the 20210A allele is 2.8 (95% confidence interval [CI], 1.4–5.6). Even after exclusion of patients with APC resistance and circulating lupus anticoagulants, the unmatched excess risk for thrombosis remains high at 2.7. The prothrombin mutation has been associated with increased prothrombin concentrations, suggesting a potential prothrombotic phenotype.

A subsequent review of 99 unselected patients with venography verified DVT and 282 controls identified the 20210A allele in 7.1% of the patient group vs. 1.8% in the control group (Spencer and Becker, 1999). After adjustment for age, sex, and FVL mutation carrier status, the relative risk of venous thrombosis was 3.0 (95% CI, 1.1–13.2). Of note, 2% of the patients were carriers of the FVL mutation; therefore, 34% of these unselected patients were carriers of an inherited thrombophilia. Further investigation is required to understand the prothrombin mutation and its association with venous thromboembolism. Defects in the thrombomodulin molecule have been isolated among patients with venous thromboembolism (Öhlin and Marlar, 1997).

Malignancy

An association between malignancy and thromboembolic events was recognized by Armand Trousseau late in the 19th century (Trousseau, 1865). Currently, a large body of clinical evidence suggests that coagulation abnormalities may represent an epiphenomenon of disseminated malignancy or exist as a primary abnormality with profound clinical implications.

A wide variety of thrombotic disorders have been described, including recurrent superficial and DVT, pulmonary embolism, MI and other arterial thrombotic events, and nonbacterial (marantic) endocarditis with peripheral embolism. Spontaneous or recurrent thrombosis is particularly common among patients with pancreatic carcinoma, adenocarcinoma of the gastrointestinal tract, and bronchogenic carcinoma (Weick, 1978).

A large amount of information has been gathered that links malignancy and thromboembolic events. Some investigators propose that chronic DIC with platelet activation and fibrin deposition is the primary abnormality. Although this entity may certainly be a contributing factor in some patients, the thromboembolic tendency is likely multifactorial in origin. The long list of potential contributors includes increased activated platelet (King and Kelton, 1984; Schernthaner et al., 1970), elevated fibrinogen concentrations, increased coagulation factors Va, Xa, and VIIIa, and decreased AT levels. Increased thrombin generation is supported by an observed increase in fibrinopeptide A, thrombin–antithrombin complexes, and prothrombin fragment 1.2 concentrations.

There is increasing evidence that procoagulant activity can be expressed by tumor cells directly or by shed membrane-bound vesicles. Indeed, both have been shown to express tissue factor activity and to activate factor X and the prothrombinase complex, leading to fibrin generation and thrombus formation.

Myeloproliferative Disorders

The myeloproliferative disorders include polycythemia vera, essential thrombocythemia, myelofibrosis, chronic myelogenous leukemia, and myeloid metaplasia. Hemorrhagic and thrombotic events occur not uncommonly, the latter typified by recurrent venous thrombosis, pulmonary embolism, stroke, MI, and microvascular thrombi. Although increased plasma and/or whole-blood viscosity may be a contributing feature, particularly in polycythemia vera and essential thrombocythemia, qualitative platelet abnormalities with increased adhesion, aggregation, and activation are centrally involved in the observed thrombotic tendency. Reduced fibrinolytic activity as a result of PAI-1 excess may also contribute.

Paroxysmal Nocturnal Hemoglobinuria

Paroxysmal nocturnal hemoglobinuria is an acquired hemolytic disorder characterized by the proliferation of an abnormal clone of stem cells that is susceptible to complement-mediated cellular membrane damage. Microcirculatory thrombosis is common, as is recurrent venous thrombosis involving the hepatic, splenic, portal, cerebral, and deep peripheral veins. Arterial thrombosis occurs rarely.

Hyperhomocysteinemia

Homocysteine is a sulfhydryl amino acid derived from the metabolism of methionine, which occurs via one of three enzymatic pathways:

1. Remethylation to methionine catalyzed by methionine synthase; the methyl group is donated by methyltetrahydrofolate; cobalamin (vitamin B_{12}) serves as cofactor.
2. Remethylation to methionine catalyzed by betaine-homocysteine methyltransferase; betaine is the methyl donor.
3. Transsulfuration by cystathionine β–synthase into cystathionine; pyridoxal 5′ phosphate (vitamin B6) is the cofactor.

Several inherited or acquired conditions affecting these pathways can result in varying degrees of hyperhomocysteinemia: severe (>100 μmol/L), moderate (30–100 μmol/L), and mild (15–30 μmol/L).

Homocystinuria is an inborn error of metabolism with variable expression caused by a deficiency of cystathionine β–synthetase. In its homozygous form, accumulation of homocysteine in the tissues and vasculature is responsible for typical symptoms and physical findings that include premature vascular occlusive events. In addition, however, heterozygous homocystinemia may also be a cause of premature peripheral occlusive and ischemic cerebrovascular diseases. Fatal MI has been described as well, reflecting thrombus formation at a site of endothelial injury.

Vasculitis

The vasculitides are characterized by various states of inflammation, involving small, medium-, or large-caliber vessels (depending on the disorder). Inflammation with accompanying structural and functional endothelial abnormalities and shear stress, increasing as a result of changes in luminal dimension, foster platelet adherence, activation, and fibrin deposition. Although some systemic disorders may be associated with circulating procoagulant factors (e.g., antiphospholipid antibodies), the majority exhibit a thrombotic tendency, primarily on the basis of focal abnormalities involving the vessel wall. Active vasculitis can cause arterial thrombosis, including MI. In addition, however, healed vasculitis involving the coronary arteries can cause accelerated atherosclerosis, itself a procoagulant state. Overall, the vasculitic disorders most commonly causing arterial thrombosis are polyarthritis nodosa and giant cell arteritis.

Antiphospholipid Syndrome

Antiphospholipid antibodies (APAs) are autoantibodies of either the IgG or IgM variety that can be detected in either plasma or serum using a solid-phase immunoassay in which negatively charged phospholipids serve as an antigen. Antiphospholipid antibodies commonly cross-react with cardiolipin, phosphatidylserine, phosphatidylinositol, phosphatidylethanolamine, and phosphatidylcholine as well as endothelial cell and platelet surface membranes.

Antiphospholipid antibodies are typically identified in individuals with auto-immune disorders, particularly systemic lupus erythematosus (SLE); however, they may occur in other disorders as well, including acute and chronic viral infections and malignancy. Occasionally, they develop in individuals without an underlying systemic disorder (primary antiphospholipid syndrome) or following ingestion of one of several drugs, such as chlorpromazine, procainamide, hydralazine, pheny-toin, or quinidine.

Antiphospholipid antibodies have been associated with the development of transient ischemic attacks, cerebrovascular accidents, spontaneous abortion, livedo reticularis, and thromboembolic events. Arterial thrombosis has been documented in the retinal, intracranial, mesenteric, peripheral, and coronary arteries. Venous thrombosis occurs as well, involving the renal, hepatic, mesenteric, cerebral, reti-nal, and superficial and deep veins of the lower extremities.

The potential mechanism for pathologic thrombosis in patients with circulat-ing APAs is currently under investigation. Cross-reactivity with phospholipids in endothelial cell and platelet surface membranes may be directly involved, prevent-ing prostacyclin release and increasing platelet aggregability, respectively. Increased von Willebrand factor (vWF) activity and decreased fibrinolytic potential, resulting from prekallikrein inhibition and decreased plasminogen activator release, have also been described. However, a number of interesting observations have been made recently. The binding of APAs occurs only in plasma or serum, suggesting that a cofactor is required. Indeed, the cofactor β_2-glycoprotein 1 (β_2-GP1), a single-chain polypeptide of 50,000 kd, has been recognized for its pathobiologic impor-tance. $\beta2$-GP1 binds and neutralizes negatively charged macromolecules that may activate either platelets or the intrinsic coagulation pathway. Therefore, if $\beta2$-GP1 serves as an antigenic cofactor for APA binding, its own neutralization may explain, at least in part, the observed thrombotic tendency.

Although variable, several investigators have identified the presence of APAs in patients with coronary heart disease. They have also been reported in patients at risk for saphenous vein occlusion following coronary bypass surgery and among young survivors of MI in whom their presence predicts an increased likelihood of recurrent cardiac events. Although in these settings the presence of circulating APAs may reflect a secondary immune response to either an acute or chronic in-flammatory state rather than a primary disorder, their presence may nonetheless serve as a clinically useful prognostic marker.

Lupus Anticoagulant

The lupus anticoagulant (LA) was originally described in two patients with SLE who were noted to have a prolonged prothrombin time (PT) and whole-blood clot-ting time. An antiphospholipid antibody with the ability to prolong phospholipid-dependent coagulation tests (most often the activated partial thromboplastin time [aPTT]) was subsequently identified. The term *lupus anticoagulant* is a misnomer, stemming from this in vitro property. In fact, patients with the LA are at increased risk for thromboembolic events. Although occasionally associated with arterial thrombosis, the LA more commonly predisposes to venous thrombosis. Like APA thrombosis syndrome, a wide variety of venous systems may be affected (although DVT of the lower extremities and pulmonary embolism remain the most common manifestations). The prevalence of LA in the general population has not been clearly defined; however, it has been estimated that 6% to 8% of otherwise healthy patients with LA will experience thromboembolism.

Drug-Induced Disorders

Heparin-Induced Thrombocytopenia with Thrombosis

Heparin (unfractionated) is a heterogeneous mucopolysaccharide that accelerates the inhibitory interaction of AT with a number of circulating coagulation proteins, primarily factors IIa (thrombin) and Xa. Thrombocytopenia is a well-recognized complication of heparin administration, occurring within 3 to 10 days in 10% to 15% of the patients receiving heparin from porcine intestinal mucosa and bovine lung, respectively (King and Kelton, 1984).

Platelet-associated IgG is frequently elevated in patients with heparin-induced thrombocytopenia. As it is commonly elevated in patients with other drug-induced thrombocytopenia as well, platelet-associated IgG lacks specificity. At present, functional assays including heparin-induced platelet aggregation (washed platelets with low and high heparin concentrations) and heparin-dependent platelet c-serotonin release are considered the diagnostic tests of choice (high specificity); however, enzyme-linked immunosorbent assays (ELISAs) for the platelet factor 4 (PF4)– heparin antibody complex are important diagnostic tools as well (high sensitivity).

As many as 18% of patients receiving intravenous heparin experience a moderate reduction in the platelet count within the first 2 days. Heparin-associated thrombocytopenia (HAT), formerly known as heparin-induced thrombocytopenia (HIT) type I, is caused by a direct platelet–heparin interaction. The binding of heparin to platelets is determined by molecular weight and the degree of sulfation. Thus, unfractionated heparin causes the greatest degree of thrombocytopenia.

In contrast to HAT, HIT (formerly type II) is immune-mediated and occurs between 5 and 20 days of heparin therapy (although it can occur within several hours if there has been a prior exposure). Despite a declining platelet count, bleeding is uncommon; however, thrombosis (venous, arterial) does occur. The platelet FC receptor plays a key role; heparin-induced antibodies bind and activate platelets via the FC receptor. These antibodies also bind to heparan sulfate and activate endothelial cells. Activated platelets release PF4, which has high affinity to heparin. The large complex (heparin–PF4) acts as a major antigen that binds antibodies (predominantly IgG) to form immune complexes, which then activate platelets through FC receptors. The same complexes form on endothelial cells (heparin-like molecules on endothelial surface). Thus, concomitant activation of platelets and endothelial cells are responsible for thrombotic events.

Antifibrinolytic Agents

The synthetic antifibrinolytic drugs ε-aminocaproic acid (Amicar) and tranexamic acid (Cyklokapron) impede fibrinolysis by impairing plasminogen activation and the binding of both plasminogen and plasmin to fibrin and fibrinogen substrate. They are generally avoided in the presence of active intravascular clotting processes, in which a shift toward coagulation could promote further thrombus formation and serious clinical consequences.

Prothrombin Complex Concentrates

Prothrombin complex concentrates (Konyne) contain high concentrations of the vitamin K–dependent coagulation factors II, VII, IX, and X. They also contain phospholipids. Therefore, intravenous administration promotes coagulation and may, at times, cause pathologic thrombosis, particularly in patients with abnormal liver function in whom the clearance of activated factors is decreased.

Estrogens and Hormone Replacement Therapy

The use of oral contraceptives and hormone replacement therapy (HRT) leads to an increased incidence of venous thrombosis (three- to fourfold increase), MI, stroke, and peripheral vascular occlusive events, the risks of which are highest during the first year of use (Rosendaal et al., 2003). Women with inherited thrombophilias (or other acquired thrombophilias) are at increased risk for thrombotic events when they take oral contraceptives or HRT. The prevalence of thrombophilias among women who experience venous thromboembolism (VTE) during gestation is outlined in Table 24.2.

Location of Thrombi

In patients with inherited thrombophilias, thrombi are usually located in the venous circulation, not infrequently involving unusual sites such as the mesenteric,

Table 24.2 Prevalence of Thrombophilia in Women with VTE during Gestation

Factor V Leiden mutation	30–50%
Prothrombin G20210A mutation	10–20%
MTHFR 677 TT	10–20%
Antiphospholipid antibodies	10–20%
Protein S deficiency	2–10%
Protein C deficiency	1–5%

MTHFR, methylenetetrahydrofolate reductase, VTE, venous thromboembolism.

Table 24.3 Approach to Suspected Thrombophilia*

Thrombophilic (hypercoagulable) states should be suspected with *one or more* of the following:
   Venous thromboembolism before age 55
   Arterial thromboembolism before age 45
   Recurrent spontaneous venous thrombosis
   Thrombosis in unusual site (e.g., mesenteric vein, cerebral sinus)
   Family history of thromboembolism
   Relatives of patients with thrombophilic condition
   Skin necrosis, particularly if secondary to warfarin
   Unexplained neonatal thrombosis
   Recurrent fetal loss
   Unexplained prolongation of aPTT
First-Line Laboratory Evaluation (for Venous Thrombosis)

APC resistance	Functional (screening) test
Factor V Leiden mutation	Genetic test (if APC resistance screening test abnormal)
Prothrombin G20210A mutation	Genetic test
Anticardiolipin antibodies (IgG, IgM)	Immunologic test
Lupus anticoagulant	Functional test (multistep)
Homocysteine	Direct measurement
Protein C activity	Functional test
Protein S (total/free)	Direct measurement
Antithrombin activity	Functional test

First-Line Laboratory Evaluation (for Arterial Thrombosis)
   Anticardiolipin antibodies (IgG, IgM)
   Lupus anticoagulant
   Homocysteine
   Activated protein C resistance (followed by factor V Leiden genotype if abnormal) (patients <50 yr of age)

*The ideal time to perform a comprehensive evaluation is 3–6 mo after the event (particularly for laboratory tests such as protein C, protein S, and antithrombin). Protein C and S levels are decreased by warfarin. The antithrombin level is decreased by heparin (UFH, LMWH).
aPTT, activated partial thromboplastin time; APC, activated protein resistance; Ig, immunoglobulin; LMWH, low-molecular-weight heparin; UFH, unfractionated heparin.

adrenal, dural, or retinal veins, with a few important exceptions. Patients with hyper-homocysteinemia may have early-onset arterial as well as venous thrombosis. A meta-analysis of studies investigating the impact of FVL, prothrombin 20210, and methylenetetrahydrofolate reductase mutations on arterial thrombosis (MI, stroke, peripheral) found a modest association in patients greater than 50 years of age. The association was somewhat stronger for younger individuals, particularly among women who smoke (Kim and Becker, 2003).

When Is the Best Time to Perform Thrombophilia Studies?

Acute thrombosis, an accompanying acute-phase response, and anticoagulant therapy can influence functional assays. Accordingly, only genetic studies can be performed with reliable results in the initial stages of venous and/or arterial events. The preferred time to embark upon a formal evaluation (when indicated) is 3 to 6 months later (Table 24.3).

Summary

The evaluation of patients with suspected thrombophilias begins with a thorough history including family members and first-degree relatives. The decision to embark upon a comprehensive laboratory evaluation requires careful, thorough, experience, and consideration of pretest likelihood of disease and the impact of acute thrombosis on test results.

References

Becker RC, Corrao JM, Bovill EG, et al. Intravenous nitroglycerin-induced heparin resistance: a qualitative antithrombin III abnormality. *Am Heart J* 1990;119:1254–1261.

Bertina RM, Reitsma PH, Rosendaal FR, et al. Resistance to activated protein C and factor V Leiden as risk factors for venous thrombosis. *Thromb Haesmost* 1995;74: 449–453.

Bovill EG, Bauer KA, Dickerman JD, et al. The clinical spectrum of heterozygous protein C deficiency in a large New England kindred. *Blood* 1989;73:712–717.

Clouse LH, Comp PC. The regulation of hemostasis: the protein C system. *N Engl J Med* 1986;314:1298–1304.

de Fouw NJ, Haverkate F, Bertina RM, et al. The cofactor role of protein S in the acceleration of whole blood clot lysis by activated protein C in vitro. *Blood* 1986;67: 1189–1192.

Esmon CT. Protein C: biochemistry, physiology, and clinical implications. *Blood* 1983; 62:1155–1158.

Hacker SM, Williamson BD, Lisco S, et al. Protein C deficiency and acute myocardial infarction in the third decade. *Am J Cardiol* 1991;68:137–138.

Innerfield I, Goldfischer JD, Reicher-Reiss H, et al. Serum antithrombin in coronary artery disease. *Am J Clin Pathol* 1976;65:64–68.

Kim RJ, Becker RC. Clinical investigations. Association between factor V Leiden, prothrombin G20210A and methylenetetrahydrofolate reductase C677T mutations and events of the arterial circulatory system: a meta-analysis of published studies. *Am Heart J* 2003;146:948–957.

King DJ, Kelton JG. Heparin-associated thrombocytopenia. *Ann Intern Med* 1984;100: 535–540.

Kyrle PA, Minar E, Hirschl M, et al. High plasma levels of factor VIII and the risk of recurrent venous thromboembolism. *N Engl J Med* 2000;343:457–462.

Lensing AW, et al. *Lancet* 1999;353:479–485.

Martinelli I, Mannucci PM, De Stefano V, et al. Different risks of thrombosis in four coagulation defects associated with inherited thrombophilia: a study of 150 families. *Blood* 1998;92:2353–2358.

Matsuda T, Ogawara M, Kodama M, et al. Changes of antithrombin (antithrombin III, a-macroglobulin) in various diseases. *Acta Haematol Jpn* 1977;40:261–266.

O'Brien JR. Antithrombin III and heparin clotting times in thrombosis and atherosclerosis. *Thromb Diath Haemorrh* 1974;32:116–123.

Öhlin A, Marlar RA. Mutations in the thrombomodulin gene associated with thromboembolic disease. *Thromb Haemost* 1997;78:1164–1166.

Poort SR, Rosendaal FR, Reitsma PH, et al. A common genetic variation in the 3-untrauslated region of the prothrombin gene is associated with elevated plasma prothrombin levels and an increase in venous thrombosis. *Blood* 1996;88:3698–3703.

Price DT, Ridker PM. Factor V Leiden mutation and the risks for thromboembolic disease: a clinical perspective. *Ann Intern Med* 1997;127:895–903.

Ridker PM, Cushman M, Stampfer MJ, et al. Inflammation, aspirin, and the risk of cardiovascular disease in apparently healthy men. *N Engl J Med* 1997;336:973–979.

Rosendaal FR, Van Hylckama Vlieg A, Tanis BC, Helmerhorst FM. Estrogens, progestogens and thrombosis. *J Thromb Haemost* 2003;1:1371–1380.

Schernthaner G, Ludwig H, Siberbauer K. Elevated plasma β–thromboglobulin levels in multiple myeloma in polycythemia vera. *Acta Haematol (Basel)* 1970;62:211–222.

Schwarz HP, Schernthaner G, Griffin JH. Decreased plasma levels of protein S in well-controlled type I diabetes mellitus. *Thromb Haemost* 1987;57:240

Spencer FA, Becker RC. The New Cardiology Management Guide. Online Education Resource for Practicing Cardiologists. Edward Arnold Publishers, 1999.

Trousseau A. Phlegmasia alba dolens Clinique medical de l'Hotel de Paris. *The New Sydenham Society,* London, England 1865;3:94.

Vigano-D'Angelo S, D'Angelo A, Kaufman J, et al. Protein S deficiency occurs in the nephrotic syndrome. *Ann Intern Med* 1987;107:42–47.

Walker FJ. Regulation of activation protein C by a new protein. A possible function for bovine protein S. *J Biol Chem* 1980;255:5521–5524.

Weick JK. Intravascular coagulation in cancer. *Semin Oncol* 1978;5:203–211.

Winter JH, Fenech A, Ridley W, et al. Familial antithrombin III deficiency. *Q J Med* 1982;51:373–395.

Part VII
Monitoring Antithrombotic Therapy

Platelet Antagonists

25

Platelet antagonists play an important role in both primary and secondary prevention of atherothrombotic events. Despite their proven benefit, individual response (and protection) varies considerably, emphasizing the importance of developing monitoring tools (tested prospectively in clinical trials) that can better determine the degree of platelet inhibition that is both safe and effective.

Determining Hemostatic Potential

Platelet function studies were developed originally for the evaluation of patients with unexplained bleeding and have contributed greatly to the understanding, diagnosis, and management of hereditary abnormalities such as von Willebrand disease and Glanzmann's thrombasthenia (platelet glycoprotein [GP] IIb/IIIa receptor deficiency). Although conventional platelet function studies (turbidimetric aggregometry) have technical limitations that preclude their routine use for gauging antithrombotic therapy, they may provide guidance when hemorrhagic complications arise and in determining pretreatment risk in individuals suspected of having an intrinsic platelet abnormality.

Bleeding Time

The bleeding time, considered an indicator of primary hemostasis (platelet plug formation), is defined as the time between making a small standardized skin incision and the precise moment when bleeding stops. The test is performed with a template, through which the medial surface of the forearm is incised under 40 mmHg standard pressure. A normal bleeding time is between 6 and 10 minutes. Although considered a "standardized" test of platelet function, the bleeding time can be influenced by a variety of factors, including platelet count, qualitative abnormalities, and features intrinsic to the blood vessel wall (George and Shattil, 1991).

Platelet Adhesion Tests

Platelet adhesion is the initiating step in primary hemostasis. Although platelet binding is an important component of this process, there are many others, including blood flow rate, endothelial cell function, adhesive proteins, and the subendothelial matrix. The original test used for assessing adhesion, platelet retention, was based on adherence to glass bead columns.

Platelet Aggregometry

The current laboratory evaluation of platelet function is based predominantly on *turbidimetric platelet aggregometry* (also known as light transmission aggregometry). This test is performed by preparing platelet-rich plasma (with platelet-poor plasma as a control) and eliciting an aggregation response with adenosine diphosphate, epinephrine, collagen, arachidonic acid, and ristocetin (Born, 1962).

Impedance platelet aggregometry (Cardinal and Flower, 1980) was introduced as an alternative to turbidimetric methods, with the potential physiologic advantage of using whole blood samples. The reproducibility of platelet aggregometry is influenced by a variety of factors, which include:

- Concentration of sodium citrate in the collecting tubes
- Adjustment of the platelet count
- Storage time
- Stirring rate
- Temperature
- pH of the blood sample

Hereditary Congenital Abnormalities Affecting Platelet Function

Abnormal platelet function (qualitative defect) is capable of causing clinical hemorrhage that, at times, can be life-threatening. The common inherited platelet disorders for which in vitro testing may be diagnostic are summarized in Table 25.1.

Acquired Platelet Defects

Quantitative or, more commonly, qualitative platelet abnormalities are encountered frequently in clinical practice and in most cases represent a desired effect from drug therapy (Figure 25.1). A variety of systemic disorders can also influence platelet function (Table 25.2).

Table 25.1 Inherited Platelet Disorders

Disease	Genetic Transmission	Specific Deficiency	Defect/Effect	Diagnosis
Glanzmann's thrombasthenia	Autosomal recessive	GPIIb/IIIa	Inability to bind fibrinogen and thus form platelet-to-platelet bridges	BT prolonged; abnormal aggregation response with all agonists; normal aggregation with ristocetin
Storage pool disease	Autosomal recessive and dominant	Storage and release of platelet granules	Important proteins for activation and aggregation inaccessible	Impaired aggregation response to various agonists
Bernard Soulier disease	Autosomal recessive	GPIb/IX	Missing ligand for vWf leads to inability of platelets to bind to subendothelium	BT may exceed 20 min; thrombocytopenia; abnormal aggregation response with ristocetin
von Willebrand disease				
Type I	Autosomal dominant	vWf–factor VIII	—	Reduced vWf antigen
Type IIa	Autosomal dominant	Qualitative defect in vWF	Decreased adhesion	Decreased response to RIPA; decreased ristocetin cofactor activity
Type IIb	Autosomal dominant	Increased affinity of vWf for GPIb/IX receptor	Decreased adhesion	Reduced vWf; high-molecular-weight multimers
Type III	Autosomal dominant	Very low or absent vWf	Decreased adhesion	Reduced vWf; high-molecular-weight multimers; increased RIPA at low levels*
Platelet type or pseudo vWd	Autosomal dominant	vWf receptor	Enhanced avidity for vWf leads to platelet consumption and low plasma vWf	Similar to type I; severe bleeding common
				RIPA with patient's platelets and normal plasma reproduce the defect; this differentiates from type IIb vWd

* Aggregation in response to very low concentrations of ristocetin (<0.6 mg/mL).
BT, bleeding time; GP, glycoprotein; RIPA, ristocetin-induced platelet aggregation; vWd, von Willebrand disease; vWf, von Willebrand factor.

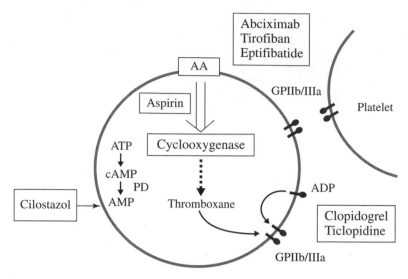

Figure 25.1 The available platelet antagonists "target" specific receptors and/or biologic events rendering the platelet "unfit" for participation in thrombus formation. AA, arachidonic acid; ADP, adenosine diphosphate; AMP, adenosine monophosphate; ATP, adenosine triphosphate; cAMP, cyclic adenosine monophosphate; GP, glycoprotein; PD, phosphodiesterase.

Flow Cytometry

Although not routinely available, flow cytometry offers a wide range of diagnostic capabilities for determining hemostatic potential and response to platelet-inhibiting therapies. Whole blood samples are used and must be processed rapidly to maintain the "physiologic" environment (Becker et al., 1994).

Bedside Assays and Instruments

Bedside assays, near-patient testing, and point-of-care monitoring instruments are attractive for several reasons. First, they provide a rapid, reliable, and reproducible means to assess hemostatic potential and treatment response. Second, the techniques involved require minimal training, reagent handling, calibration, and physical space. Third, emerging technology will likely offer a full complement of coagulation and platelet tests that can be used for management in the home, ambulatory clinic, emergency department, angioplasty suite, coronary care unit, and operating room (Becker, 1995).

Table 25.2 Acquired Platelet Disorders

Drugs
    Aspirin
    Ticlopidine
    Clopidogrel
    Cilostazol
    Glycoprotein IIb/IIIa antagonists (abciximab, tirofiban, eptifibatide)
Systemic Disorders and Disease States
    Chronic renal failure
    Myeloproliferative disorders
    Paraproteinemias
    Cardiopulmonary bypass
    Hemodialysis
    Disseminated intravascular coagulation

Platelet Function Analyzer-100

The platelet function analyzer (PFA)-100 simulates primary hemostasis under high shear stress conditions. Citrated whole blood is drawn by capillary action through a membrane coated with either collagen and epinephrine or collagen and adenosine diphosphate (ADP) (Mammen et al., 1998). An aperture in the membrane occludes following platelet adhesion and aggregation and the test results are recorded as closure time.

The assay is most useful in detecting primary hemostasis abnormalities (primary platelet function disorders and von Willebrand disease) and determining response to replacement therapy (Jennings and White, 1998).

Clot Retraction Assay

The strength of clot retraction can serve as a measure of platelet function (Greilich et al., 1995) and a hemostasis analyzer has been developed for this purpose. Citrated whole blood or platelet-rich plasma is placed in a sample chamber where calcium and thrombin are added to stimulate clot formation. As platelets bind, undergo cellular contraction, and polymerize with fibrin strands, the force developed by the platelets is measured by a probe transducer that produces an electrical output (a voltage signal converted to force reported in dynes) proportional to the amount of force generated.

The clot retraction assay provides information on the functional contribution of platelets to clot formation, and can use whole blood or plasma obtained from standard citrated blood collection tubes. Potential uses include the evaluation of hemostatic defects in uremia and following bypass surgery.

Rapid Platelet Function Assay

The rapid platelet function assay is a semi-automated turbidimetric system that is based on the ability of activated platelets to interact with fibrinogen, yielding macroscopically visible agglutination.

Fibrinogen-coated polystyrene beads, buffers, and a modified thrombin receptor–activating peptide (iso-TRAP) are incorporated into a disposable cartridge and exposed to samples of citrated whole blood. The instrument detects agglutination between quantitative digital displays. Because agglutination is proportional to the number of unblocked (unoccupied) GPIIb/IIIa receptors, this device is well suited for determining platelet inhibitory response to currently available GPIIb/IIIa receptor antagonists (Coller et al., 1991). The time required to obtain results is 2 minutes.

The semiautomated system is easy to use and correlates closely with traditional measurements of platelet function, turbidimetric platelet aggregation ($r^2 = 0.95$), and the percentage of free GPIIb/IIIa molecules ($r^2 = .96$) (Smith et al., 1999). The use of whole blood and duplicate analysis eliminates variables in sample preparation and minimizes the random errors. Results can be reported as an absolute rate of aggregation or as a percentage of baseline aggregation.

A rapid bedside assay that provides a reliable measurement of GPIIb/IIIa receptor blockage offers a broad range of medical, interventional, and surgical applications. Dose titration with intravenous agents could be performed, achieving a safe and effective degree of platelet inhibition (Kereiakes et al., 1999).

Figure 25.2 The occurrence of major adverse cardiac events (MACEs), death, myocardial infarction, and urgent target vessel revascularization, correlated with the intensity of platelet inhibition 10 minutes after initiation of glycoprotein (GP) IIb/IIIa antagonist therapy. (From Steinhubl SR, Talley JD, Braden GA, et al. Point-of-care measured platelet inhibition correlates with a reduced risk of an adverse cardiac event after percutaneous coronary intervention: results of the GOLD (AU-Assessing Ultegra) multicenter study. *Circulation* 2001;103:2572–2578.)

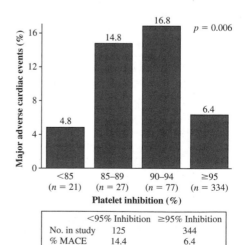

	<95% Inhibition	≥95% Inhibition
No. in study	125	344
% MACE	14.4	6.4

The intensity or level of platelet inhibition (achieved with GPIIb/IIIa antagonist therapy) required to prevent thrombotic complications following percutaneous coronary intervention (PCI) was determined in 485 patients participating in the GOLD (Au-Assessing Ultegra Multicenter) study (Steinhubl et al., 2001). One-quarter of all patients did not achieve greater than or equal to 95% inhibition (rapid platelet function assay) 10 minutes after the initiation of treatment and experienced a significant higher incidence of death, myocardial infarction (MI), or urgent target vessel revascularization (14.4% vs. 6.4%). Those with less than 70% inhibition at 8 hours were also at increased risk (25% vs. 8.1%) (Figures 25.2 and 25.3).

A reliable and readily available means to assess inhibitory response to GPIIb/IIIa receptor antagonists may also provide guidance for dose titration in patients at risk for bleeding complications, including those with thrombocytopenia, prior hemorrhagic events, and known coagulopathies (Table 25.3) (Mukherjee et al., 2001).

Summary

The recognized role of platelets as the initiating step in arterial thrombosis provides a strong basis for their targeted inhibition in the primary and secondary prevention of cardiovascular events. Traditionally, the assessment of platelet activity has been viewed as a diagnostic tool for evaluating patients with hemorrhage; however,

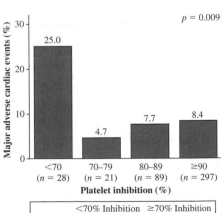

Figure 25.3 In the GOLD study, major adverse cardiac events (MACEs) correlated with the intensity of platelet inhibition 8 hours after initiation of treatment. GP, glycoprotein. (From Steinhubl SR, Ialley JD, Braden GA, et al. Point-of-care measured platelet inhibition correlates with a reduced risk of an adverse cardiac event after percutaneous coronary intervention: results of the GOLD (AU-Assessing Ultegra) multicenter study. *Circulation* 2001;103:2572–2578.)

Table 25.3 Clinical Settings in Which Platelet Monitoring Might Be Useful

Patient-Related (confirm target inhibition)
  Prior to percutaneous coronary intervention
  Patients with refractory ischemia or recurrent symptoms despite receiving
    glycoprotein (GP) IIb/IIIa receptor antagonist therapy
  Interruption of infusion
  Thrombocytopenia
  Qualitative platelet abnormality
  Renal insufficiency
  Low or high body weight
Clinically Related
  Bleeding
    Confirm intensity of inhibition
    Confirm reversal of inhibition following replacement therapy
  Emergent surgery
    Guidance to reverse platelet inhibition (if clinically necessary)
  Transition from one GPIIb/IIIa receptor antagonist to another

more readily available technology that permits rapid assessment of platelet performance stands to create opportunities for management decisions in prothrombotic settings as well.

References

Becker RC. Exploring the medical need for alternate site testing. A clinician's perspective. *Arch Pathol Lab Med* 1995;119:894–897.

Becker RC, Tracy RP, Bovill EG, Mann KG, Ault K for the TIMI-III Thrombosis and Anticoagulation Study Group. The clinical use of flow cytometry for assessing platelet
activation in acute coronary syndromes. *Coronary Artery Dis* 1994;5:339–345.

Born GVR. Qualitative investigations into the aggregation of blood platelets. *J Physiol
(London)* 1962;27:162.

Cardinal DC, Flower RJ. The electronic aggregometer: a novel device for assessing
platelet behavior in blood. *J Pharmacol Methods* 1980;3:135–158.

Coller BS, Scudder LE, Beer J, et al. Monoclonal antibodies to platelet glycoprotein
IIb/IIIa as antithrombotic agents. *Ann NY Acad Sci* 1991;614:193–213.

George JN, Shattil SJ. The clinical importance of acquired abnormalities of platelet function. *N Engl J Med* 1991;324:27–39.

Greilich PE, Carr ME, Carr SL, Chang AS. Reductions in platelet force development by
cardiopulmonary bypass are associated with hemorrhage. *Anesth Analg* 1995;80:
459–465.

Jennings LK, White MM. Expression of ligand induced binding sites on glycoprotein IIb/IIIa complexes and the effect of various inhibitors. *Am Heart J* 1998;135: S179–S183.

Kereiakes DJ, Mueller M, Howard W, et al. Efficacy of abciximab induced platelet blockade using a rapid point of care assay. *J Thromb Thrombolysis* 1999;7:265–276.

Mammen EF, Comp PC, Gosselin R, et al. PFA-100 system: a new method for assessment of platelet dysfunction. *Semin Thromb Hemost* 1988;24:195–202.

Mukherjee D, Chew DP, Robbins M, et al. Clinical application of procedural platelet monitoring during percutaneous coronary intervention among patients at increased bleeding risk. *J Thromb Thrombolysis* 2001;11:151–154.

Smith JW, Steinhubl SR, Lincoff AM, et al. Rapid platelet-function assay: an automated and quantitative cartridge-based method. *Circulation* 1999;99:620–625.

Steinhubl SR, Talley JD, Braden GA, et al. Point-of-care measured platelet inhibition correlates with a reduced risk of an adverse cardiac event after percutaneous coronary intervention: results of the GOLD (AU-Assessing Ultegra) multicenter study. *Circulation* 2001;103:2572–2578.

Anticoagulants

26

Because of the narrow therapeutic index of warfarin and unfractionated heparin (UFH), monitoring their anticoagulant effects is required. On the other hand, low-molecular-weight heparin (LMWH) and fibrinolytic agents need to be monitored only under certain circumstances. Although newer anticoagulants will not require routine monitoring for dose titration, a means to determine their systemic effects and individual (patient-specific) response to administration will likely have roles in clinical practice.

Vitamin K Antagonists

The prothrombin time is used to monitor vitamin K antagonist therapy. This test is sensitive to the plasma concentrations (activity) of clotting factors II (prothrombin), V, VII, and X. Vitamin K antagonists affect the vitamin K–dependent factors II, VII, IX, and X, as well as proteins C, S, and Z. Thus, the prothrombin time does not reflect the effect of vitamin K antagonists on some factors (IX and proteins C, S, and Z) and is sensitive to others (factor V) (not directly influenced by treatment). The prothrombin time is not an ideal test for monitoring vitamin K antagonists; however, its simplicity and widespread availability have established its place in clinical practice.

By convention, prothrombin times are now reported as international normalized ratios (INRs). This is the ratio of the patient's prothrombin time to a control prothrombin time, raised to a power—the international sensitivity index (ISI). The latter reflects the calibration of the thromboplastin used for the prothrombin time testing to an internationally agreed upon standard. In many laboratories the reagent currently used is a recombinant thromboplastin, which has an ISI of 1.0

There are several cautions related to interpreting the results of prothrombin time tests that are worth monitoring. Since the test is sensitive to the level of factor V in the plasma, improper sample storage or delayed testing may cause loss of factor V (activity) and yield prothrombin time values above the expected range. High concentrations of heparin may also prolong the prothrombin time; this usually occurs when the sample is obtained within a few minutes of administering a bolus dose. Direct thrombin inhibitors, such as hirudin, bivalirudin, argatroban, and ximelagatran, may also prolong the prothrombin time to a variable degree. Some thromboplastins are sensitive to lupus anticoagulants; prolonged prothrombin times reported under these circumstances may deceive the clinician into thinking that the patient is adequately anticoagulated. In patients known to have a lupus anticoagulant, prothrombin times should be performed with an insensitive thromboplastin. An anti-Xa assay can also be used to gauge anticoagulant response to vitamin K antagonist treatment.

Unfractionated Heparin

Unfractionated heparin is monitored with the activated partial thromboplastin time (aPTT) test. In contrast to the prothrombin time, there is no generally agreed upon standardization for the aPTT. Different laboratories use reagents with varying sensitivities to the effects of UFH. As a result, aPTT values correspond to different heparin concentrations depending on the instrument and assay employed. The activated clotting time (ACT) is used for heparin-response monitoring in the angioplasty suite and operating room. The thrombin time is also prolonged by UFH. The reptilase time is not influenced by UFH.

Low-molecular-weight heparin does not require laboratory monitoring in clinically stable patients, whether given for prophylaxis or treatment (Laposata et al., 1998). Monitoring is recommended in the following situations:

- Pediatric patients and in those who weigh less than 50 kg
- Pregnant patients
- Patients with renal failure (creatinine clearance <40 mL/min)
- Patients at high risk for bleeding
- Patients with major hemorrhagic events (particularly if neutralization or replacement therapy is administered)
- Patients with interrupted therapy or overdosing

The usual test selected for monitoring is the chromogenic anti-factor Xa (anti-Xa) assay, obtained 4 hours after a dose of LMWH.

In the ELECT (Evaluating Enoxaparin Clotting Time) study, 445 patients who had received IV or SC enoxaparin underwent elective percutaneous coronary intervention (PCI). Coagulation monitoring was undertaken with a point-of-care clotting time instrument that correlates with enoxaparin plasma concentration (enoxaparin clotting time). There was no association between enoxaparin times and ischemic events; however, the lowest overall event rates were observed with enoxaparin time between 250 and 450 seconds (compared to times outside this range). An elevated ENOX time was associated with bleeding at the time of sheath removal (1% increase for each 30-second rise) (Moliterno et al., 2003).

It is important to be aware that LMWH preparations with relatively low anti-Xa and anti-IIa properties (e.g., dalteparin) will prolong the ACT to a modest degree.

Table 26.1 Coagulation Tests for Direct Thrombin Inhibitors

Agent	Test	Therapeutic Range	Dose Adjustment
Lepirudin	aPTT at 4 h*	1.5–2.5[†] (not to exceed 90s)	Renal failure
Bivalirudin	ACT at 15 min	300–350[†]	Renal failure
Argatroban	aPTT at 2 h	1.5–3.0[††] (not to exceed 100s)	Liver failure

*Ecarin clotting time at 15-minute intervals for cardiopulmonary bypass.
[†]During percutaneous coronary intervention.
[††]Above mean normal control.
ACT, activated clotting time; aPTT, activated partial thromboplastin time.

Direct Thrombin Inhibitors

Monitoring is required when the currently available intravenous direct thrombin inhibitors (lepirudin, bivalirudin, and argatroban) are administered. Table 26.1 summarizes the tests that are used, the therapeutic range needed, and the conditions requiring dose adjustments for each agent. When lepirudin is used for cardiopulmonary bypass, the ecarin clotting time, titrated to the lepirudin plasma level, appears to be the most reliable monitoring assay (Poetzsch and Madlener, 2000). The adaptation of whole blood thrombin generation tests to point-of-care technology may have a role in the monitoring of anticoagulant therapy, but further investigation must be undertaken.

References

Laposata M, Green D, Van Cott EM, Barrowcliffe TW, Godnight SH, Sosolik RC. The clinical use and laboratory monitoring of low-molecular-weight heparin, danaparoid, hirudin and related compounds, and argatroban. *Arch Pathol Lab Med* 1998;122: 799–807.

Moliterno DJ, Hermiller JB, Keriakas DJ, et al. A novel point-of-care enoxaparin monitor for use during PCI. Results of Evaluating Enoxaparin Clotting Time (ELECT) study. *J Am Coll Cardiol* 2003;42:1132–1139.

Poetzsch B, Madlener K. Management of cardiopulmonary bypass anticoagulation in patients with heparin-induced thrombocytopenia. In: Warkentin TE, Greinacher A, eds. *Heparin-induced thrombocytopenia*. New York: Marcel Dekker: 2000;355–369.

Anticoagulation Clinics and Self-Testing

27

Oral anticoagulation is a time-tested and effective therapy for patients at risk for thromboembolism (Ansell, 1993). Because of the high risk–benefit ratio of oral vitamin K antagonists, physicians are sometimes reluctant to initiate therapy even for well-established indications (Kutner et al., 1991; McCrory et al., 1995). Furthermore, management is recognized as labor intensive. These factors can be minimized and the benefits of treatment maximized by implementation of an expert model of management that can be achieved with a coordinated and focused system of care known as a coordinated anticoagulation clinic (Ansell and Hughes, 1996). Patient self-testing (and management) may also foster more wide-scale and effective treatment of thromboembolic disorders.

Anticoagulation Clinics

The concept of a coordinated anticoagulation clinic (ACC) is not new. Programs focusing on the management of oral anticoagulation have existed in the United States since the late 1950s, and several Scandinavian and other European countries are well known for their coordinated programs (Loeliger et al., 1984), some of which oversee the care of all anticoagulated patients in their respective countries. In the United States, ACCs are growing in number and diversity of services, spurred on by increasing evidence of improved clinical outcomes and cost-effectiveness. The basic elements of a coordinated ACC include (1) a manager or team leader (physician, pharmacist), (2) support staff (nurse practitioner, pharmacist, or physician assistant), (3) standardized record keeping and a computerized database, (4) a manual of operation and practice guidelines, and (5) a formal mechanism for communicating with referring physicians and patients.

Development of Coordinated Care Program

Currently, most oral anticoagulation therapy in the United States is managed by a patient's personal physician. In essence, the monitoring and dose titration of patients with thromboembolic disease represents a relatively small proportion of the physician's overall clinical practice. This approach can be characterized as "traditional" or routine medical care. There may be no specialized system or guidelines in place to track patients or ensure their regular follow-up. An ACC uses a focused

333

and coordinated approach to managing anticoagulation (Ansell et al., 1997). What constitutes an ACC may vary depending on the individuals involved and the health care system or practice setting, but in most cases it is a specialized program of patient management focused predominantly, if not exclusively, on the management of anticoagulation. The program is often directed by a single physician (or pharmacist) who assumes no major responsibility for the primary care of the patients being managed. The actual management is usually conducted by registered nurses, nurse practitioners, pharmacists, or physician assistants. At a minimum, the goals of an ACC are to coordinate and optimize anticoagulation by doing the following:

- Helping to determine the appropriateness of care
- Managing anticoagulation dosing and treatment decisions
- Providing systematic monitoring and patient evaluation
- Providing ongoing education
- Communicating with other providers involved in the patient's care

Clinical Outcomes with Coordinated Care Program

There are several studies assessing clinical outcome when oral anticoagulation is managed under a model of routine medical care as defined previously (Gitter et al., 1995; Landefeld and Goldman, 1989; Petitti et al., 1986) (Table 27.1). Although the information is limited, the available data suggest that a rate of major hemorrhage of 7% to 8% per patient year of therapy is expected. There is a similar rate of thromboembolism in these patients for an overall serious adverse event rate of 15% to 20% per patient year of therapy. Many studies indicate that the high adverse event rates are a direct consequence of poor therapeutic control, with hemorrhage or thrombosis occurring as a consequence of excessive and subtherapeutic anticoagulation, respectively.

The observed outcomes from routine medical care can be contrasted to the rates identified in a large number of retrospective and some prospective studies of outcomes with an ACC (Bussey et al., 1989; Conte et al., 1986; Errichetti et al., 1984; Kornblit et al., 1990; Palareti et al., 1996) (Table 27.2). Although the studies performed to date are observational in design, they suggest a 50% reduction for both major hemorrhagic and thrombotic events.

A summary of studies examining management strategies in which coordinated care was measured against a control group of routine medical care (Bussey et al., 1996; Cohen et al., 1985; Cortelazzo et al., 1993; Garabedian-Ruffalo et al., 1985; Hamilton et al., 1985; Wilt et al., 1995) is presented in Table 27.3. These predominantly nonrandomized, retrospective analyses have assessed the care provided to patients before and after enrollment in an ACC; despite methodologic limitations, they do provide evidence for benefit in favor of coordinated care.

Table 27.1 Frequency of Thromboembolism and Hemorrhage with Routine Anticoagulation Management

Study	Patients (No.)	Patient Years	Target PTR/INR	Major Hemorrhage	Minor Hemorrhage	Fatal Events[a]	Thromboembolism[b]
Petitti et al. (1986)	2,442	NA	NA	18.0	NA	NA	NA
Landefeld and Goldman (1989)	565	876	NA	7.4	7.4	10	NA
Gitter et al. (1995)	261	221	NA	8.1	14.5	1	8.1

[a]Fatal events expressed as individual events.
[b]Results expressed as percent per patient year of therapy.
INR, international normalized ratio; NA, not available or not applicable; PTR, prothrombin time ratio.

Table 27.2 Frequency of Thromboembolism and Hemorrhage with Anticoagulation Service Management

Study[a]	Patients (No.)	Patients Years	Target PTR/INR	Major Hemorrhage	Minor Hemorrhage	Fatal Events[b]	Thromboembolism[c]
Davis et al. (1977)	263	254	1.5–3.0	4.3	4.3	0	NA
Fofar (1982)	541	1,362	1.8–2.6	4.2	NA	2	NA
Errichetti et al. (1984)	144[d]	105	1.3–2.0	6.6	24.7	NA	NA
Conte et al. (1986)	141[d]	153	NA	2.6	58.0	NA	8.4
Petty (1988)	321[d]	385	NA	7.3	NA	3	NA
Charney et al. (1988)	73	77	1.5–2.5	0	42.0	0	5.0
Bussey et al. (1989)	82	199	NA	2.0	15.5	NA	3.5
Kornbilt et al. (1990)	177	148[e]	NA	5.4	30.5	1	NA
Seabrook et al. (1990)	9.3	158	1.5–2.0	3.8	6.9	0	4.4[f]
Fihn et al. (1993)	1,103[d]	1,950	1.3–1.8	13.4	54.9	4	7.5
Van der Meer et al. (1993)	6,814	6,085	2.4–5.3 (INR)	3.3	13.8	39	NA
Cannegieter et al. (1995)	1608 (INR)	6,475	2.0–4.9	2.5	NA	22	0.7
Palareti et al. (1996)	2,745	2,011	2.0–4.5 (INR)	1.4	6.2	5	NA
TOTAL	**14,105**	**19,362**		**4.4** **(0–13.4)**	**25.7** **(4.3–50.0)**		**4.8** **(0.7–8.4)**

[a]Mixed indications for anticoagulation (i.e., venous and arterial disease), except the study by Cannegieter et al. (1995), which included prosthetic heart valves only.
[b]Fatal events expressed as individual events.
[c]Results expressed as percent per patient years of therapy.
[d]Courses of therapy listed rather than number of patients.
[e]Patient years of therapy not provided, but calculated from average duration of follow-up.
[f]Arterial events only.
INR, international normalized ratio; NA, not available or not applicable; PTR, prothrombin time ratio.

Table 27.3 Frequency of Thromboembolism and Hemorrhage with Routine Medical Care vs. Anticoagulation

Study[a]	Type of Care	Patients (No.)	Patient Years	Target PTR/INR	Major Hemorrhage	Minor Hemorrhage	Fatal Events[b]	Thromboembolism[c]
Hamilton et al. (1985)	RMC	49	73.25	NA	6.8	21.0	NA	8.0
	ACC	41	91.75	6.5	23.0	8.0	0	NA
Cohen et al. (1985)	RMC	17	NA	1.5–2.5	9.0[d]	NA	0	
	ACC	18			6.9[d]			6.2
Garabedian	RMC	26	64.3	1.5–2.5	12.4	NA	NA	
Ruffalo et al. (1985)	ACC	26	41.9	2.4	0			
Cortelazzo et al. (1993)	RMC	271	677	3.0–4.5	4.7	NA	0	6.6
	ACC	271	669		0.1		0	0.6
Wilt et al. (1995)	RMC	NA	34.97	NA	28.6	14.3	NA	48.6
	ACC		80.38		0	13.7		0
Bussey et al. (1996)	RMC	117	92	NA	4.3	NA	NA	11.7
	ACC	146	110		0.9			3.6
TOTAL	**RMC**	**480+**	**941.52+**		**10.9 (4.3–26.8)**	**17.6 (14.3–21.0)**		**16.2 (6.2–48.6)**
	ACC	**562+**	**993.03+**		**2.8 (0–6.9)**	**18.3 (13.7–23.0)**		**2.4 (0–8.0)**

[a]Mixed indications for anticoagulation (i.e., venous and arterial disease) except the studies by Hamilton et al. (1985) and Cortelazzo et al. (1993), which included prosthetic heart valves only.

[b]Fatal events expressed as individual events.

[c]Results expressed as percent per patient years of therapy.

[d]Combined major and minor hemorrhage.

ACC, anticoagulation clinic; INR, international normalized ratio; NA, not available or not applicable; PTR, prothrombin time ratio; RMC, routine medical care.

337

Cost-Effectiveness

The favorable cost-effectiveness profile of ACC is derived from a reduction in adverse clinical events and reduced use of hospital services (Table 27.4). Gray and colleagues (1985) estimated a benefit–cost ratio of 6.5, or a savings of $860 per patient year of therapy due to a reduction in hospital days per patient year. Wilt and colleagues (1995), in a relatively small study, identified an extraordinary cost savings in favor of ACC's reduction in hospital or emergency room visits. Bussey and colleagues (1996) reported their estimates of cost savings through a coordinated approach compared to routine care with 11 vs. 34 hospital or emergency room visits for complications (either excessive or inadequate), respectively, resulting in approximately $1,000 saved per patient year of therapy. Lee and Schommer (1996) also found a reduction in hospital admissions with coordinated care, but did not estimate the dollars saved.

The savings from an ACC can also be estimated by comparing the rates of major bleeding and thromboembolism as presented in Table 27.3. If one excludes the report by Wilt and colleagues (1995), which had disproportionately high complication rates, the reduction of major bleeding is roughly five events per 100 patient years by coordinated care. Eckman and colleagues (1995) estimated the inpatient cost of major hemorrhage as being between $3,000 and 12,000, depending on outcome. Thus, using a median value of $7,500, the annual savings achieved by preventing five major events would be $33,750 for 100 patients, or $337 per patient year. Similarly, the decreased incidence of thromboembolism achieved by coordinated care is approximately five events per 100 patient years. Eckman and colleagues estimated the inpatient hospital cost of a thromboembolism between $5,000 and $18,000, depending on outcome. Therefore, using a median cost of $11,500, the data would indicate an annual savings of $57,500 per 100 patient years, or $575 per patient year. Based on these assumptions, neither of which take

Table 27.4 Cost Savings Due to Reduced Hospital and Emergency Department Use Achieved by Anticoagulation Clinic Management[a]

Gray et al. (1985)	0.48 vs. 3.22 hospital days per patient year
	$860/patient year of therapy
Wilt et al. (1995)	0 vs. 21 hospital or ED visits
	$4,072/patient year of therapy
Bussey et al. (1996)	11 vs. 34 hospital or ED visits
	~ $1,000/patient year of therapy
Lee et al. (1996)	3 vs. 15 hospital admissions
	$ savings not determined

[a]*Rates for coordinated care vs. routine medical care.*
ED, emergency department.

into account the long-term morbidity or costs of complications, the combined savings of coordinated care by lowering the incidence of both major bleeding and thromboembolism is approximately $912 per patient year. Therefore, the available data indicate that coordinated care will not only reduce the incidence of adverse outcomes, but will also reduce health care costs.

Patient Self-Testing and Patient Self-Management

Portability of instrumentation means that prothrombin time measurements are no longer confined to the physician's office, a private laboratory, or a nearby hospital, but can be moved into the patient's home or even taken with the patient when traveling. Standardization of reagents and instruments as well as reliance on the international normalized ratio (INR) reduce the inaccuracies of multiple reagents and laboratories, and the simplicity of the actual procedure creates the possibility of patient self-testing (or in selected cases, self-management).

Since the late 1980s, a number of instruments have been developed (Leaning and Ansell, 1996). In general, these instruments are based on a clot detection methodology that uses thromboplastin to initiate clot formation, but the endpoint of clot detection varies from instrument to instrument.

Patient Self-Testing

Patient self-testing represents a logical step in the application of point-of-care technology. A number of studies have demonstrated the ability of patients to perform self-testing and obtain an accurate result (Ansell et al., 1989). White and colleagues (1989) showed the potential value of having patients perform their own monitoring following discharge. In the randomized study, 23 patients instructed in the use of a fingerstick sampling method and a portable coagulation monitor were discharged and asked to perform their own testing, reporting the results to their physicians for dose adjustments. Compared to a standard treatment group, patients self-testing spent a greater percentage of time within the therapeutic range (93% vs. 75%; $p = .003$) and were less likely to be in a subtherapeutic range during the follow-up period (63% vs. 23%; $p < .001$). There were no significant differences in other parameters studied, including above target range prothrombin times and hemorrhagic or thromboembolic complications.

Anderson and colleagues (1993) confirmed the feasibility of patient self-testing in 40 patients over a period of 6 to 24 months and demonstrated a high degree of patient satisfaction as well. In a relatively large study, Byeth and Landefeld (1997) followed 325 elderly patients, 163 of whom were managed by a single investigator based on INR results from home self-testing, and compared outcomes with 162 patients managed by their private physicians. Over a 6-month period, the investigators recorded a rate of major hemorrhage of 12% in the latter group and 5.7% in the self-testing group. This finding was based on an intention-to-treat analysis; for those actually performing self-testing, there was only a 1.2% incidence of major hemorrhage.

Home coagulation monitoring, in essence, is analogous to home glucose monitoring, which raises the possibility of self-management as patients with diabetes have done for years. Although coagulation monitoring is not as intense as glucose monitoring for insulin therapy, relatively frequent assessment of its biologic effect and regular dose adjustments are still required. The concept of self-management is not new. In a study by Erdman and colleagues (1974), a protocol for patient self-adjustment of warfarin dosing based on physician-derived guidelines was tested. The prothrombin times were obtained on plasma samples by routine laboratory instrumentation. Overall, there was a greater proportion of patients within the target range of anticoagulation (98% of 195 patients enrolled) compared with a retrospective survey of patients managed in a routine fashion (71% success rate). Patients performing self-management experienced two hemorrhagic and two thromboembolic events during the observation period. Using a similar protocol, Schachner and colleagues (1992) compared self-management patients ($n = 59$) and standard-care patients ($n = 61$). The self-management group experienced four episodes of thromboembolism, compared to 24 episodes in the standard-care group ($p < .0005$). Similarly, the self-management group experienced fewer total hemorrhagic events (5.7% per patient year) compared to the standard-care group (7.5% per patient year; $p < .05$). Ansell and colleagues (1995) updated the results of an earlier pilot study of patient self-testing and self-management using point-of-care methodology in 20 patients followed for 7 years. Patients ranged from 7 to 87 years of age, had a wide variety of indications for anticoagulation-performed home testing, and adjusted their warfarin doses according to specified guidelines. The study group was compared to matched controls managed by an established anticoagulation service. Self-managed patients were found to be in the predetermined target range for 88.6% of prothrombin time determinations vs. 68% of prothrombin time determinations in the controls ($p < .001$). In addition, fewer dose changes were required by study patients than by controls (10.7% vs. 28.2%; $p < .001$). Complication rates did not differ between the groups and study patients were satisfied with this mode of therapy (based on their responses to a survey questionnaire).

Bernardo (1996) published the experience from her work in Germany, where patient self-management has become widespread. A report based on 216 self-monitored and self-managed patients over a 4-year period concluded that a majority (83.1%) of the prothrombin time results were within target range; perhaps even more impressive, there were no serious adverse events recorded during the observation period.

Horstkotte and colleagues (1996) published the results from a randomized prospective study of 150 patients with prosthetic heart valves managing their own warfarin therapy ($n = 75$) who were compared to a control group ($n = 75$) managed by their private physicians. The self-managed patients tested themselves approximately every 4 days and achieved the target 92% of the time. The physician-managed patients were tested approximately every 19 days and only 59% of the INRs were found to be in the prespecified range. They also experienced adverse clinical events more often than patients who were self-managed, with an 11% incidence of any type of bleeding. In a related study, the investigators demonstrated that a frequency of INR testing of every 4 days was optimal for a majority of patients (Piper et al., 1996). Sawicki randomized 179 patients receiving long-term oral anticoagulation treatment to structured teaching and self-management programs or conventional care (provided by family physicians and specialists as required). Deviation of INR values from the target range was significantly lower in the intervention group at 3- and 6-month follow-up. They were also more likely to be within the target range and have higher quality of life measures (Sawicki, 1999).

The Early Self-Controlled Anticoagulation Trial (ESCAT II) included 3,300 patients with mechanical heart valve replacement who performed INR self-testing and anticoagulation management (Koertke et al., 2003). An interim report (1,818 patients) revealed that greater than 70% of patients were within the prespecified target INR range, with clinical events (thromboembolism, bleeding) in less than 1% (per patient year of treatment) (Figure 27.1).

Based on the available information, point-of-care coagulation monitoring offers the potential to (1) lower the risk–benefit profile on warfarin therapy, (2) improve patient satisfaction and possibly patient compliance, and (3) by reducing the labor intensity of physician management, facilitate the more widespread use of warfarin.

Anticoagulation Clinics of the Future

The development of new anticoagulants, some of which that do not require routine monitoring, will encourage diversity within the realm of anticoagulation clinics. Patient selection, education, periprocedural management, and evaluation to determine the best-suited drug and strategy will remain the cornerstone of optimal care. An opportunity to treat a larger number of patients with thrombotic disorders will create added responsibility for caregivers, which can be best met through the establishment of coordinated programs for specialized services.

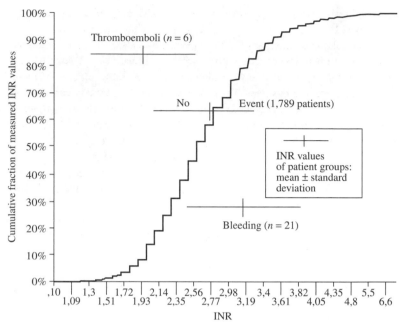

Figure 27.1 Internation normalized ratio (INR) values of aortic valve replacement patients practicing anticoagulation self-management, who were able to keep large percentages of their INR values within the target range. The clinical event rates were low as well. (From Koertke H, Minami K, Boethig D, et al. INR self-management permits lower anticoagulation levels after mechanical heart valve replacement. *Circulation* 2003;108:II75–II78.)

References

Anderson D, Harrison L, Hirsch J. Evaluation of portable prothrombin time monitor for home use by patients who require long-term oral anticoagulant therapy. *Arch Intern Med* 1993;153:1441–1447.

Ansell J, Holden A, Knapic N. Patient self-management of oral anticoagulation guided by capillary fingerstick whole blood prothrombin times. *Arch Intern Med* 1989; 149:2509–2511.

Ansell JE. Oral anticoagulant therapy—50 years later. *Arch Intern Med* 1993;153: 586–596.

Ansell J, Becker D, Andrew M, et al. Accurate and precise prothrombin time measurement in a multicenter anticoagulation trial employing patient self-testing. *Blood* 1995;86(Suppl 1):864a.

Ansell JE, Hughes R. Evolving models of warfarin management: anticoagulation clinics, patient self-monitoring, and patient self-management. *Am Heart J* 1996;132:1095–1100.

Ansell JE, Oertel LB, Wittkowsky AK, eds. *Managing oral anticoagulation: clinical and operational guidelines.* Gaithersburg. Md.: Aspen Publishers, Inc., 1997.

Bernardo A. Experience with patient self-management of oral anticoagulation. *J Thromb Thrombolysis* 1996;2:321–325.

Bussey HI, Rospond RM, Quandt CM, et al. The safety and effectiveness of long-term warfarin therapy in an anticoagulant clinic. *Pharmacotherapy* 1989;9:214–219.

Bussey HI, Chiquette E, Amato MG. Anticoagulation clinic care versus routine medical care: a review and interim report. *J Thromb Thrombolysis* 1996;2:315–319.

Byeth RJ, Landefeld CS. Prevention of major bleeding in older patients treated with warfarin: results of a randomized trial. *J Gen Intern Med* 1997;12:66.

Cannegieter SC, Rosendaal FR, Wintzen AR, van der Meer FJM, Vandenbroucke JP, Briet E. Optimal oral anticoagulant therapy in patients with mechanical heart valves. *N Engl J Med* 1995;33:11–17.

Charney R, Leddomado E, Rose DN, Fuster V. Anticoagulation clinics and the monitoring of anticoagulant therapy. *Int J Cardiol* 1988;18:197–206.

Cohen IA, Hutchison TA, Kirkling DM, et al. Evaluation of a pharmacist-managed anticoagulation clinic. *J Clin Hosp Pharm* 1985;10:167–175.

Conte RR, Kehoe WA, Nielson N, et al. Nine-yr experience with a pharmacist-managed anticoagulation clinic. *Am J Hosp Pharm* 1986;43:2460–2464.

Cortelazzo S, Finazzi G, Viero P, et al. Thrombotic and hemorrhagic complications in patients with mechanical heart valve prostheses attending an anticoagulation clinic. *Thromb Haemost* 1993;69:316–320.

Eckman MH, Levine JH, Pauker SG. Making decisions about antithrombotic therapy in heart disease. *Chest* 1995;108(Suppl):457S–470S.

Erdman S, Vidne B, Levy MJ. A self-control method for long-term anticoagulation therapy. *J Cardiovasc Surg* 1974;15:454–457.

Errichetti AM, Holden A, Ansell J. Management of oral anticoagulant therapy: experience with an anticoagulation clinic. *Arch Intern Med* 1984;144:1966–1968.

Fihn SD, McDonell M, Martin D, et al. Risk factors for complications of chronic anticoagulation: a multicenter study. *Ann Intern Med* 1993;118:511–520.

Forfar JC. A seven year analysis of haemorrhage in patients on long-term anticoagulant treatment. *Br Heart J* 1979;42:128–32.

Garabedian-Ruffalo SM, Gray DR, Sax MJ, et al. Retrospective evaluation of a pharmacist-managed warfarin anticoagulation clinic. *Am J Hosp Pharm* 1985;42:304–308.

Gitter MJ, Jaeger TM, Petterson TM, Gersh BJ, Silverstein MD. Bleeding and thromboembolism during anticoagulant therapy: a population-based study in Rochester, Minnesota. *Mayo Clin Proc* 1995;70:725–733.

Gray DR, Garabedian-Ruffalo SM, Chretien SD. Cost-justification of a clinical pharmacist-managed anticoagulation clinic. *Drug Intell Clin Pharm* 1985;19:575–580.

Hamilton GM, Childers RW, Silverstein MD. Does clinic management of anticoagulation improve the outcome of prosthetic valve patients. *Clin Res* 1985;33:832A.

Horstkotte D, Piper C, Wiemer M, Schulte HD, Schultheiss H-P. Improvement of prognosis by home prothrombin estimation in patients with life-long anticoagulant therapy. *Eur Heart J* 1996;17(Suppl):230.

Koertke H, Minami K, Boethig D, et al. INR self-management permits lower anticoagulation levels after mechanical heart valve replacement. *Circulation* 2003;108(Suppl II): II75–II78.

Kornblit P, Senderoff J, Davis-Ericksen M, Zenk J. Anticoagulation therapy: patient management and evaluation of an outpatient clinic. *Patient Education* 1990;15:21–32.

Kutner M, Nixon G, Silverstone F. Physicians' attitudes toward oral anticoagulants and antiplatelet agents for stroke prevention in elderly patients with atrial fibrillation. *Arch Intern Med* 1991;151:1950–1953.

Landefeld CS, Goldman L. Major bleeding in outpatients treated with warfarin: incidence and prediction by factors known at the start of outpatient therapy. *Am J Med* 1989;87:144–152.

Leaning KE, Ansell JE. Advances in the monitoring of oral anticoagulation: point-of-care testing, patient self-monitoring and patient self-management. *J Thromb Thrombolysis* 1996;3:377–383.

Lee YP, Schommer JC. Effect of a pharmacist-managed anticoagulation clinic on warfarin-related hospital readmissions. *Am J Health Sys Pharm* 1996;53:1580–1583.

Loeliger EA, van Dijk-Wierda CA, van den Besselaar AMHP, Broekmans AW, Roos J. Anticoagulant control and the risk of bleeding. In: Meade TW, ed. *Anticoagulants and myocardial infarction: a reappraisal.* Chichester, UK: John Wiley & Sons, Ltd., 1984: 135–177.

McCrory DC, Matchar DB, Samsa G, Sanders LL, Pritchett ELC. Physician attitudes about anticoagulation for nonvalvular atrial fibrillation in the elderly. *Arch Intern Med* 1995;155:277–281.

Palareti G, Leali N, Coccheri S, et al. Bleeding complications of oral anticoagulant treatment: an inception-cohort, prospective collaborative study (ISCOAT). *Lancet* 1996; 348:423–428.

Petitti DB, Strom BL, Melmon KL. Duration of warfarin anticoagulant therapy and the probabilities of recurrent thromboembolism and hemorrhage. *Am J Med* 1986;81: 255–259.

Petty GW, Lennihan L, Mohr JP, et al. Complications of long-term anticoagulation. *Ann Neurol* 1988;23:570–574.

Piper C, Horstkotte D, Wiemer W, Schulte HD, Schultheiss H-P. Optimization of oral anticoagulation following valve replacement: results of a prospective randomized study. *Eur Heart J* 1996;17(Suppl):230.

Sawicki PT. A structured teaching and self-management program for patients receiving oral anticoagulation. A randomized controlled trial. *JAMA* 1999;281:145–150.

Schachner A, Deviri E, Shabat S. Patient-regulated anticoagulation. In: Butchart EG, Bodnar E, eds. *Thrombosis embolism and bleeding.* London: ICR Publishers, 1992;318–324.

Seabrook GR, Karp D, Schmitt DD, Bandyk DF. An outpatient anticoagulation protocol managed by a vascular nurse-clinician. *Am J of Surg* 1990;160:501–504.

White RH, McCurdy SA, von Marensdorff H, Woodruff DE, Leftgoff L. Home prothrombin time monitoring after initiation of warfarin therapy. *Ann Intern Med* 1989; 111:730–737.

Wilt VM, Gums JG, Amhed OI, Moore LM. Outcome analysis of a pharmacist-managed anticoagulation service. *Pharmacotherapy* 1995;15:732–739.

Part VIII
Complications of Treatment
and Their Management

Platelet Antagonists

28

Antithrombotic and fibrinolytic drugs impair normal hemostasis and, as a result, increase the risk for hemorrhage. It is important to consider that many treatment strategies include agents of differing classes (platelet antagonists, anticoagulants, fibrinolytics) and categories (aspirin, clopidogrel, glycoprotein [GP] IIb/IIIa receptor antagonists), creating a multisite and/or hemostatic phase defect.

Platelet Antagonists

Platelet antagonists, by impairing primary hemostasis, are associated most often with hemorrhage involving the skin and mucous membranes; however, the gastrointestinal and genitourinary tracts may occasionally be involved.

GPIIb/IIIa Receptor Antagonists

Fixed-dose unfractionated heparin (UFH) therapy is a modifiable risk factor associated with hemorrhage in patients receiving GPIIb/IIIa receptor antagonists. The Evaluation of c7E3 Fab in Preventing Ischemic Complications of High-Risk Angioplasty (EPIC) trial was a prospective, randomized, placebo-controlled trial examining the efficacy of treatment with abciximab (EPIC Investigators, 1994). A total of 2,099 patients were scheduled for coronary angioplasty or direct atherectomy and were considered to be at high risk for abrupt closure. The primary composite endpoint of the study at 30 days was death from any cause, nonfatal myocardial infarction (MI), coronary artery bypass grafting (CABG) or repeat percutaneous coronary intervention (PCI), or placement of an intraaortic balloon pump to relieve refractory ischemia. All patients received therapy with 325 mg of aspirin and bolus dosing of UFH between 10,000 and 12,000 U followed by additional boluses of 3,000 U every 15 minutes to maintain an activated clotting time (ACT) between 300 and 350 seconds. Patients were randomized to receive either abciximab 0.25 mg/kg as a bolus followed by placebo infusion, or a placebo bolus and infusion. A significant increase in the incidence of major hemorrhage was demonstrated in patients receiving abciximab bolus and infusion compared to placebo bolus and infusion. A total of 14% of patients receiving abciximab bolus and infusion experienced a major bleeding complication as compared to 7% in the placebo bolus and infusion group ($p = .001$). Analysis of major hemorrhage in patients treated with abciximab bolus and infusion as a function of UFH dose revealed a dose-dependent increased risk. In patients treated with UFH doses between 70 and 120 U/kg, a 3.75-fold increased risk of major hemorrhage was observed in patients treated with abciximab bolus and infusion as compared to placebo bolus and infusion.

Subgroup analyses of the EPIC trial prompted investigators to assess abciximab therapy with lower doses of UFH. The Evaluation in Percutaneous Transluminal Coronary Angioplasty (PTCA) to Improve Long-Term Outcome with Abciximab GPIIb/IIIa Blockade (EPILOG) was a prospective, randomized, placebo-controlled trial in 2,792 patients undergoing PCI (EPILOG Investigators, 1997). The primary composite endpoint was death from any cause, MI, reinfarction, or severe myocardial ischemia requiring urgent CABG or repeated PTCA within 30 days after randomization. Patients were enrolled if they had greater than or equal to 60% stenosis of one coronary artery. All patients received 325 mg of aspirin. Patients were randomized to receive either 0.25 mg/kg abciximab as a bolus followed by abciximab infusion of 0.125 µg/kg/min and 100 U/kg UFH (standard dose) followed by weight-adjusted boluses (target ACT 300 seconds); bolus abciximab of 0.25 mg/kg followed by infusion of abciximab 0.125 µg/kg/min and 70 U/kg of UFH (low dose) followed by weight-adjusted boluses (target ACT 200 seconds); or placebo and 100 U/kg of UFH followed by weight-adjusted boluses (target ACT 300 seconds).

The median preintervention ACT was 329 seconds in the placebo group, 283 seconds in the abciximab plus low-dose UFH group, and 361 seconds in the abciximab and standard-dose UFH group. The incidence of major hemorrhage in the placebo group was 3.1% compared to 2.0% in the abciximab plus low-dose UFH group ($p = .19$) and 3.5% in the abciximab plus standard-dose UFH group ($p = .7$). The findings from EPIC and EPILOG highlighted the importance of UFH dosing and subsequently led to weight-based dosing recommendations from the American College of Cardiologists and American Heart Association (ACC/AHA) (Smith et al., 2001).

In addition to UFH dosing, renal insufficiency is another risk factor for bleeding. Limited information exists on GPIIb/IIIa inhibitor use for patients with renal dysfunction. Frilling and colleagues (2002) compiled a registry of 1,040 patients with varying renal function who were treated with abciximab. The investigators studied the effects of renal impairment on the incidence of hemorrhage. Renal insufficiency was defined as serum creatinine greater than or equal to 1.3 mg/dL. Procedural success was defined as residual stenosis less than 50%, TIMI grade 3 flow, and no subsequent death, stroke, MI, emergent CABG, or repeat PCI. Major bleeding was defined as bleeding that required transfusion. The incidence of major bleeding was 4.5% in the renal insufficiency group vs. 0.6% in patients with normal renal function ($p = .003$).

Approach to Hemorrhagic Complications

Emergent reversal of GPIIb/IIIa receptor inhibitors is closely linked to the pharmacokinetics of the specific agent. Abciximab exhibits strong binding affinity to the GPIIIb/IIIa receptor. Since little free abciximab circulates in the plasma, an infusion of platelets would replenish the number of viable GPIIb/IIIa receptors, allowing for a return to normal hemostasis (Mascelli et al., 1998).

Bleeding with tirofiban and eptifibatide are managed differently. These agents undergo significant renal elimination. Thus, patients with normal renal function are expected to return to baseline platelet function within 4 to 8 hours of discontinuing the infusion. For patients requiring immediate reversal, data in human subjects are sparse. Recalling that hundreds of tirofiban or eptifibatide molecules per GPIIb/IIIa receptor circulate in patients' plasma, platelet infusions alone may not be adequate to reverse the antiplatelet effects (Li et al., 2001). Accordingly, cryoprecipitate or fresh frozen plasma as rich resources of fibrinogen followed by platelet transfusions is a preferred approach to hemorrhagic complications (Table 28.1).

Thrombocytopenia

Thrombocytopenia ($<100,000/mm^3$) is observed in approximately 3% to 4% of patients receiving GPIIb/IIIa receptor antagonists and occurs more commonly following abciximab administration (particularly following reexposure). Episodes of profound thrombocytopenia ($<20,000/mm^3$) have been reported within several hours of (early onset) to weeks after (late onset) drug administration (Tables 28.2 and 28.3).

Aspirin

Aspirin has modest platelet-inhibiting properties; however, its effect on prostaglandin metabolism (seen to a greater extent with increasing doses) amplifies the inherent risk for bleeding in the upper gastrointestinal tract.

Although minor bleeding of the skin (petechia, ecchymoses) and mucous membranes (epistaxes) is the most common complication, anaphylactic and anaphylactoid (angioedema) reactions have been reported, as well as asthma (particularly in patients with nasal polyps and/or reactive airway disease).

The circulating half-life of aspirin is short; however, its biologic effect is long (7 ± 2 days). Platelet transfusions and desmopressin (DDAVP) can be used to attenuate the biologic effect of aspirin.

Table 28.1 Approach to Hemorrhagic Complications Associated with Antithrombotic Therapy

Agent	Category	Mechanism of Action	Antidote	Available Substrate for Attenuating Effects
Asprin	Platelet antagonist	Cyclooxygenase inhibition	DDAVP	Platelet transfusion
Clopidogrel	Platelet antagonist	ADP-receptor inhibition	None	Platelet transfusion
Ticlopidine	Platelet antagonist	ADP-receptor inhibition	None	Platelet transfusion
Abciximab	Platelet antagonist	GPIIb/IIIa receptor inhibition	None	Platelet transfusion, FFP, cryoprecipitate
Tirofiban	Platelet antagonist	GPIIb/IIIa receptor inhibition	None	Cryoprecipitate, FFP, platelet transfusion
Eptifibatide	Platelet antagonist	GPIIb/IIIa receptor inhibition	None	Cryoprecipitate, FFP, platelet transfusion
UFH	Anticoagulant	Thrombin inhibition (indirect)	Protamine	FFP
LMWH	Anticoagulant	Thrombin inhibition (indirect)	Protamine (60%)	Factor VIIa (recombinant)
Lepirudin	Anticoagulant	Thrombin inhibition (direct)	None	FFP, plasmapheresis
Argatroban	Anticoagulant	Thrombin inhibition (direct)	None	FFP, plasmapheresis
Bivalirudin	Anticoagulant	Thrombin inhibition (direct)	None	FFP, plasmapheresis
Warfarin	Anticoagulant	Clotting factor inhibitor	Vitamin K	FFP
Alteplase, Reteplase Tenecteplase	Fibrinolytic	Fibrinolysis/Fibrinogenolysis	Aminocaproic acid	Cryoprecipitate, FFP Platelet transfusion

ADP, adenosine 5'diphosphate; DDAVP, Desmopressin; FFP, fresh frozen plasma; GP, glycoprotein; LMWH, low-molecular-weight heparin; UFH, unfractionated heparin.

Table 28.2 Acute Thrombocytopenia Management Algorithm following GPIIb/IIIa Antagonist Administration

Platelet Count	Bleeding	Recommended Treatments
Acute <10,000/mm³	No Bleeding	1. Transfuse 6–10 pooled random platelet donor packs or one single donor plateletpheresis pack. 2. Reverse heparin with protamine, warfarin with vitamin K.
	Minor to moderate bleeding (including mucous membrane)	1. Transfuse platelets. 2. Reverse heparin with protamine, warfarin with vitamin K.
	Severe bleeding[a]	1. Provide conventional critical care. 2. Transfuse platelets. 3. Reverse heparin with protamine, warfarin with vitamin K. 4. Transfuse PRBCs as indicated.
Acute 10,000–50,000/mm³	None	1. Careful observation. 2. Discontinue heparin, warfarin. 3. Consider platelet transfusions if invasive procedure of surgery required.
	Minor to moderate bleeding (including mucous membrane)	1. Transfuse platelets. 2. Reverse heparin with protamine, warfarin with vitamin K.
	Severe bleeding[a]	1. Provide conventional critical care. 3. Transfuse platelets. 5. Reverse heparin with protamine, warfarin with vitamin K. 6. Transfuse PRBCs as indicated.
Acute 50,000–100,000/mm³		1. Careful observation 2. Consider discounting anticoagulants.

[a]In cases of severe, life-threatening bleeding that does not respond to steps 1 to 4, consider plasmapheresis.
GP, glycoprotein; PRBC, packed red blood cell.

From Giugliano RP. Drug-induced thrombocytopenia: is it a serious complex for GPIIb/IIIA receptor inhibitors? J Thromb Thrombolysis 1998;5:191–202.

Table 28.3 Delayed Thrombocytopenia Management Algorithm[a]

Platelet Count	Bleeding	Recommended Treatments
Delayed <10,000/mm³	No bleeding or minor to moderate bleeding	1. Transfuse platelets. 2. Reverse heparin with protamine, warfarin with vitamin K. 3. Consider IV steroitd and IgG.
	Severe bleeding[b]	1. Provide conventional critical care. 2. Transfuse platelets. 3. Reverse heparin with protamine, warfarin with vitamin K. 4. Transfuse PRBCs as indicated. 5. Administer IV steroids and IgG.
Delayed 10,000–50,000/mm³	Minor to moderate bleeding (including mucous membrane)	1. Careful observation 2. Discontinue heparin, or other anticoagulant. 3. Consider platelet transfusions. 4. Consider IV steroids and IgG.
	Severe bleeding[b]	1. Provide conventional critical care. 2. Transfuse platelets. 3. Reverse heparin with protamine, warfin with vitamin K. 4. Transfuse PRBCs as indicated. 5. Administer IV steroids and IgG.
Delayed >50,000/mm³		1. Careful observation 2. Consider discontinuing anti-coagulants.

[a]*Immune-mediated thrombocytopenia should be suspected if (1) platelet–antibody test is positive and/or (2) timing of thrombocytopenia is well after the start of the study drug (e.g., after day 5).*
[b]*In cases of severe, life-threatening bleeding that does not respond to steps 1–5, consider emergent plasmapheresis.*
Ig, immunoglobulin; PRBC, packed red blood cell.

From Giugliano RP. Drug-induced thrombocytopenia: is it a serious complex for GPIIIb/IIIA receptor inhibitors? J Thromb Thrombolysis *1998;5:191–202.*

Thienopyridines

Ticlopidine and clopidogrel, like aspirin (with which they are used frequently in combination), have short circulating half-lives but impair platelet performance for their lifespan. Platelet transfusions can attenuate their inhibitory effects. The impact of red blood cell transfusions (providing a source of adenosine 5' diphosphate [ADP]) has not been studied in clinical practice but is known to reduce bleeding times.

Thrombotic thrombocytopenic purpura (TTP) is a life-threatening, multisystem disease characterized by thrombocytopenia, fever, neurologic abnormalities, renal failure, and microangiopathic hemolytic anemia. The estimated incidence of TTP with ticlopidine is one in 1,600 patients treated with a 33% mortality rate. The incidence with clopidogrel is much lower, on the order of one in 50,000. Symptoms can be seen from 2 to 12 weeks following initiation of therapy (typically within 2–3 weeks) for clopidogrel and later with ticlopidine.

The management of TTP includes prompt drug discontinuation and initiation of plasma exchange therapy (Bennet et al., 1998, 2000).

Factor VIIa (recombinant; NovoSeven) represents an important treatment alternative in patients with life-threatening hemorrhage secondary to platelet-related coagulopathies.

References

Bennet CL, Kiss JE, Ewinberg PD, et al. Thrombotic thrombocytopenic purpura after stenting and ticlopidine. *Lancet* 1998;352:1036–1037.

Bennet CL, Connors JM, Carwile JM, et al. Thrombotic thrombocytopenic purpura associated with clopidogrel. *N Engl J Med* 2000;342:1773–1777.

EPIC Investigators. Use of a monoclonal antibody directed against the platelet glycoprotein IIb/IIIa receptor in high-risk coronary angioplasty. The EPIC Investigation. *N Engl J Med* 1994;300:956–961.

EPILOG Investigators. Effect of the platelet glycoprotein IIb/IIIa receptor inhibitor ab ciximab with lower heparin dosages in ischemic complications of percutaneous coronary revascularization. The EPILOG Investigation. *N Engl J Med* 1997;336: 1689–1696.

Frilling B, Zahn R, Fraiture B, et al. Comparison of efficacy and complication rates after percutaneous coronary interventions in patients with and without renal insufficiency treated with abciximab. *Am J Cardiol* 2002;89:450–452.

Giugliano RP. Drug-induced thrombocytopenia: is it a serious complex for GPIIIb/IIIA receptor inhibitors? *J Thromb Thrombolysis* 1998;5:191–202.

Li YF, Spencer FA, Becker RC. Comparative efficacy of fibrinogen and platelet supplementation on the in vitro reversibility of competitive glycoprotein IIb/IIIa (alpha IIb/beta3) receptor-directed platelet inhibition. *Am Heart J* 2001;142;204–210.

Mascelli MA, Lance ET, Damaraju L, et al. Pharmacodynamic profile of short-term abciximab treatment demonstrates prolonged platelet inhibition with gradual recovery from GP IIb/IIIa receptor blockade. *Circulation* 1998;97:1680–1688.

Smith SC Jr, Dove JT, Jacobs AK, et al. ACC/AHA guidelines for percutaneous coronary intervention (revision of the 1993 OTC/a guidelines)—executive summary: a report of the American College of Cardiology/American Heart Association task force on practice guidelines (committee to revise the 1993 guidelines for percutaneous transluminal coronary angioplasty) endorsed by the Society of Cardiac Angiography and Interventions. *Circulation* 2001;103:3019–3041.

Anticoagulants

29

Anticoagulant therapy, particularly when used in combination with fibrinolytics and less often platelet antagonists, can cause life-threatening hemorrhage. This supports the importance of coagulation proteases in several phases of thrombus development; paradoxically, several anticoagulants can also cause microvascular and macrovascular thrombotic disorders.

Warfarin

Hemorrhage is the most common adverse effect associated with warfarin administration. To predict the risk of bleeding, Beyth and colleagues (1998) developed a 5-point scoring system, with 1 point given for each of the following:

- Age greater than 65
- History of stroke
- History of gastrointestinal bleeding
- Specific comorbid conditions (recent myocardial infarction [MI], elevated serum creatinine, hematocrit <30%, or diabetes)

Low-risk patients have a score of 0; intermediate-risk patients, 1 or 2; and high-risk, 3 or 4. The risk of bleeding in these three groupings at 12 months was 3%, 8%, and 30%, respectively.

Drug Interactions

Many commonly used medications have significant interactions with warfarin (Table 29.1). In 1994, Wells and colleagues (1994) reviewed all reports of warfarin–drug interactions and found original reports totaling 186. Potentiation of warfarin effect was observed with six antibiotics, five cardiac drugs, two antiinflammatory agents, two histamine$_2$-blockers, and alcohol in persons with concomitant liver disease. Inhibition of warfarin effect was noted with three antibiotics, three central nervous system (CNS) drugs, cholestyramine, and sucralfate. An important interaction between acetaminophen and warfarin has also been recognized (Hylek et al., 1998), and certain herbal remedies, such as ginkgo biloba, ginseng, and garlic, may enhance the effects of warfarin.

Table 29.1 Drug–Warfarin Interactions

Drug	Potentiate	Inhibit
Antibiotics	Cotrimoxazole Erythromycin Fluconazole Isoniazid Metronidazole Miconazole Ciprofloxacin	Griseofulvin Rifampin Nafcillin
Cardiac drugs	Clofibrate Propafenone Propranolol Sulfinpyrazone	—
Antipyretics Antiinflammatories	Acetaminophen Phenybutazone Piroxicam	—
Histamine$_2$-blockers	Cimetidine Omeprazole	—
Central nervous system agents	—	Barbiturates Carbamazepine Chlordiazepoxide
Other	Lovastatin Simvastatin	Cholestyramine Androgens Sucralfate

Management of Warfarin-Induced Bleeding

The first step in the management of bleeding is to stop the drug; however, recovery of clotting factor levels may take several days, depending upon the vitamin K content of the patient's diet and rate of intrinsic metabolism. To rapidly raise coagulant factor concentrations in patients with life-threatening hemorrhage, clotting factor concentrates are given (Makris et al., 1997). The older concentrates were plasma-derived and consisted mainly of activated prothrombin complex factors. They had the disadvantages of thrombogenicity and potential for transmission of infectious agents. More recently, recombinant factor VIIa (NovoSeven) has been used with excellent control of bleeding, although thrombosis risk remains a very real concern (as well as cost). Fresh frozen plasma is an alternative therapy, but may not completely correct the prothrombin time.

Doses of 15 to 18 mL/kg are needed to raise clotting factor levels above 20% of normal; these doses carry a substantial risk of causing circulatory overload. After an initial bolus of 200 mL, plasma may be given as a continuous infusion of 100 mL/hour with monitoring of venous pressure and administration of diuretics. Recently, plasma treated to inactive infectious agents has become available.

Patients with warfarin-induced bleeding should also receive vitamin K, but the doses should be adjusted according to the international normalized ratio (INR) and presence or absence of bleeding (Table 29.2) and intensity of anticoagulation.

Adverse Reactions Other Than Bleeding

Skin and muscle necrosis is a dreaded complication of warfarin therapy. The pathogenesis is related to the effect of warfarin on proteins C and S. Because these anticoagulant proteins disappear at a faster rate than prothrombin, an imbalance between procoagulant and anticoagulant proteins transiently develops. The clinical manifestations of this disorder are necrosis of skin and fat, especially in areas such as the breast and abdominal wall. In addition, the veins of the lower extremities may thrombose, leading to venous gangrene.

This devastating syndrome is prevented by avoiding warfarin use in patients with low baseline levels of proteins C and S, including those with inherited deficiencies (detected by a positive personal or family history of thrombosis). In patients with hereditary deficiencies of protein C or S, warfarin is introduced slowly when therapeutic levels of heparin or low-molecular-weight heparin (LMWH) have been achieved and maintained for several days. In patients who are receiving warfarin, the syndrome may be recognized by the development of skin discoloration and pain in a well-localized body area and should be suspected strongly if the prothrombin time elevates rapidly following a single dose of warfarin (suggesting extreme sensitivity of the vitamin K–dependent proteins to the vitamin K antagonist).

Table 29.2 Management of Prolonged INR Associated with Warfarin Therapy[a]

INR	<6.0	6.0–10.0	<10.0	>20.0
Clinical profile[a] Recommended approach	No bleeding Omit next 1–2 doses of warfarin	No bleeding Vitamin K 1–2 mg SC ↓ Repeat INR in 8 h ↓ Consider additional vitamin K	No bleeding Vitamin K 3 mg SC ↓ Repeat INR in 6 h ↓ Consider additional vitamin K	No bleeding Vitamin K 5–10 mg SC ↓ Repeat INR in 6 h ↓ Consider additional vitamin K

[a]For rapid reversal of anticoagulant effect because of life-threatening hemorrhage, fresh frozen plasma or prothrombin concentrates should be administered. Concomitant administration of vitamin K (3–5 mg IV) is also recommended.

INR, international normalized ratio.

Another complication of warfarin treatment is the "purple toe" syndrome. Patients with this syndrome typically have severe aortoiliac atheromatous disease; warfarin administration promotes plaque destabilization with distal embolization of cholesterol crystals, especially to the toes. Cessation of warfarin therapy generally resolves the problem, but vascular surgery may be necessary if there is tissue hypoperfusion.

The teratogenicity of warfarin is well recognized. The greatest risk is from week 6 to week 12 of gestation, but central nervous system malformations may occur later (second trimester). During the third trimester, there is a risk of intracranial bleeding in the fetus. Therefore, warfarin should be discontinued when pregnancy is confirmed, followed by institution of an alternative anticoagulant.

Heparin and Low-Molecular-Weight Heparin

The use of unfractionated heparin (UFH) and LMWH is associated with a variety of complications; as with warfarin, the most frequent is bleeding. However, other serious adverse effects also occur, including heparin-induced thrombocytopenia (HIT), osteoporosis, and, less commonly, eosinophilia, alopecia, and transaminitis.

Management of Bleeding Due to Heparins

Bleeding in patients receiving UFH is managed initially by discontinuing the agent. Often this approach is effective because the short half-life of the drug (90 minutes) ensures that the anticoagulant effect will disappear rapidly. However, if serious bleeding begins immediately after a dose is given or the patient has delayed heparin clearance (because of renal or hepatic disease), it may be necessary to neutralize the heparin with protamine. The dose is 1 mg for each 100 U of heparin given in the past 4 hours. In practice, giving half this dose may be effective and can be repeated if necessary. Large protamine doses may cause hypotension and even bleeding; allergic (anaphylactic or prophylactic) reactions to the drug have also been reported.

Reversal of LMWH is more challenging given its longer half-life and reduced susceptibility to inactivation by protamine. In a study of comparative neutralizing effects, Wolzt and colleagues (1995) found that a dose of 1 mg/100 anti-Xa U of LMWH almost completely reversed prolongation of the activated partial thromboplastin time (aPTT) and thrombin time, but had a modest effect on anti-Xa activity. In general, protamine effectively neutralizes the anti-IIa effects, but has no impact on LMWH-mediated factor X inhibition.

Factor VIIa (recombinant; NovoSeven) represents a treatment option in patients with life-threatening hemorrhage.

Heparin-Induced Thrombocytopenia

Heparin-induced thrombocytopenia is an uncommon but clinically significant complication of heparin therapy that is important for three reasons. First, it is a drug-related immunohematologic reaction. Second, it can be complicated by life- and limb-threatening complications. Third, the optimal treatment approach, although still uncertain, is gradually being defined with greater accuracy.

Etiology

The HIT syndrome is due to the development of an antibody, usually IgG, that binds to and activates platelets in the presence of heparin. The pathogenic antibody is directed at an immunogenic complex formed by heparin (or other mucopolysaccharides) and a basic protein, most commonly platelet factor 4 (PF4) (Amiral et al., 1992). The immune complex formed by IgG, heparin, and protein then binds to and clusters the platelet Fcγ receptor (FcγRIIa), initiating platelet activation (Visentin et al., 1994). Rarely, HIT can be caused by alternative mechanisms, including IgA and/or IgM anti-PF4/heparin antibodies or antibodies directed against PF4-related chemokines (Chong, 1995). Platelet activation is associated with generation of procoagulant platelet microparticles (Warkentin et al., 1994). Additional evidence suggests that the antibody can also bind to endothelial cells (and PF4 on their surface), leading to endothelial cell damage or activation with expression of tissue factor (stimulating the extrinsic coagulation pathway) (Cines et al., 1987). It is hypothesized that the intense surge of procoagulant activity overwhelms heparin's anticoagulant effect, predisposing to intravascular thrombosis (Figure 29.1).

Incidence

The true incidence of HIT is uncertain but has probably been underestimated. Well-designed prospective studies suggest that the incidence varies from greater than 1% to 3% of patients exposed to UFH, whereas the incidence is significantly lower in patients exposed only to LMWH (Warkentin et al., 1995). Assays used to measure heparin-related antibodies vary widely in their sensitivity. Earlier studies in unselected patients receiving UFH demonstrated a 5% to 10% incidence of antibodies, whereas more recent work employing sensitive immunoassays directed at PF4 heparin have identified antibodies in upward of 50% of individuals with selected clinical conditions such as cardiopulmonary bypass surgery. This more recent finding supports a vast clinical spectrum in the expression of HIT, ranging from asymptomatic antibody formation to antibody formation associated with thrombocytopenia to antibody formation associated with isolated thrombocytopenia and thrombosis. The clinical significance of heparin-induced antibodies without thrombocytopenia remains unclear, but is the subject of ongoing investigation.

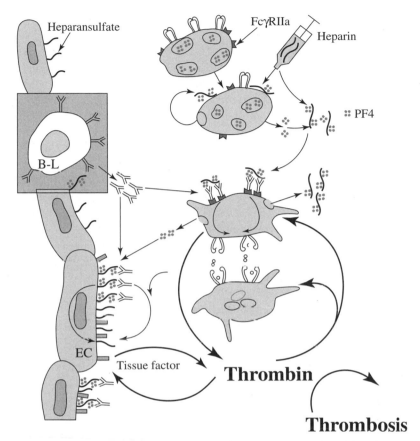

Figure 29.1 Proposed explanation for the presence of both thrombocytopenia and thrombosis in heparin-sensitive subjects who are treated with heparin. According to Visentin et al., injected heparin reacts with platelet factor 4 (PF4) that is normally present on the surface of endothelial cells or released in small quantities from circulating platelets (1) to form PF4–heparin complexes. Specific IgG antibodies react with these conjugates to form immune complexes that (2) bind to Fc receptors on circulating platelets. Fc-mediated platelet activation (3) releases PF4 from alpha granules in platelets (4). Newly released PF4 binds to additional heparin, and the antibody forms more immune complexes, establishing a cycle of platelet activation. PF4 released in excess of the amount that can be neutralized by available heparin binds to heparin-like molecules (glycosamino-glycans) on the surface of endothelial cells (EC) to provide targets for antibody binding. This process leads to immune-mediated EC injury (5) and heightens the risk of thrombosis and disseminated intravascular coagulation. (From Aster RN, *N Engl J Med* 1995;332:1374–1376.)

Clinical Manifestations

The major clinical manifestations of HIT are thrombocytopenia and thrombosis (Table 29.3). The onset of thrombocytopenia and/or thrombosis usually occurs 5 to 12 (range 4–20) days after treatment initiation among patients who are exposed to the drug for the first time. Symptoms may occur more rapidly (within 24 hours or less) in patients who have had previous exposure to heparin, particularly if the exposure has occurred within the prior 3 months. Rarely, the onset of thrombocytopenia and/or thrombosis may be delayed and occur after several weeks of exposure.

Patients with HIT usually develop mild to moderate thrombocytopenia with the nadir platelet counts ranging from 20 to 150 × 10^9/L. However, HIT should be suspected whenever an unexplained decrease of greater than 50% from the baseline platelet count occurs during heparin therapy (even if the platelet count remains in the reference range) or if the count falls below 100 × 10^9/L.

Thromboembolic complications involve both the arterial and venous circulating systems and can affect either large vessels (e.g., intracranial, coronary, mesenteric arteries) or microcirculation. Although venous thromboembolism is more common than arterial thrombosis, the latter is more devastating due to the associated tissue injury. Thrombotic events herald a turning point in the syndrome, with mortality rates approaching 50%. The diagnosis should also be suspected in patients

Table 29.3 Clinical Events Associated with Heparin-Induced Thrombocytopenia

---

Platelet Count Abnormalities
  Thrombocytopenia
  Falling platelet count does not reach thrombocytopenic levels (generally, ≥50% platelet count
    fall beginning after day 5 of heparin use)
Venous Thrombotic Complications
  Deep vein thrombosis (usually proximal vein thrombosis)
  Pulmonary embolism
  Adrenal hemorrhagic infarction (secondary to adrenal vein thrombosis)
  Cerebral vein cerebral dural sinus thrombosis
Arterial Thrombotic or Thromboembolic Complications
  Lower limb arterial thrombosis
  Thrombotic stroke
  Myocardial infarction
  Aortic thrombosis (may cause spinal cord infarction)
  Vascular graft occlusion
Skin Reaction at Heparin Subcutaneous Injection Sites
  Erythematous plaques
  Skin necrosis
Sequelae That Can Occur Shortly after IV Heparin Bolus Use in Patients with HIT-IgG
  Acute systemic reactions (inflammatory or respiratory)
  Transient global amnesia

HIT, heparin-induced thrombocytopenia; Ig, immunoglobulin.

who develop skin necrosis (particularly at subcutaneous injection sites). Similarly, when a patient develops skin necrosis while on both heparin and an oral anticoagulant, HIT should be considered in the absence of protein C deficiency. There are several less common but important manifestations of HIT that clinicians must be aware of that include fever, anaphylactoid, and life-threatening anaphylactic reactions developing within 30 to 60 minutes of heparin administration. Transient global amnesia is a rare feature of HIT. Erythematous plaques and skin necrosis are localized skin reactions that indicate HIT in patients receiving subcutaneous heparin injections (Warkentin et al., 1998).

Patients receiving heparin should be monitored for the development of HIT. Because HIT can occur with any form of heparin administration, including use of heparin-coated indwelling vascular catheters, all patients exposed to heparin are potentially at risk. Proposed diagnostic criteria for the diagnosis of HIT are as follows:

1. Onset of otherwise unexplained thrombocytopenia or thrombosis following initiation of heparin therapy
2. Positive test for presence of heparin-dependent antibodies by a sensitive and specific diagnostic assay

In addition, recovery of the platelet count into the reference range within several days of heparin cessation supports a diagnosis of HIT. A comprehensive laboratory evaluation should be considered to differentiate HIT from other causes of thrombocytopenia, including nonimmune heparin-induced thrombocytopenia (formerly call HIT type I). Nonimmune heparin-induced thrombocytopenia is more common than HIT and is associated with a more modest decrease in the platelet count and a lack of thrombotic manifestations. Tests for heparin-dependent antibodies are negative in patients with the nonimmune form of HIT.

Laboratory Testing

Specific testing for HIT can be grouped into two types of assays: (1) platelet-based or functional assays and (2) antibody recognition of the heparin–PF4 complex. Platelet-based assays depend on activation or lysis of platelets in the presence of a test sample and heparin. Washed normal platelets provide a sensitive test system when $C_{serotonin}$ release platelet aggregation is used as an endpoint. The $C_{serotonin}$ release assay has been evaluated in a prospective clinical study and a positive assay was strongly associated with HIT (odds ratio, 78.2; 95% confidence interval [CI] 12.0–818.8; $p < .001$) with a specificity of 96%. The specificity of these assays may be improved by performing the assay at low (0.1–0.3 U/mL) and high (10–100 U/mL) concentrations of heparin–PF4 complexes from the platelet surface and may interfere with HIT antibody interaction with platelet FcγRIIa and subsequent platelet activation. Thus, platelet activation or lysis, manifested by platelet aggregation or

$C_{serotonin}$ release, at low but not high concentrations of heparin is regarded as diagnostic of HIT (Favaloro et al., 1992; Isenhart and Brandt, 1993).

Experience with these test systems has also confirmed the need for careful selection of platelet donors and the use of weakly positive HIT control samples. Substantial variation in the sensitivity of FcγRIIa-mediated platelet activation may be found among normal donors. Thus, it is essential to use donor platelets known to be responsive to HIT samples. The difficulties with platelet-washing procedures and the inconvenience of using radioactive material have prompted many laboratories to use platelet-rich plasma-based aggregation assays. It has been suggested that platelet aggregation, using platelet-rich plasma, is less sensitive than the washed platelet system; however, comparisons of optimized test systems have demonstrated comparability. It is possible that, with appropriate attention to detail, platelet-rich plasma assays provide a convenient and more rapid method for diagnosis of HIT. Some hospital laboratories perform a heparin-induced platelet aggregation (HIPA) assay. Although the assay has a high specificity, it is only 70% sensitive; therefore, a negative result does not exclude the diagnosis of HIT. The test is labor intensive and prior notification of the laboratory is often required.

The second laboratory approach to the diagnosis of HIT uses assays that detect antibodies to the heparin–PF4 macromolecular complex. Enzyme-linked immunosorbent assays (ELISAs) have been developed to permit identification of antibodies reacting with heparin–PF4. Microtiter plate wells are coated with heparin–PF4 and allowed to incubate with a patient sample. Bond antibody can then be detected by appropriate antisera to IgG, IgA, or IgM by standard techniques. Although the concordance between platelet-based activation and ELISAs is high (high sensitivity), the results are discordant in approximately 10% to 20% of cases (80–90% specificity). Several factors may contribute to this discordance. First, the ELISA may detect IgA and IgM antibodies that are incapable of mediating FcγRIIa-induced platelet activation. Second, some antibodies are directed at complexes of heparin and other proteins such as interleukin-8 and neutrophil activating peptide-2. Third, the ELISA method may detect low titer (or avidity) antibodies that are not associated with clinical manifestations. To date, there are no data from prospective clinical trials delineating the performance of these two approaches to the laboratory confirmation of HIT. Therefore, it is difficult to recommend one technique over another, although, as previously mentioned, there is level one evidence correlating the serotonin release assay with clinical HIT.

Management of Heparin-Induced Thrombocytopenia

Once a diagnosis of HIT has been established (high clinical suspicion with or without laboratory confirmation), it is important that all sources of heparin, including heparin-coated catheters, be discontinued immediately. An alternative anticoagulant strategy should be used if the patient requires anticoagulation for the management of thromboembolism. Although it was initially thought that LMWH would be an effective treatment option, clinical studies have shown a high rate of laboratory-based cross-reactivity (60–70%) with existing antibodies. Heparinoids, such as danaparoid sodium (Orgaran), may be very effective and have a low rate of cross-reactivity (Magnani, 1993); however, they are difficult to titrate and neutralize (when bleeding occurs). In addition, the drug is not available in the United States. The direct thrombin inhibitors hirudin (Greinacher et al., 1999) and argatroban are the most attractive alternatives for anticoagulation in patients with HIT (Table 29.4) (Warkentin et al, 1998).

It is important to remember that anticoagulation therapy may, in fact, be required for the management of HIT even in the absence of thrombotic events. The rationale is based on several considerations. First, thrombosis occurs in 20% to 30% of patients with heparin-related antibodies and thrombocytopenia. Second, the risk of thrombosis presents for days or weeks after the termination of heparin treatment. Third, the natural history of HIT with thrombosis may not be modifiable in the absence of aggressive therapy.

Clinicians are reminded that warfarin administration should be avoided in patients with HIT because of its prothrombotic potential (rapid decrease in protein C levels). If warfarin is required for long term treatment of thromboembolism, an alternative anticoagulant (danaparoid sodium, hirudin) should be administered for several days before starting treatment.

Table 29.4 Anticoagulant Therapy in Patients with Heparin-Induced Thrombocytopenia

Agent	Dose and Monitoring
Lepirudin	IV bolus of 0.4 mg/kg Continuous infusion of 0.15 mg/kg/h Monitor with aPTT; do baseline and repeat 4 h after initiation: ratio to normal should be 1.5–2.5 Check aPTT at least twice daily during therapy Reduce dose by 50% or more if renal failure present
Argatroban	Continuous IV infusion of 2 μg/kg/min Check aPTT 2 h after initiation and adjust dose until target aPTT of 1.5–3.0 times control is attained (not to exceed 100 sec) Reduce dose to 0.5 μg/kg/min if hepatic impairment
Danaparoid[†]	IV bolus of 2,500 U Then, 400 U/h × 4; 300 U/h × 4 h Then, 200 U/h as continuous infusion Monitor platelet count; if renal failure, obtain anti-Xa level during treatment (should not exceed 1 U/mL)

aPTT, activated partial thromboplastin time.
[†] *limited availability.*

References

Amiral J, Bridey F, Dreyfus M, et al. Platelet factor 4 complexed to heparin is the target for antibodies generated in heparin-induces thrombocytopenia. *Thromb Haemost* 1992;68:95–96.

Beyth RJ, Quinn LM, Landefeld CS. Prospective evaluation of an index for predicting the risk of major bleeding in outpatients treated with warfarin. *Am J Med* 1998; 105:91–99.

Chong BH. Heparin-induced thrombocytopenia. *Br J Haematol* 1995;89:431–439.

Cines DB, Tomaski A, Tasnnenbaum S. Immune endothelial-cell injury in heparin-associated thrombocytopenia. *N Engl J Med* 1987;316:581–589.

Favaloro EJ, Bernal-Hoyes E, Exner T, Koutts J. Heparin-induced thrombocytopenia: laboratory investigation and confirmation of the diagnosis. *Pathology* 1992;24: 177–183.

Greinacher A, Janssens MD, Berg G, et al. for the Heparin-Associated Thrombocytopenia (HAT) Investigators. Lepirudin (recombinant hirudin) for parenteral anticoagulation in patients with heparin-induced thrombocytopenia. *Circulation* 1999;100: 587–593.

Hylek EM, Heiman H, Skates SJ, Shehan MA, Singer DE. Acetaminophen and other risk factors for excessive warfarin anticoagulation. *JAMA* 1998;279:567–662.

Isenhart CE, Brandt JT. Platelet aggregation studies for the diagnosis of heparin-induced thrombocytopenia. *Am J Clin Pathol* 1993;99:324–330.

Magnani HN. Heparin-induced thrombocytopenia (HIT): an overview of 230 patients treated with Orgaran (Org 10172). *Thromb Haemost* 1993;70:554–561.

Makris M, Greaves M, Phillips WS, Kitchen S, Rosendaal FR, Pteston FE. Emergency oral anticoagulant reversal: the relative efficacy of infusion of fresh frozen plasma and clotting factor concentrate on correction of the coagulopathy. *Thromb Haemost* 1997;77:477–480.

Visentin DP, Ford SE, Scott JP, Aster RH. Antibodies from patients with heparin-induced thrombocytopenia/thrombosis are specific for platelet factor 4 complexed with heparin or bound to endothelial cells. *J Clin Invest* 1994;93:81–88.

Warkentin TE, Hayward CPM, Boshkov LK, et al. Sera from patients with heparin-induced thrombocytopenia generate platelet-derived microparticles with procoagulant activity: an explanation for the thrombotic complications of heparin-induced thrombocytopenia. *Blood* 1994;84:3691–3699.

Warkentin TE, Levine MN, Hirsh J, et al. Heparin-induced thrombocytopenia in patients treated with low-molecular-weight or unfractionated heparin. *N Engl J Med* 1995;332:1330–1335.

Warkentin TE, Bhong BH, Greinacher A. Heparin-induced thrombocytopenia: towards consensus. *Thromb Haemost* 1998;79:1–7.

Wells PS, Holbrook AM, Crowther NR, Hirsh J. Interactions of warfarin with drugs and food. *Ann Intern Med* 1994;121:676–683.

Wolzt M, Weltermann A, Nieszpaur-Los M, et al. Studies on the neutralizing effects of protamine on unfractionated and low molecular weight heparin (Fragmin) at the site of activation of the coagulation system in man. *Thromb Haemost* 1995;73:4 39–443.

Fibrinolytic Agents

30

The generation of plasmin from plasminogen by plasminogen activators (fibrino-lytic agents) induces a variety of effects in addition to dissolving fibrin strands, de-grading fibrinogen, and inhibiting tissue factor pathway and factor VIII. It also, in high concentrations, causes platelet activation. Thus, fibrinolytic agents have both prothrombotic and antihemostatic properties—the latter of which is often augmented by the concomitant use of anticoagulants and platelet antagonists (see Chapter 12).

Hemorrhagic Complications

Bleeding is the most common complication of fibrinolytic (and adjunctive anti-thrombotic) therapy. The most important predictors of nonintracranial hemorrhage are older age, invasive procedures, low body weight, and female sex (Table 30.1) (de Jaegre et al, 1992; GISSI 2 Investigators, 1990; GUSTO-III Investigators, 1997; INJECT Investigators, 1995). Predictors of intracranial hemorrhage include age (>65 years), low body weight (<70 kg), hypertension on admission, and alteplase (vs. streptokinase) (Table 30.2) (GUSTO-III Investigators, 1997).

Management of Fibrinolytic-Induced Bleeding

The approach to patient management in cases of fibrinolytic-induced bleeding is summarized in Figure 30.1. It is important to consider antithrombotic agents that may concomitantly increase hemorrhagic potential. Factor VIIa (recombinant; NovoSeven) represents a treatment alternative for life-threatening hemorrhagic complications.

References

de Jaegre PP, Arnold AA, Balk AH, Simoons ML. Intracranial hemorrhage in association with thrombolytic therapy: incidence and clinical predictive factors. *J Am Coll Cardiol* 1992;19:289–294.

Global Use of Strategies to Open Occluded Infarct Arteries (GUSTO-III) Investigators. An international, multicenter, randomized comparison of reteplase and tissue

Table 30.1 Hemorrhage Rates (Other than Intracranial) in Comparative Fibrinolytic Therapy

Trial	n	Major* Hemorrhage (n)	n	Major* Hemorrhage[†] (n)	Difference
		Streptokinase		*Alteplase*	*Alteplase vs. streptokinase*
GISSI-2	10,386	0.9% (96)	10,372	0.6% (64)	−0.3%
ISIS-3	13,607	0.9% (118)	13,569	0.8% (109)	−0.1%
GUSTO-1	20,196	12.9% (2611)	10,366	11.1% (1155)	−1.8%
		Streptokinase		*Reteplase*	*Reteplase vs. streptokinase*
INJECT	3,006	1.0%	3,004	0.7%	−0.3%
		Alteplase		*Reteplase*	*Reteplase vs. streptokinase*
GUSTO-III	4,921	6.8%	10,138	6.9%	+0.2%

Major hemorrhage is defined as receiving or requiring transfusion.
[†]*Alteplase 100 mg over 3 h in GISSI-2, duteplase 0.6 MU/kg over 4 h in ISIS-3, alteplase 100 mg over 90 min in GUSTO-1.*

Table 30.2 Intracranial Hemorrhage Rates in Comparative Trials of Fibrinolytic Therapy

Trial	n	Rate (n)	n	Rate (n)	Difference
		Streptokinase		*Alteplase*[†]	*Alteplase vs. streptokinase*
GISSI-2 International Study	10,396	0.29% (30)	10,372	0.42% (64)	+0.23%
ISIS-3	12,848	0.30% (39)	12,841	0.72% (92)	+0.42%
GUSTO-1	20,213	0.51% (104)	10,376	0.70% (73)	+0.19%
		Streptokinase		*Reteplase*	*Reteplase vs. streptokinase*
INJECT	3,006	0.37% (11)	3,004	0.77% (23)	+0.40%
		Alteplase		*Reteplase*	*Reteplase vs. streptokinase*
GUSTO-III	4,921	0.87%	10,138	0.91%	+0.04%

[†]*Alteplase 100 mg over 3 h in GISSI-2, duteplase 0.6 MU/kg over 4 h in ISIS-3, alteplase 100 mg over 90 min in GUSTO-1.*

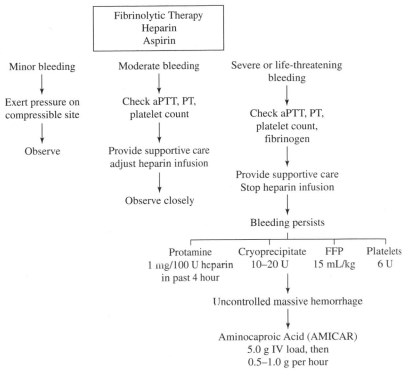

Figure 30.1 A recommended approach to the management of patients with bleeding complications following fibrinolytic (and adjunctive) therapy. aPTT, activated partial thromboplastin time; FFP, fresh frozen plasma; PT, prothrombin time. Supportive Care: oxygen as needed; blood transfusion as needed; vasopressors for hypotension; compression, or surgical intervention for site of bleeding.

plasminogen activator for acute myocardial infarction. *N Engl J Med* 1997;337: 1118–1123.

Gruppo Italiano per lo Studio della Sopravvivenza nell'Infarto Miocardico. GISSI-2: a factorial randomised trial of alteplase versus streptokinase and heparin versus no heparin among 12,490 patients with acute myocardial infarction. *Lancet* 1990; 336:65–71.

International Joint Efficacy Comparison of Thrombolytics (INJECT) Investigators. Randomised, double-blind comparison of reteplase double-bolus administration with streptokinase in acute myocardial infarction (INJECT): trial to investigate equivalence. *Lancet* 1995;346:329–336.

Appendixes

Agent	General Class	Route of Administration	Onset of Antithrombotic Effect	Offset of Antithrombotic Effect
Abciximab (ReoPro)	Platelet GPIIb/IIIa receptor antagonist	IV	Rapid (within minutes); 90% ADP inhibition at 30 min	50% ADP inhibition at 24 h after termination
Acetylsalicylic acid (aspirin)	Platelet antagonist	Oral, rectal, IV[a]	Rapid (within 30 min when administered orally)	Delayed (days)
Aggrenox (aspirin, ER dipyridamole)	Platelet antagonist	Oral		Delayed (days)
Argatroban	Anticoagulant	IV	Rapid (within minutes of IV administration)	Rapid (hours)
Clopidogrel bisulfate[b] (Plavix)	Platelet antagonist	Oral	Delayed (2–3 d); with 6 h following higher doses (300–600 mg oral loading, 3–4 h)	Delayed (days)
Dalteparin (Fragmin)	Anticoagulant	SC	Intermediate (peak anticoagulant effect 4–6 h after SC administration)	Intermediate (hours)

Clinical Indication	Dose	Adverse Effects	Cost (USD)
PCI, refractory UA when PCI planned within 24 h	0.25 mg/kg IV bolus (10–60 min before start of PCI) 0.125 μg/kg/min to maximum of 10 μg/kg/min for 12 h 0.25 mg/kg IV bolus, 0.125 μg/kg/min (maximum 10 μg/min) for 18–24 h (concluding 1 h after PCI) in patients with refractory unstable angina	Bleeding, thrombocytopenia	$1,400.00 (12-h infusion)
ACS, primary prevention (high-risk patients), secondary prevention, PCI, coronary stents, mechanical heart valves (high-risk patients), bypass grafts (greatest benefit during first post-operative year), atrial fibrillation (low-risk patients), cerebrovascular disease (TIA, stroke)	160–325 mg daily	Bleeding, bronchospasm, GI intolerance, allergic reactions (including anaphylaxis)	$3.14 (per mo)
Secondary prevention (stroke, TIA)	25/200 mg bid	Bleeding , flushing, nausea, hypotension	—
HIT, PCI in patients with suspected HIT			
Secondary prevention of atherosclerotic vascular events; ACS; post-PCI with stenting; postbrady therapy	75 mg qd	Bleeding, rash diarrhea, dyspepsia, TTP (rare)	$86.76 (per mo)
DVT (prophylaxis), ACS	5,000 U SC qd (prophylaxis) 120 V/kg (≤10,000 U) SC bid (unstable angina, non–ST-segment elevation MI)		$0.49 (per 100 ant-XaU)

continued

Agent	General Class	Route of Administration	Onset of Antithrombotic Effect	Offset of Antithrombotic Effect
Danaparoid sodium (Orgaran)	Anticoagulant	IV or SC	Rapid (within minutes of IV administration)	Rapid (hours)
Enoxaparin (Lovenox)	Anticoagulant	SC	Intermediate (peak anticoagulant effect 3–5 h after SC administration	Rapid (hours)
1 mg/kg SC			Rapid (peak anticoagulant effect within 5–10 min after IV administration)	
Eptifibatide (Integrilin)	Platelet GPIIb/IIIa receptor antagonist	IV	Rapid (within minutes); 90% ADP inhibition at 30 min	Very rapid (50% ADP inhibition at 4 h)
Hirudin (lepirudin; Refluden)	Anticoagulant	IV (can be given SC)	Rapid (within minutes of IV administration	Rapid (hours)
r PA (retavase)	Fibrinolytic agent	IV	20–30 min	12–24 h
Streptokinase	Fibrinolytic agent	IV	30–60 min	11–24 h
Ticlopidine HCl (Ticlid)	Platelet antagonist	Oral	Delayed (2–3 d); with 6 h following higher doses (500–1,000 mg)	Delayed (days)

Clinical Indication	Dose	Adverse Effects	Cost (USD)
DVT (prophylaxis, treatment), HIT	750 U SC bid (prophylaxis) 2,250 U SC (load), 1,250–1,500 SC q8–12h (treatment)	Bleeding, allergic reactions, cross-reactivity with heparin-induced antibodies	$195.00 (per day), prophylaxis $448.40 (per day with bid SC dosing), treatment
Venous thromboembolism (prophylaxis, treatment), non–ST-segment elevation ACS	30 mg SC or 40 mg qd (DVT prophylaxis) 1 mg/kg SC bid (DVT treatment) or 1 mg/kg SC bid (UA/non–ST-segment elevation MI) or 2,250 U IV (load), 400 U/h × 4 h, then 300 U/h × 4 h, then 150–200 U/h	Bleeding, allergic reactions, thrombocytopenia (rare)	$0.38 (per mg) $526.40 (per day with IV dosing), treatment
ACS, PCI	180 µg/kg bolus, 2 µg/kg/min up to 72 h (ACS) 135 µg/kg bolus, 0.5 µg/kg/min for 20–24 h (PCI)	Bleeding, thrombocytopenia	$325.00 (24-h treatment)
HIT, venous/arterial thrombotic disorders in patients unable to receive heparin, DVT (prophylaxis)[c]	0.4 mg/kg (up to 110 mg) over 15–20 sec (bolus)[c] 0.15 mg/kg (up to 110 mg) infusion; target aPTT 1.5–2.5 × control[c]	Bleeding, allergic reactions, liver function abnormalities	$536.40 (24-h treatment)
Acute MI (ST-segment elevation, bundle branch block)	10 U over 2 min, wait 30 min, 10 U over 2 min	Bleeding	$1,086.00 (per vial)
Acute MI (ST-segment elevation, bundle branch block), acute PE	1.5 million U over 60 min (for MI), 250,000 U/h × 24 h	Bleeding, hypotension, anaphylaxis	$400.00
ACS (with aspirin allergy), stroke (high-risk patients), coronary stents, bypass grafts (with aspirin allergy)	250 mg	Bleeding, rash, nausea/vomiting, neutropenia (bone marrow suppression), TTP	$113.93 (per mo)

continued

Agent	General Class	Route of Administration	Onset of Antithrombotic Effect	Offset of Antithrombotic Effect
Tirofiban (Aggrastat)	Platelet GPIIb/IIIa receptor antagonist	IV	Rapid (within minutes); 90% ADP inhibition at 30 min	Very rapid (50% ADP inhibition at 30 min)
TNK-tPA (tenecteplase)	Fibrinolytic agent	IV	20–30 min	12–24 h
tPA (alteplase)	Fibrinolytic agent	IV	20–30 min	12–24 h
Unfractionated heparin	Anticoagulant	IV or SC	Rapid (within minutes of IV administration)	Rapid (hours)
Urokinase	Fibrinolytic agent	IV	30–60 min	11–24 h
Warfarin	Anticoagulant	Oral, IV	Maximum plasma concentration reached within 2–3 h	Delayed (days)

[a]*Intravenous acetylsalicylic acid not available in the United States.*
[b]*Not tested in randomized clinical trials.*
[c]*Reduce does if creatinine ≥1.5 mg/dL (algorithm for dosing in renal insufficiency is available).*
[d]*Cost variable.*

Clinical Indication	Dose	Adverse Effects	Cost (USD)
ACS with or without PCI (not stents)	0.4 µg/kg/min × 30 min, 0.1 µg/kg/min for 48–108 h 12–24 h after PCI	Bleeding, thrombocytopenia	$325.00 (24-h treatment)
Acute MI (ST-segment elevation, bundle branch block)	0.53 mg/kg slow IV bolus; maximum 50 mg	Bleeding	$2,400.00
Acute MI (ST-segment elevation, bundle branch block), acute ischemic stroke, PE	1.5 mg IV bolus; 0.75 mg/kg over following 60 min 0.9 mg/kg maximum 90 mg), 10% as bolus remainder over following 60 min (for acute ischemic stroke) 100 mg given over 2 h (for PE)	Bleeding	$2,400.00
ACS, venous thromboembolism (prophylaxis, treatment) PCI, heart–lung bypass	5,000 U SC bid/tid (DVT prophylaxis) Treatment (of venous/arterial allergic reactions thromboembolism) (50–60 U/kg/h); target aPTT 1.5–2.5 × control value; ACT >200 for PCI	Bleeding, thrombocytopenia (with/without thrombosis), (including anaphylaxis), hypoaldosteronism	$20.00 (per day) (including infusion
Acute PE, AV fistula (venous catheter occlusion peripheral arterial occlusion)	4,400 u/kg over 10 min, 4,400 U/kg/h × 12–24 h (for PE)		$389.00 (25,000 U)
Venous thromboembolism, atrial fibrillation, secondary prevention following MI, mechanical prosthetic heart valves, high-risk patients with tissue prosthetic heart valves	Titrated to desired anticoagulant effects (target INR)	Bleeding, skin necrosis atheroembolism	$55.00 (100 5 mg tablets)

ACS, acute coronary syndromes; ACT, activated clotting time; ADP, adenosine 5'diphosphate; aPTT, activated partial thromboplastin time; AV, arteriovenous; DVT, deep vein thrombosis; ER, extended release; GI, gastrointestinal; GP, glycoprotein; HIT, heparin-induced thrombocytopenia; INR, international Normalized Ratio; MI, myocardial infarction; PCI, percutaneous coronary interventions; PE, pulmonary embolism; rPA, recombinant plasminogen activator; TIA, transient ischemic attack; tPA, tissue plasminogen activator; TTP, thrombotic thrombocytopenic purpura; UA, unstable angina; USD (United States dollars).

Appendix B Drug Dosing with Renal Insufficiency

Drug	Normal Dose	CrCl 30–50 mL/min	CrCl 10–30 mL/min	CrCl <10 mL/min	Hemodialysis	Continuous Hemoperfusion CAVHD/CVVHD	Notes
Abciximab (ReoPro)	0.25 mg/kg IV bolus, then 0.125 mcg/kg/min × 12 hrs	No change		No change	No change Abciximab may not be cleared by dialysis	No change Abciximab may not be cleared by dialysis	Monitor platelets 4 h into the infusion
Alteplase (Activase)	**>67 kg** 15 mg IV bolus, 50 mg over 30 min, then 35 mg over the next 60 min **≥67 kg** 15 mg IV bolus, 0.75 mg/kg over 30 min (up to 50 mg), then 0.50 mg/kg over the next 60 min (up to 35 mg)	No change	No change Administer if benefits outweigh risks	No change Administer if benefits outweigh risks	No guidelines determined Administer if benefits outweigh risks	No guidelines determined Administer if benefits outweigh risks	Maintain aPTT with heparin at 1.5–2 × control (50–70 sec) for 48 h
Anistreplase (Eminase)	IV bolus of 30 U infused over 5 min	No change	No change	No change	No guidelines determined	No guidelines determined	
Aspirin	81–325 mg PO q24h	No change	No change	Use if benefits outweigh risks	Dose after dialysis	No change	May increase bleeding risk in uremic patients with dysfunctional platelets
Clopidogrel (Plavix)	Loading doses of 300 mg × 1 may be given followed by 75 mg PO q24h	No change	No change	No change	No guidelines determined Administer if benefits outweigh risks	No guidelines determined Administer if benefits outweigh risks	Monitor for signs and symptoms of TTP

(continued)

381

Appendix B (*continued*)

Drug	Normal Dose	CrCl 30–50 mL/min	CrCl 10–30 mL/min	CrCl <10 mL/min	Hemodialysis	Continuous Hemoperfusion CAVHD/CVVHD	Notes
Dalteparin (Fragmin)	**Prophylaxis** 2,500–5,000 U SC q24h **Acute coronary syndromes** 120 U/kg SC q12h	No change	No guidelines determined	No guidelines determined	No guidelines determined	No guidelines determined	ACS doses not recommend for use in patients with CrCl <30 mL/min unless monitoring anti-Xa levels
Danaparoid (Orgaron)	Prophylaxis: 750 U SC q12h	No change	No guidelines determined	No guidelines determined	No guidelines determined	No guidelines determined	
Dipyridamole (Persantine)	50–100 mg PO q6–8h	No change	No change	No change	No guidelines determined	No guidelines determined	
Enoxaparin (Lovenox)	**DVT prophylaxis** 30 mg SC q12h or 40 mg SC q24h **DVT treatment and acute coronary syndromes** 1 mg/kg SC q12h or 1.5 mg/kg SC q24h for in-patient treatment of DVT	No change	No guidelines determined	No guidelines determined	No guidelines determined	No guidelines determined	DVT treatment and ACS doses not recommended for use in patients with CrCl <30 mL/min unless monitoring anti-Xa levels
Eptifibatide (Integrilin)	**Medical management** 180 μg/kg IV bolus, then 2 μg/kg/min **Catheterization lab** 180 μg/kg IV bolus, then 2 μg/kg/min	**SCr ≤2mg/dL** 180 μg/kg bolus, then 2 μg/kg/min infusion **2 mg/dL <SCr <4 mg/dL** 135 μg/kg bolus, then 0.5 μg/kg/min infusion			No data available Eptifibatide may be cleared by dialysis	No data available Eptifibatide may be cleared by dialysis	If heparin is used, maintain aPTT in the range of 50–70 sec. Continue eptifibatide 12–24 h postangioplasty unless specified otherwise

Drug	Dosing					Comments
Unfractionated heparin	followed by a second 180 μg/kg/min IV bolus 10 min into the maintenance infusion **DVT Prophylaxis** 5,000 U SC q8–12h **Acute coronary syndromes** 60 U/kg (maximum 4,000 U) IV bolus followed by 12 U/kg/h (max 1,000 U/h) for patients receiving fibrinolytics or GPIIb/IIIa receptor antagonists	No change	No change	No change	No change	Maintain aPTT in the range of 50–70 sec for patients receiving fibrinolytics or GPIIb/IIIa receptor antagonists
Lepirudin (Refludan)	**Heparin induced thrombocytopenia** 0.4 mg/kg IV bolus over 15–20 sec (max bolus 44 mg), infuse at 0.15 mg/kg/h (max infusion 16.5 mg/h)	0.2 mg/kg IV bolus, infuse at: 0.075 mg/kg/h for CrCl 45–60 mL/min or 0.045 mg/kg/h for CrCl 30–44 mL/min or 0.0225 mg/kg/h for CrCl 15–29 mL/min	0.1 mg/kg IV bolus, monitor aPTT and rebolus when aPTT is <1.5 × control	0.1 mg/kg IV bolus, monitor aPTT and rebolus when aPTT is <1.5 × control	0.1 mg/kg IV bolus, monitor aPTT and rebolus when aPTT is <1.5 × control	Dosage adjustments are based on aPTT monitoring
tPA (Retavase)	Two 10 U IV boluses, administered over 2 min, 30 min apart	No change Administer if benefits outweigh risks	No change Administer if benefits outweigh risks	No guidelines determined Administer if benefits outweigh risks	No guidelines determined Administer if benefits outweigh risks	Maintain aPTT with heparin at 1.5–2 × control (50–70 sec for 48 h)

(continued)

Appendix B (*continued*)

Drug	Normal Dose	CrCl 30–50 mL/min	CrCl 10–30 mL/min	CrCl <10 mL/min	Hemodialysis	Continuous Hemoperfusion CAVHD/CVVHD	Notes
Streptokinase (Kabikinase, Streptase)	Acute MI: 1.5 million U IV over 60 min	No change	No change	No change	No guidelines determined Administer if benefits outweigh risks	No guidelines determined Administer if benefits outweigh risks	Antigenic: allergic reactions 2–4% (shivering, rash) Hypotension may respond to slowing the infusion rate
Ticlopidine (Ticlid)	250 mg PO q12h taken with food	No change Reduce dose or discontinue if hemorrhagic problems are encountered	No change Reduce dose or discontinue if hemorrhagic problems are encountered	No change Reduce dose or discontinue if hemorrhagic problems are encountered	Administer if benefits outweigh risks Reduce dose or discontinue if hemorrhagic problems are encountered	No change Reduce dose or discontinue if hemorrhagic problems are encountered	Monitor CBC q2w for the first 3 mo Also monitor for signs and symptoms of TTP
Tinzaparin (Innohep)	DVT treatment: 175 IU/kg SC q24h	No change	No guidelines determined	No guidelines determined	No guidelines determined	No guidelines determined	Not recommended for use in patients with CrCl <30 mL/min
Tirofiban (Aggrastat)	0.4 µg/kg/min IV bolus over 30 min, followed by 0.1 µg/kg/min × 48	No change	0.2 µg/kg/min IV bolus over 30 min, followed by 0.05 µg/kg/min × 48–108 h	0.2 µg/kg/min IV bolus over 30 min, followed by 0.05 µg/kg/min × 48–108 h	No data available Tirofiban is removed by hemodialysis	No data available Tirofiban is removed by hemodialysis	If heparin is used, maintain aPTT in the range of 50–70 sec Continue tirofiban 12–24 h postangioplasty unless specified otherwise

Drug	Dosing					
TNK-tPA (Tenecteplase)	<60 kg: 30 mg; ≥60 kg but <70 kg: 35 mg; ≥70 kg but <80 kg: 40 mg; ≥80 kg but <90 kg: 45 mg; ≥90 kg: 50 mg	No change	Benefits should be weighed against risks with hemostatic defects secondary to renal disease	Benefits should be weighed against risks in patients with hemostatic defects secondary to renal disease	Benefits should be weighed against risks in patients with hemostatic defects secondary to renal disease	Benefits should be weighed against risks in patients with defects — Maintain aPTT with heparin at 1.5–2 × control (50–70 sec) for 48 h
Urokinase (Abbokinase)	4,400 U/kg IV bolus over 10 min, then 4,400 U/kg/h for 12 h	No change	No change	No change	No guidelines determined	No guidelines determined
Warfarin (Coumadin)	Initiate at 3–5 mg PO qd and increase or decrease doses based on goal INR	No change	No change	No change; May require lower doses	No change; May require lower doses	No change; May require lower doses

---

Creatinine clearance based on the Cockcroft-Gault equation (males) = $[(140 - \text{age}) \times IBW]/SCr \times 72$

Creatinine clearance based on the Cockcroft-Gault equation (females) = Male CrCl × 0.85

IBW = Ideal body weight (Males) = [50 kg + 2.3 (every inch greater than 60 inches) Ideal body weight (females) = [45 kg + 2.3 (every inch greater than 60 inches)]

If actual body weight is lower than ideal body weight, use the actual body weight to calculate the creatinine clearance.

ACS, acute coronary syndrome; aPTT, activated partial thromboplastin time; CAV-D, continuous arteriovenous hemodialysis; CBC, complete blood cell; CrCl, creatinine clearance; CVVHD, continuous venovenous hemodialysis; DVT, deep vein thrombosis; GP, glycoprotein; INR, international normalized ratio; MI, myocardial infarction; SCr, serum creatinine; TTP, thrombotic thrombocytopenic purpura.

Index

Page numbers followed by f indicate figures, those followed by t indicate tables.

Coventry University Library